Urinary Bladder Pathology

Haijun Zhou • Charles C. Guo
Jae Y. Ro
Editors

Urinary Bladder Pathology

Springer

Editors
Haijun Zhou
Department of Pathology
and Genomic Medicine
Houston Methodist Hospital
Houston, TX
USA

Weill Cornell Medical College
Houston Methodist
Houston, TX
USA

Jae Y. Ro
Department of Pathology
and Genomic Medicine
Houston Methodist Hospital
Houston, TX
USA

Weill Cornell Medical College
Houston Methodist
Houston, TX
USA

Charles C. Guo
Department of Pathology
MD Anderson Cancer Center
Houston, TX
USA

ISBN 978-3-030-71508-3 ISBN 978-3-030-71509-0 (eBook)
https://doi.org/10.1007/978-3-030-71509-0

This Springer imprint is published by the registered company Springer Nature Switzerland AG
The registered company address is: Gewerbestrasse 11, 6330 Cham, Switzerland

To my wife Catherine and our daughters Ava and Olivia for their support and love!

Haijun Zhou, MD, PhD

To my loving wife Cathy and my wonderful son Brian.

Charles C. Guo, MD

To my wife Jungsil and my son's family (Bobby, Kim, Avery, and Christian) for their love and support!

Jae Y. Ro, MD, PhD

Preface

Bladder diseases are common in clinical practice. While many inflammatory conditions and other abnormalities are usually managed clinically, tissue diagnosis is often needed if neoplastic lesions or non-neoplastic tumoral conditions are suspected. Bladder cancer is one of the top ten most common cancers in the United States (fourth in men and twelfth in women). Accurate diagnosis of bladder cancer plays a central role in daily pathology practice, clinical management, and prognosis. The variety of tumor histologic types and corresponding mimickers complicate bladder cancer pathologic diagnosis. Familiarity with common and uncommon bladder pathologic entities is vital for successful diagnosis of bladder cancers and subsequent patient management.

The focus of this book is bladder cancer pathology, including primary bladder malignancies and other tumor varieties involving the bladder, with an emphasis on diagnostic pitfalls and clinical relevance. This book also describes normal bladder histology, benign abnormalities with cancer mimickers, and cancer carcinogenesis – important subject matter for understanding bladder cancers, correct diagnosis, and differential diagnoses. Advances in immunohistochemistry and molecular pathology have enhanced the accuracy of cancer pathology diagnoses. In addition to covering the anatomic and histologic features of bladder tumors, this book also reviews recent molecular and immunohistochemical advances in these areas. Recently updated clinical management information is also presented in this book.

Many experienced genitourinary pathologists, surgical pathologists, molecular pathologists, and clinical oncologists have contributed to this book, in addition to many fellows and residents.

We hope this book will be a useful resource for practicing pathologists, pathology trainees, and other health professionals who treat patients with bladder cancers.

Houston, TX, USA Haijun Zhou
Houston, TX, USA Charles C. Guo
Houston, TX, USA Jae Y. Ro

Acknowledgment

This book is a result of teamwork with tremendous help and support from numerous colleagues. We thank our trainees and colleagues for providing insights in our practice of diagnostic genitourinary pathology and acknowledge the clinical teams in taking care of bladder cancer patients with their expertise and passion.

We would like to thank Adrienne Winston and Sasha Pejerrey for their assistance with scientific and editorial working in the preparation of our book.

Contents

1 **Introduction to Urinary Bladder Pathology** 1
Haijun Zhou, Charles C. Guo, and Jae Y. Ro

2 **Normal Anatomy and Histology of the Urinary Bladder with Pathologic Correlates** 7
Ziad M. El-Zaatari and Jae Y. Ro

3 **Flat Urothelial Lesions** 21
Gang Wang

4 **Papillary and Inverted Tumors** 35
Haijun Zhou, Charles C. Guo, and Jae Y. Ro

5 **Invasive Urothelial Carcinoma with Molecular Types** 45
Charles C. Guo, Jae Y. Ro, and Bogdan Czerniak

6 **Morphological Variants of Invasive Urothelial Carcinoma** 63
Kyung En Park, Qihui "Jim" Zhai, and Fang-Ming Deng

7 **Other Types of Carcinoma** 83
Kosuke Miyai, Hussam Abu-Farsakh, and Jae Y. Ro

8 **Mesenchymal Tumors** 97
Michael J. Hwang and Pheroze Tamboli

9 **Neuroendocrine Tumors of the Urinary Bladder** 113
Ahmed N. Shehabeldin and Jae Y. Ro

10 **Bladder Lymphoma and Leukemia** 129
Jie Xu, Shaoying Li, and M. James You

11 **Secondary Tumors in the Bladder** 141
Miao Zhang

12 **Urine Cytology** 147
Haijun Zhou

13 **Diagnostic Values of Immunohistochemistry in Bladder Cancer** 159
Qihui "Jim" Zhai and Fang-Ming Deng

14 **Molecular Pathology** 175
Dilek Ertoy Baydar

15 Surgical Treatment in Urinary Bladder Cancer 189
Dalsan You, Bumjin Lim, and Choung-Soo Kim

16 Medical Treatment with Targeted Therapy for Metastatic Urothelial Bladder Carcinoma 199
Omar Alhalabi and Jianjun Gao

17 Bladder Cancer: Specimen Handling and Reporting 211
Yong Mee Cho and Jae Y. Ro

18 AJCC Staging of Bladder Cancers 229
Euno Choi, Sanghui Park, and Jae Y. Ro

19 Conclusion and Remarks 249
Haijun Zhou, Charles C. Guo, and Jae Y. Ro

Index 253

Contributors

Hussam Abu-Farsakh, MD, FCAP Department of Pathology, First Medical Lab, Amman, Jordan

Omar Alhalabi, MD Department of Genitourinary Medical Oncology, University of Texas MD Anderson Cancer Center, Houston, TX, USA

Dilek Ertoy Baydar, MD Department of Pathology, Koc University Hospital, Istanbul, Turkey

Yong Mee Cho, MD, PhD Department of Pathology, Asan Medical Center, University of Ulsan College of Medicine, Seoul, South Korea

Euno Choi, MD Department of Pathology, Ewha Womans University/Mok-dong Hospital, Seoul, South Korea

Bogdan Czerniak, MD, PhD Department of Pathology, The University of Texas MD Anderson Cancer Center, Houston, TX, USA

Fang-Ming Deng, MD, PhD Department of Pathology, New York University Langone Health, New York, NY, USA

Ziad M. El-Zaatari, MD Department of Pathology and Genomic Medicine, Houston Methodist Hospital, Houston, TX, USA

Jianjun Gao, MD, PhD Department of Genitourinary Medical Oncology, The University of Texas MD Anderson Cancer Center, Houston, TX, USA

Charles C. Guo, MD Department of Pathology, The University of Texas MD Anderson Cancer Center, Houston, TX, USA

Michael J. Hwang, MD, PhD Department of Pathology and Laboratory Medicine, Indiana University School of Medicine, Indianapolis, IN, USA

Choung-Soo Kim, MD, PhD Department of Urology, Asan Medical Center, Seoul, South Korea

Shaoying Li, MD Department of Hematopathology, The University of Texas MD Anderson Cancer Center, Houston, TX, USA

Bumjin Lim, MD Department of Urology, Asan Medical Center, Seoul, South Korea

Kosuke Miyai, MD, PhD National Defense Medical College, Department of Basic Pathology, Saitama, Japan

Kyung En Park, MD Department of Pathology, New York Langone Medical Health, New York, NY, USA

Sanghui Park, MD, PhD Department of Pathology, Ewha Womans University/Mok-dong Hospital, Seoul, South Korea

Jae Y. Ro, MD, PhD Department of Pathology and Genomic Medicine, Weill Medical College of Cornell University/Houston Methodist Hospital, Houston, TX, USA

Ahmed N. Shehabeldin, MD Department of Pathology and Genomic Medicine, Houston Methodist Hospital, Houston, TX, USA

Pheroze Tamboli, MBBS Department of Pathology, The University of Texas MD Anderson Cancer Center, Houston, TX, USA

Gang Wang, MD, PhD Department of Pathology and Laboratory Medicine, British Columbia Cancer Vancouver Centre, Vancouver, BC, Canada

Jie Xu, MD, PhD Department of Hematopathology, The University of Texas MD Anderson Cancer Center, Houston, TX, USA

Dalsan You, MD, PhD Department of Urology, Asan Medical Center, University of Ulsan College of Medicine, Seoul, South Korea

M. James You, MD, PhD Department of Hematopathology, The University of Texas MD Anderson Cancer Center, Houston, TX, USA

Qihui "Jim" Zhai, MD Lab Medicine and Pathology, Mayo Clinic Florida, Jacksonville, FL, USA

Miao Zhang, MD, PhD Department of Pathology, MD Anderson Cancer Center, Houston, TX, USA

Haijun Zhou, MD, PhD Department of Pathology and Genomic Medicine, Weill Medical College of Cornell University/Houston Methodist Hospital, Houston, TX, USA

Introduction to Urinary Bladder Pathology

1

Haijun Zhou, Charles C. Guo, and Jae Y. Ro

The urinary bladder is a sac-like organ that functions in urine storage and urination. From the innermost epithelium (urothelium) to the outer muscle layer, many diseases and conditions can originate from the bladder. Inflammatory conditions, such as cystitis, are the most common, with a clinical presentation of urinary urgency and frequency. Congenital and acquired anomalies, such as diverticulum, exstrophy, vesicoureteral reflux, and urachal cysts, are also common clinically. Hematuria, obstruction, and radiologically abnormal findings would prompt further evaluation with cytology and cystoscopy with pathologic examination to rule out potential malignant processes. Pathological evaluation is critical for further clinical management and is key to differentiate benign or reactive processes from malignant conditions. Pathological findings can range from inflammatory or metaplastic changes to low-grade neoplasms or high-grade malignancies. These pathologic features from different entities will be discussed in the following chapters.

Bladder Cancer Epidemiology

Globally, bladder cancer is the tenth most common type of cancer, with approximately 550,000 new cases diagnosed worldwide in 2018 [1]. The prevalence of bladder cancer is considerably higher in the Western countries than in the developing world [2]. In the United States, the lifetime risk of receiving a diagnosis of bladder cancer is 3.9% for males and 1.2% for females, respectively [3]. An estimated of 81,400 new cases of bladder cancer will be diagnosed and an estimated 17,980 people will die from bladder cancer in 2020: 13,050 males and 4930 females, respectively, in the United States [4].

Multiple risk factors have been established for bladder cancer. Cigarette smoking is the most significant environmental risk factor for bladder cancer, and it is estimated to cause up to half of all cases in the United States [4], and smokers have two to five times greater risk of developing bladder cancer than the general population [5]. The risk of bladder cancer is also increased among persons with hazardous industrial exposures to aniline dyes and aromatic amines [6], as well as among persons who have consumed

H. Zhou (✉) · J. Y. Ro
Department of Pathology and Genomic Medicine, Weill Medical College of Cornell University/Houston Methodist Hospital, Houston, TX, USA
e-mail: hzhou@houstonmethodist.org; JaeRo@houstonmethodist.org

C. C. Guo
Department of Pathology, The University of Texas MD Anderson Cancer Center, Houston, TX, USA
e-mail: ccguo@mdanderson.org

H. Zhou et al. (eds.), *Urinary Bladder Pathology*, https://doi.org/10.1007/978-3-030-71509-0_1

a high level of arsenic in their drinking water [7]. Certain bladder congenital defects, parasitic infection (schistosomiasis), or long-term urinary tract irritation (such as catheters or stone) are also risk factors.

Bladder Urothelial Carcinogenesis

Bladder cancer is a heterogeneous group of neoplasms. More than 90% bladder cancer cases are urothelial (transitional cell) carcinoma, which arise from the bladder urothelial epithelium. Other primary tumors, such as adenocarcinoma, squamous cell carcinoma, and small cell carcinoma, and mesenchymal tumors are less common.

Bladder urothelial neoplasms morphologically originate from two distinct precursor lesions: low-grade noninvasive papillary tumors and flat noninvasive urothelial carcinoma (carcinoma in situ (CIS)), respectively.

Low-grade papillary tumors arise from a hyperplastic carcinogenesis pathway that accounts for about 80% of urothelial tumor cases [8]. This pathway initiates from urothelial hyperplasia and then progresses to low-grade papillary urothelial carcinoma (LGUC). In this pathway, the most frequent genetic abnormalities are mutations of fibroblast growth factor receptor 3 (FGFR3) [9, 10], H-ras oncogene [11–13], and phosphatidylinositol-4,5-bisphosphate 3-kinase catalytic subunit alpha (PIK3CA) genes [9, 14]. These hyperplastic pathway papillary tumors are genetically stable with nonaggressive behavior and a characteristically high recurrence rate [15].

Flat noninvasive urothelial carcinoma/CIS originates from the dysplastic pathway, which is less common than the hyperplastic pathway and is responsible for approximately 20% of urothelial carcinoma cases. This pathway starts with dysplasia and then leads to high-grade urothelial carcinoma (HGUC), including high-grade papillary carcinoma or flat urothelial CIS. HGUC can progress to muscle-invasive, high-stage tumors with regional lymph node involvement and/or distant metastases. This pathway is associated with many tumor suppressors [16, 17], including p53 [18, 19], retinoblastoma gene (RB) [18], and phosphatase and tensin homolog (PTEN) [19]. This pathway is genetically unstable, and inactivating mutations of *TP53* are identified in about 60% of these tumors. Of note, approximately 10–15% of low-grade papillary tumors can progress to high-grade invasive carcinoma, which is often preceded by the development of flat CIS within papillary lesions or in the adjacent urothelial mucosa of papillary tumors [20].

Early genetic events, such as loss of heterozygosity (LOH), predispose the urothelium to develop neoplasms. LOH of chromosome 9q21 locus of the cyclin-dependent kinase inhibitor 2A gene (CDKN2A) that encodes the p16INK4A protein is one of the earliest molecular changes seen in the development of both noninvasive papillary carcinoma and flat urothelial CIS [21–23]. A variety of chromosomal abnormalities have been reported in association with urothelial carcinoma [24]. Aneuploidy of chromosomes 3, 7, and 17 and the loss of the 9p21 locus have been incorporated into a FISH test in urine (UroVysion), which may be used alone or coupled with cytology for bladder cancer screening and surveillance.

Multifocal occurrence is a common characteristic of urothelial malignancy, which is explained by two proposed theories: the monoclonal theory and the field cancerization theory [20, 21, 25–27]. Understanding monoclonal versus oligoclonal early tumor development is important for determining treatment strategies and the detection of recurrent or residual disease when molecular diagnostic information is used.

The dual-track molecular carcinogenesis theory is supported by in vitro studies and animal models; however, it is still unclear how molecular alterations contribute to the development of these two morphologically distinct bladder cancer types [20]. This model may be oversimplified compared to the genomic complexity of urothelial cancer. More detailed information can be found in Chap. 14.

Bladder Cancer Clinical Course and Management

The majority of bladder cancer patients experience either gross or microscopic hematuria. Other symptoms, including increased frequency or urgency of urination or dysuria, can be seen alone or in combination in a significant proportion of patients.

Urine cytology and cystoscopy should be initiated for the evaluation of bladder mucosal lesions. Visible small lesions (such as papillary tumors) and flat lesions suspected of CIS under cystoscopy are sampled with cold-cup biopsy forceps. Tumor grading and invasiveness are evaluated microscopically. The presence of muscularis propria is important for tumor staging and management and should be included in biopsies whenever possible [28].

Surgical resection is the most common treatment option for bladder cancer patients, as approximately 75% of new urothelial carcinoma cases are nonmuscle-invasive. Suspicious lesions should be resected transurethrally as completely as possible at initial clinical evaluation. Pathology-confirmed early-stage nonmuscle-invasive carcinoma (Ta/Tis/T1 lesions) may be treated by removing the tumor and then administering immunotherapy [bacillus Calmette-Guérin (BCG)] or chemotherapy drugs directly into the bladder (intravesical therapy). More advanced muscle-invasive tumors (T2 and above) may require cystectomy either with or without regional lymph node dissections and neoadjuvant or adjuvant chemotherapy. Metastatic bladder cancer patients are typically treated with chemotherapy. Outcomes in patients with muscle-invasive urothelial carcinoma are improved with the use of neoadjuvant chemotherapy before cystectomy. Immunotherapy and targeted therapy drugs are new options for patients with an advanced stage of urothelial carcinoma in conjunction with chemotherapy and/or radiation.

The 5-year relative survival rate for bladder cancer is 77%, and for noninvasive urothelial carcinoma cases, the 5-year survival rate is 96% [4]. Tumor recurrence is a significant risk factor for cancer progression [29, 30] and is common in urothelial cancer. Therefore, timely follow-up care is extremely important for all bladder cancer patients. Subsequent bladder cancer can typically be identified during surveillance due to the multifocal features of bladder cancer carcinogenesis.

Pathology Prospective

Pathologic evaluation plays a central role in the screening, diagnosis, treatment, and surveillance of bladder cancer. Urine cytology and cystoscopy-based biopsy are critical in the initial evaluation of the disease. Morphologic evaluation gives vital firsthand information: normal with variation versus disease, nonneoplastic versus neoplastic, benign changes versus malignancy, noninvasive versus invasive, flat versus papillary, urothelial versus non-urothelial tumor, nonmuscle-invasive versus muscle-invasive, and primary malignancy versus secondary metastasis. All pertinent morphologic information will determine the next steps for the management of the patient. The pathologic evaluation of resection cystectomy specimens will help to determine the precise pathology stage and the efficacy of neoadjuvant chemotherapy. Subsequent surveillance will rely on scheduled cytology and biopsy.

The advances of pathology techniques help to further classify urothelial carcinomas. Immunohistochemical markers have been used to classify urothelial carcinoma into luminal carcinomas (CK20+, GATA3+, CK5/6-) and basal-like carcinomas (CK5/6+, CD44+, CK20-) [31]. Luminal carcinomas share a similar gene expression profile with superficial papillary tumors. Basal-like carcinomas express genes more characteristic of urothelial basal cells and have a significantly worse prognosis than luminal carcinomas but may be more responsive to neoadjuvant chemotherapy. Luminal type can be subdivided into a p53-like tumor type, which is resistance to chemotherapy [32].

With the advance of immune checkpoint inhibitor therapy in the treatment of bladder cancer, the evaluation of the expression levels of programmed cell death-1/programmed cell death-1 ligand (PD-1/PD-L1) in tissue blocks with immunohistochemical stains is now critical for qualifying patients for immunotherapy (using drugs such as atezolizumab, pembrolizumab, nivolumab, durvalumab, and avelumab) [33, 34]. The suggested pathology cutoffs for evaluating available PD-L1 immunostaining are drug-specific and will be discussed in Chap. 13.

Summary

With advances of molecular technologies, morphology-based molecular diagnostics will be incorporated into bladder cancer treatment; however, solid morphologic diagnostic skills are still fundamental for practicing pathologists and pathology trainees alike. This chapter illustrates many aspects of bladder pathologic diagnostics to aid in pathological diagnosis, facilitate clinical management, and impact patients' survival and quality of life.

References

1. Global cancer observatory: cancer today. International agency for research on cancer. 2018. Available from: https://gco.iarc.fr/today. Cited 01 May 2020.
2. Richters A, Aben KKH, Kiemeney L. The global burden of urinary bladder cancer: an update. World J Urol. 2020;38(8):1895–1904.
3. Howlader N NA, Krapcho M, Miller D, Brest A, Yu M, Ruhl J, Tatalovich Z, Mariotto A, Lewis DR, Chen HS, Feuer EJ, Cronin KA (eds). SEER Cancer Statistics Review, 1975–2017, National Cancer Institute. Bethesda, MD, https://seer.cancer.gov/csr/1975_2017/, based on November 2019 SEER data submission, posted to the SEER web site, April 2020.: National Cancer Institute. Bethesda, MD,; 2020.
4. Cancer Facts and Statistics. American cancer society Atlanta, GA: American cancer society; 2020.
5. Zeegers MP, Kellen E, Buntinx F, van den Brandt PA. The association between smoking, beverage consumption, diet and bladder cancer: a systematic literature review. World J Urol. 2004;21(6):392–401.
6. Droller MJ. Bladder cancer. J Urol. 1997;157(4):1266–7.
7. Kirkali Z, Chan T, Manoharan M, Algaba F, Busch C, ChengL,etal.Bladdercancer:epidemiology,stagingand grading, and diagnosis. Urology. 2005;66(6 Suppl 1): 4–34.
8. Knowles MA, Hurst CD. Molecular biology of bladder cancer: new insights into pathogenesis and clinical diversity. Nat Rev Cancer. 2015;15(1):25–41.
9. Lopez-Knowles E, Hernandez S, Malats N, Kogevinas M, Lloreta J, Carrato A, et al. PIK3CA mutations are an early genetic alteration associated with FGFR3 mutations in superficial papillary bladder tumors. Cancer Res. 2006;66(15):7401–4.
10. van Rhijn BW, Montironi R, Zwarthoff EC, Jobsis AC, van der Kwast TH. Frequent FGFR3 mutations in urothelial papilloma. J Pathol. 2002;198(2):245–51.
11. Boulalas I, Zaravinos A, Karyotis I, Delakas D, Spandidos DA. Activation of RAS family genes in urothelial carcinoma. J Urol. 2009;181(5):2312–9.
12. Mo L, Zheng X, Huang HY, Shapiro E, Lepor H, Cordon-Cardo C, et al. Hyperactivation of Ha-ras oncogene, but not Ink4a/Arf deficiency, triggers bladder tumorigenesis. J Clin Invest. 2007;117(2):314–25.
13. Oxford G, Theodorescu D. The role of Ras superfamily proteins in bladder cancer progression. J Urol. 2003;170(5):1987–93.
14. Wu XR. Urothelial tumorigenesis: a tale of divergent pathways. Nat Rev Cancer. 2005;5(9):713–25.
15. Amin MB, Smith SC, Reuter VE, Epstein JI, Grignon DJ, Hansel DE, et al. Update for the practicing pathologist: The International Consultation On Urologic Disease-European association of urology consultation on bladder cancer. Mod Pathol. 2015;28(5):612–30.
16. Cancer Genome Atlas Research Network. Comprehensive molecular characterization of urothelial bladder carcinoma. Nature. 2014;507(7492):315–22.
17. Robertson AG, Kim J, Al-Ahmadie H, Bellmunt J, Guo G, Cherniack AD, et al. Comprehensive Molecular Characterization of Muscle-Invasive Bladder Cancer. Cell. 2017;171(3):540–56.e25.
18. Zhang ZT, Pak J, Shapiro E, Sun TT, Wu XR. Urothelium-specific expression of an oncogene in transgenic mice induced the formation of carcinoma in situ and invasive transitional cell carcinoma. Cancer Res. 1999;59(14):3512–7.
19. Puzio-Kuter AM, Castillo-Martin M, Kinkade CW, Wang X, Shen TH, Matos T, et al. Inactivation of p53 and Pten promotes invasive bladder cancer. Genes Dev. 2009;23(6):675-80.
20. Guo CC, Czerniak B. Bladder Cancer in the Genomic Era. Arch Pathol Lab Med. 2019;143(6):695–704.
21. Hartmann A, Rosner U, Schlake G, Dietmaier W, Zaak D, Hofstaedter F, et al. Clonality and genetic divergence in multifocal low-grade superficial urothelial carcinoma as determined by chromosome 9 and p53 deletion analysis. Lab Invest. 2000;80(5):709–18.
22. Hartmann A, Schlake G, Zaak D, Hungerhuber E, Hofstetter A, Hofstaedter F, et al. Occurrence of chromosome 9 and p53 alterations in multifocal dysplasia and carcinoma in situ of human urinary bladder. Cancer Res. 2002;62(3):809–18.
23. Humphray SJ, Oliver K, Hunt AR, Plumb RW, Loveland JE, Howe KL, et al. DNA sequence

and analysis of human chromosome 9. Nature. 2004;429(6990):369–74.
24. Saran KK, Gould D, Godec CJ, Verma RS. Genetics of bladder cancer. J Mol Med (Berl). 1996;74(8):441–5.
25. Saran KK, Gould D, Godec CJ, Verma RS. Genetics of bladder cancer. J Mol Med (Berl). 1996;74(8):441–5.
26. Cheng L, Cheville JC, Neumann RM, Bostwick DG. Natural history of urothelial dysplasia of the bladder. Am J Surg Pathol. 1999;23(4):443–7.
27. Stoehr R, Hartmann A, Hiendlmeyer E, Murle K, Wieland W, Knuechel R. Oligoclonality of early lesions of the urothelium as determined by microdissection-supported genetic analysis. Pathobiology. 2000;68(4-5):165–72.
28. Esrig D, Freeman JA, Stein JP, Skinner DG. Early cystectomy for clinical stage T1 transitional cell carcinoma of the bladder. Semin Urol Oncol. 1997;15(3):154-60 Esrig D, Freeman JA, Stein JP, Skinner DG. Early cystectomy for clinical stage T1 transitional cell carcinoma of the bladder. Semin Urol Oncol. 1997;15(3):154–60.
29. Sylvester RJ, van der Meijden AP, Oosterlinck W, Witjes JA, Bouffioux C, Denis L, et al. Predicting recurrence and progression in individual patients with stage Ta T1 bladder cancer using EORTC risk tables: a combined analysis of 2596 patients from seven EORTC trials. Eur Urol. 2006;49(3):466-5; discussion 475–7.
30. Tanaka N, Kikuchi E, Matsumoto K, Miyajima A, Nakagawa K, Oya M. Frequency of tumor recurrence: a strong predictor of stage progression in initially diagnosed nonmuscle invasive bladder cancer. J Urol. 2011;185(2):450–5.
31. Choi W, Porten S, Kim S, Willis D, Plimack ER, Hoffman-Censits J, et al. Identification of distinct basal and luminal subtypes of muscle-invasive bladder cancer with different sensitivities to frontline chemotherapy. Cancer Cell. 2014;25(2):152–65.
32. McConkey DJ, Choi W, Shen Y, Lee IL, Porten S, Matin SF, et al. A Prognostic Gene Expression Signature in the Molecular Classification of Chemotherapy-naive Urothelial Cancer is Predictive of Clinical Outcomes from Neoadjuvant Chemotherapy: A Phase 2 Trial of Dose-dense Methotrexate, Vinblastine, Doxorubicin, and Cisplatin with Bevacizumab in Urothelial Cancer. Eur Urol. 2016;69(5):855–62.
33. Hsu FS, Su CH, Huang KH. A Comprehensive Review of US FDA-Approved Immune Checkpoint Inhibitors in Urothelial Carcinoma. J Immunol Res. 2017;2017:6940546.
34. Powles T, Smith K, Stenzl A, Bedke J. Immune Checkpoint Inhibition in Metastatic Urothelial Cancer. Eur Urol. 2017;72(4):477–81.

2 Normal Anatomy and Histology of the Urinary Bladder with Pathologic Correlates

Ziad M. El-Zaatari and Jae Y. Ro

Urinary Bladder Anatomy

Basic Anatomic Structure

The urinary bladder is a hollow viscus pelvic organ shaped like an inverted pyramid. The urinary bladder's function is the storage of urine and participating in the expulsion of urine during micturition. Anatomically, the urinary bladder is divided into three main portions: the dome, the midportion, and the base. The dome is located superiorly and is lined by peritoneum on its outer surface. The dome's tip, known as the apex, is located anterior-superiorly. The median umbilical ligament, a remnant of the fetal urachus, attaches to the bladder apex. The urachus is a tract present during fetal life that connects the bladder and umbilicus. Failure of the urachus to obliterate may lead to anomalies known as urachal remnants (see section "Urachal Remnants"). The base of the bladder is located posteriorly and inferiorly. Within the base is an area known as the trigone: a triangular area between the right and left ureteral orifices laterally and the urethral opening inferiorly. The mucosal surface of the trigone appears smooth and flat, unlike the remainder of the bladder mucosa, which normally displays mucosal folds. The bladder neck is the region opening into the urethra and merges with the prostate tissue below in males. The bladder neck rests anteriorly and laterally on the internal obturator and levator ani muscles, in addition to the pubic bone. Invasion of these structures with carcinoma may render the patient's tumor inoperable [1]. The midportion of the bladder occupies the majority of the bladder area and is located between the dome and the apex. The midportion consists of anterior and posterior and lateral (left and right) walls.

The bladder is situated among other pelvic organs, including the distal bowels (rectum) and organs from the male and female genital tracts. In males, the seminal vesicles and the ampullae of the vasa deferentia are located between the bladder and the rectum, and the prostate is located inferior to the bladder. In females, the uterine cervix and the upper vagina are between the bladder and the rectum. The anterior surface of the uterine corpus lies against the superior-posterior surface of the bladder. Knowledge of organs adjacent to the bladder is important for staging bladder tumors, which may extend to and invade surrounding structures. Any tumor which invades beyond the bladder wall and adjacent fat into adjacent organs is designated as T4 stage.

Z. M. El-Zaatari (✉)
Department of Pathology and Genomic Medicine, Houston Methodist Hospital, Houston, TX, USA
e-mail: zmel-zaatari@houstonmethodist.org

J. Y. Ro
Department of Pathology and Genomic Medicine, Weill Medical College of Cornell University/Houston Methodist Hospital, Houston, TX, USA
e-mail: JaeRo@houstonmethodist.org

H. Zhou et al. (eds.), *Urinary Bladder Pathology*, https://doi.org/10.1007/978-3-030-71509-0_2

Involvement of the prostate by carcinoma originating from the bladder may occur via direct extension through the bladder wall and/or perivesical adipose tissue or in a pagetoid fashion along the continuous bladder and the prostatic urethra mucosa. In the latter, the tumor is staged separately according to the urethral/prostatic urethral system and constitutes T2 disease [2].

Vascular Supply and Lymphatic Drainage

The major arterial supply of the urinary bladder comes from the inferior vesical arteries, which are branches of the internal iliac arteries. Other arteries participate in the bladder blood supply and include branches of the umbilical arteries, obturator arteries, inferior gluteal arteries, and uterine and vaginal arteries in females. Veins draining the bladder collect into the internal iliac veins and form the vesical venous plexus, which communicates with the prostatic venous plexus in males and the vaginal venous plexus in females. Lymphatics of the bladder drain mainly into the external and internal iliac nodes. Portions of the bladder also drain into the sacral or common iliac nodes [1]. N-stage in the current AJCC system denotes metastasis to regional lymph nodes, including the internal iliac (hypogastric), obturator, external iliac, presacral, and common iliac lymph nodes. N3 stage denotes metastasis to common iliac lymph nodes. Excluding the common iliac lymph nodes, N1–N2 stage denotes metastasis to any of the regional lymph nodes, with N1 representing a single metastasis and N2 denoting multiple metastases. Any metastasis to non-regional lymph nodes comprises M1 disease (distant metastasis) [2–4].

Functional Anatomy and Innervation

The urinary bladder receives urine from the kidney via the ureters and acts as a reservoir for urine until it is expelled via the urethra. The urinary bladder can accommodate 400–500 mL of urine without an increase in its intraluminal pressure. The bladder is fixed by ligaments at the bladder neck, but the rest of the bladder is free to expand superiorly into the abdomen when filled with urine. A fibromuscular sheath intermingles with the detrusor muscle of the bladder and is fused to the intramural portion of the ureter. This arrangement leads to the closure of the ureter orifice when the bladder is distended, thus preventing the reflux of urine [1, 5].

Innervation of the bladder comes from a plexus of both sympathetic and parasympathetic nerves; however, only the parasympathetic nerves play a role in micturition. Parasympathetic nerves stimulate the contraction of the detrusor muscle and involuntarily open the internal sphincter during micturition. However, initiation of micturition is a voluntary process that occurs by relaxation of the perineal muscles and the external sphincter. The sensation of pain when the bladder is overdistended is due to the presence of sensory nerves [1, 5].

Gross Evaluation and Handling of Bladder Specimens

Recommendations for the gross evaluation and handling of bladder specimens were communicated by the European Society of Uropathology and the Uropathology Working Group in 2004 [6] and in the most recent College of American Pathologists' (CAP) Protocols [3, 7]. Types of specimens that may be encountered include transurethral resection of the bladder (TURB), partial cystectomy, total cystectomy, cystoprostatectomy, and pelvic exenterations, in addition to resections of diverticula and excision of urachal carcinomas [3, 6, 7]. In all of these specimens, an adequate number of sections should be submitted so that the depth of tumor invasion and tumor characteristics can be assessed. In TURB specimens, at least one section per centimeter of tumor should be submitted, and the possibility of submitting the entire tumor can be considered. In cystectomy specimens, representative sections of the tumor, including the full depth of the bladder wall and especially the area of deepest macroscopic invasion should be submitted. Additionally, sections should include representative mucosa from various areas (e.g., lateral walls, dome, and trigone), including away from the grossly visible carcinoma. The rationale for including these sections is to assess for microscopic invasive or in situ carcinoma and multifocality, which is common in urothelial neoplasms. The ureteral and urethral margins of cystectomies should also be submitted, in addition to sections from the midportions of a long segment of the ureter, if present. In cystoprostatectomy specimens, sections of the prostatic urethra with surrounding prostatic parenchyma should be submitted. This is, again, to assess for possible invasion and/or multifocality and to detect pagetoid mucosal extension of bladder cancer to the prostatic urethra or to the prostatic ducts or acini. Incidental prostatic carcinoma may also be found and is actually more common in cystoprostatectomy specimens for urothelial carcinoma. In cases of more complex pelvic exenteration specimens, including the rectum, vagina, and/or uterus, targeted sections should be taken in areas where tumor appears to infiltrate into these organs [6, 7].

Another note when handling urinary bladder specimens is to pay careful attention to the margins. The margins should be totally submitted, or at least representative sections of the margins grossly closest to the tumor. Margins include deep soft tissue margins and peritoneal surfaces, soft tissue margins of partial cystectomies, ureter and urethral margins, and other margins in pelvic exenterations, such as vaginal cuff margins. In urachal adenocarcinoma, excision of the urachal tract and umbilicus is performed, necessitating attention to the soft tissue margin surrounding the urachus and to the margin of skin around the umbilicus [6, 7].

We also recommend the following useful practices when grossing cystectomy specimens. The smooth peritoneal surface covering most of the posterior bladder surface can serve as a landmark for proper orientation of cystectomy specimens during gross evaluation [8]. After opening the bladder, careful assessment of the entire bladder mucosa should be performed, and any erythematous or fibrotic areas should be well sampled. We suggest using a "Y-shaped" incision on the anterior wall of the bladder made in an inferior-superior direction to visualize the entire mucosa [8]. Also, the interureteric ridge, an anatomic structure with the appearance of a slightly raised curve resembling a lip with bulges at either end, can be used to locate the left and right ureteric orifices on the mucosal surface. The orifices will be within the left and right bulges at either end of the "lip" and can be probed [8]. Finally, sequential sections of the bladder in one direction (our preference is in the superior to inferior direction) should be taken to include the entire thickness of the bladder wall and surrounding adipose tissue for proper gross assessment of the depth of tumor invasion [8].

Histology

Urothelium

The urothelium is the epithelial lining of the urinary bladder, ureters, renal pelvis, and portions of the urethra. It consists of three layers: superficial "umbrella" cells, intermediate cells, and basal cells (Fig. 2.1). The urothelium varies in thickness

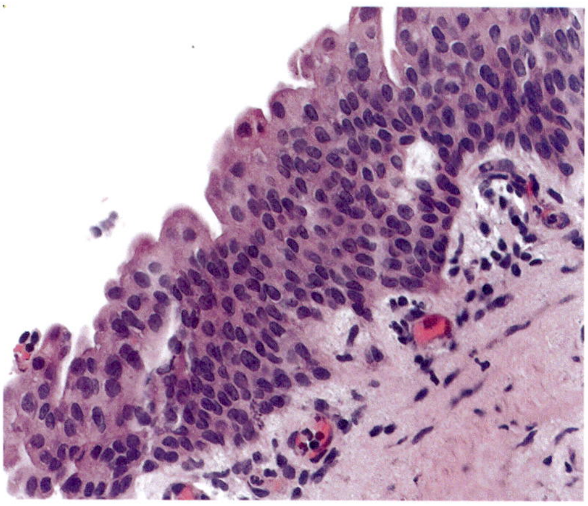

Fig. 2.1 Normal urothelium. Cells lining the urothelium are superficially umbrella cells, followed by a layer of intermediate cells and a basal cell layer. Intermediate cells are oval-round with nuclear grooves and a vertical orientation. Umbrella cells have abundant cytoplasm, are horizontally oriented, and cover more than one of the intermediate cells. Basal cells are situated on the basement membrane immediately above the lamina propria

from 2 to 7 layers, depending on the location and functional status with the degree of distension within the urinary tract. In histologic sections, the urothelium may appear artificially thickened due to an oblique plane of sectioning.

Superficial cells comprise the innermost layer of the urothelium. They are larger than other urothelial cells and lie horizontally over intermediate cells in an umbrella-like fashion. They have abundant eosinophilic cytoplasm and can be binucleated. Superficial cells are particularly susceptible to denudation and may thus appear in urine cytology specimens, in which case they must be distinguished from cells of high-grade urothelial carcinoma [9]. Umbrella cells may also become displaced from the surface in histologic sections, mimicking carcinoma in situ. Key differentiating factors for recognizing umbrella cells in this situation include the presence of abundant eosinophilic cytoplasm, binucleation, low nuclear to cytoplasmic ratio, and lack of hyperchromasia [10]. Intravesical chemotherapy (thiotepa and mitomycin C) may induce atypia of the umbrella cells in the form of nuclear enlargement, multinucleation, smudging of chromatin, and cytoplasmic vacuoles. These changes should not be overinterpreted as carcinomatous change [10].

Intermediate cells lie perpendicular to the umbrella cells, are oval or slightly elongated, and are polarized in an orderly vertical arrangement toward the surface in the normal urothelium. Their chromatin is finely stippled with no or inconspicuous nucleoli, and they often display nuclear grooves. Changes from these characteristic features of intermediate cells should prompt consideration of abnormalities as either reactive or dysplasia/urothelial carcinoma in situ. Basal cells lie on the basement membrane and are smaller than the overlying intermediate cells. They are cuboidal with condensed chromatin that suggests a lower degree of transcriptional activity compared to intermediate cells [11]. Mitoses are overall absent or at most very difficult to locate in normal urothelium [11], whereas reactive urothelium or in situ carcinoma may show numerous mitotic figures [10].

Overall, the histology of normal urothelium can be summarized with the triad of the presence of (1) umbrella cells, (2) oval-round intermediate cells with vertical polarization, and (3) nuclear grooves.

Lamina Propria, Muscularis Mucosa, and Muscularis Propria

Immediately beneath the urothelial basement membrane is a layer of loose connective tissue containing abundant vessels, lymphatics, sensory nerve endings, and some elastic fibers [1]. This layer is referred to as "submucosa" or "lamina propria" interchangeably; however, because of the lack of a well-defined muscularis mucosa in most bladders, the latter term is preferred [12]. A variable amount of smooth muscle constitutes the muscularis mucosa and was first described in 1983 by Dixon and Gosling. The 1983 description noted irregularly arranged bundles of smooth muscle located approximately midway between the urothelium above and the detrusor muscle below [13]. In 1987, Ro et al. provided a more detailed description of the muscularis mucosa, particularly in the context of the staging and treatment of urinary bladder carcinoma. In their study, the muscle fibers in the lamina propria formed a distinct muscularis mucosa layer in only 3 of 100 cases, whereas more commonly, these muscle fibers were interrupted or discontinuous (20/100 cases) and most commonly dispersed or scattered forming thin bundles (71/100 cases). A complete absence of muscle fibers was also observed in a minority of cases (6/100). Their description was based on adequate sampling of all areas of the bladder, including the dome, anterior, lateral, and posterior walls, and the trigone. All bladder locations had similar morphology and frequency of smooth muscle distribution, with the exception of the trigone where the detrusor muscle is closely adherent to the overlying urothelial layer. The authors also described the presence of vessels that run along the length of the lamina propria in either a continuous or an interrupted pattern and are closely associated with fibers of the muscularis mucosa.

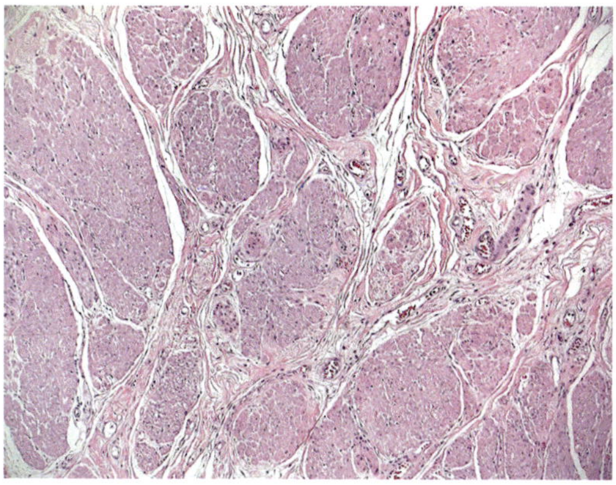

Fig. 2.2 Muscularis propria. Thick muscle bundles characterize the muscularis propria of the urinary bladder. It is important to differentiate muscularis propria from hypertrophic muscularis mucosa, as only invasion of the former constitutes T2 pathologic stage

The importance of the above findings is to differentiate the muscle fibers of the muscularis mucosa from that of the detrusor because only invasion of the latter by carcinoma necessitates cystectomy, with the consequential morbidity inherent in this procedure. Complicating the distinction between muscularis mucosa and propria is the occurrence of hyperplastic muscularis mucosa, which may more closely mimic the thick muscle bundles of the muscularis propria (Fig. 2.2). Hyperplastic muscularis mucosa, defined as muscle bundles greater than three layers thick, was found in 30–36% of samples from different bladder locations (the trigone was the exception with only 17% showing hyperplastic muscularis mucosa fibers) [14]. Beyond these initial descriptions, a more detailed description of muscularis mucosa morphology, including hyperplastic forms, is provided in the 2007 paper by Paner et al. [15].

Immunostaining for smoothelin protein may be useful to differentiate muscularis mucosa from muscularis propria [16–22]. The available studies have shown that smoothelin usually stains positively in muscularis propria and negatively in muscularis mucosa. Although some overlap in this staining pattern has been observed, when only intense staining for muscularis propria and very weak or absent staining for muscularis mucosa are considered, the specificity of smoothelin is close to 100% for discriminating muscularis mucosa from muscularis propria. Vimentin immunostaining has also been studied and increased the specificity of distinguishing muscularis propria and muscularis mucosa when used with smoothelin [21]. Despite the above findings, smoothelin immunostaining has not been widely validated using different protocols and techniques. Because of this and other limitations cited in the current literature, the International Society of Urological Pathology (ISUP) 2013 Consensus Conference did not reach a recommendation for the use of smoothelin or vimentin for subclassifying muscle types in routine practice [23].

Perivesical Adipose Tissue

The thick muscle fibers of the muscularis propria merge with the surrounding perivesical adipose tissue. T3 disease consists of invasion of bladder tumors beyond the muscularis propria and into the perivesical adipose. However, adipose tissue may be present in any layer of the bladder, which may confound the distinction of true T3 disease from a less invasive stage. In a study by Philip et al., adipose tissue was found in the muscularis propria in all of 139 cystectomies studied and was found, albeit less frequently, in more superficial layers of the bladder up to the lamina propria [24]. In addition, the perivesical adipose tissue was not well delineated from the deep muscularis propria, which haphazardly merged with the perivesical fat [24]. Recognition of these histologic variations is, therefore, crucial for the pathologist. Caution must be taken not to overdiagnose T3 disease in biopsy or transurethral tumor resections where orientation of the specimen with respect to the layers of the bladder wall is difficult. In such cases, the true depth of any adipose tissue invasion cannot be accurately assessed for the assignment of pT stage.

Developmental and Anatomic Anomalies

Urachal Remnants

Urachal remnants occur because of incomplete regression of the fetal urachus, the tract between the urinary bladder dome and the umbilicus. These remnants vary in form, from cysts between the bladder and umbilicus, to diverticula connected to the bladder dome, to urachal sinus openings at the umbilicus but disconnected from the bladder, to a fully patent urachus with a complete persistent tract opening at the umbilicus connecting to the bladder. Urachal cysts typically show a urothelial lining of cuboidal to columnar epithelium and/or denuded and inflamed cyst walls [25] (Fig. 2.3). Urachal remnants may lead to complications, such as infection necessitating surgical intervention [26]. Urachal carcinoma is a rare tumor that occurs most often in the bladder dome and is associated with the presence of urachal remnants, although the absence of urachal remnants does not necessarily rule out the diagnosis of urachal carcinoma [27].

Diverticula

A diverticulum is an outward bulge of the inner epithelial lining of the bladder through a defect in its muscular layer. It can be present since birth or acquired later in life due to various causes. There are two peak times of occurrence of diverticula: one presenting at 10 years and the other at 55–70 years. In children, diverticula are usually congenital, and very often there will only be a single outpouching. In adults, it is acquired and there may be several diverticula. Diverticula can be classified as true diverticula, which do not include muscularis propria tissue, and pseudodiverticula, which include muscularis propria in their outpouching. Diverticula form in response to increased intravesical pressure due to obstruction or weakness of Waldeyer fascia and weakness of the detrusor muscle [28].

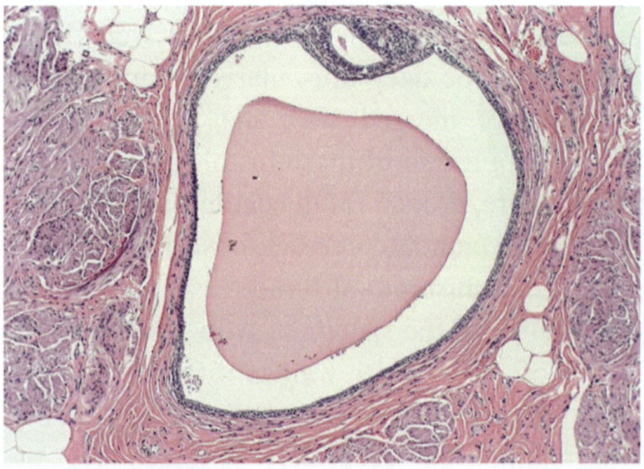

Fig. 2.3 Urachal cyst. A cystic urachal remnant lined by cuboidal epithelium. Urachal remnants can also have a benign urothelial lining

A wide array of histologic findings occurs in diverticula either primarily or in association with other conditions and pathologies present simultaneously in the urinary bladder. These include both malignancies and benign findings: chronic inflammation, acute inflammation, granulomatous inflammation, cystitis glandularis, intestinal metaplasia, keratinizing and non-keratinizing squamous metaplasia, nephrogenic adenoma, ulceration, polypoid cystitis, papillary hyperplasia, reactive urothelial atypia, carcinoma in situ, high-grade urothelial carcinoma including variant morphologies, papillary urothelial carcinoma, primary squamous carcinoma, and secondary melanoma [28, 29].

Bladder Exstrophy

Bladder exstrophy is a rare congenital defect characterized by eversion of the bladder and related structures through the ventral wall of the abdomen between the umbilicus and the symphysis pubis. This results in the bladder mucosa being fused to the adjacent skin [25]. The prevalence is estimated at around 2 per 100,000 births and is approximately twice common in males than in females [30]. Exstrophy is associated with other congenital defects of the urogenital tract, including epispadias and undescended testes in males and bifid clitoris and divergent labia in females [30]. Microscopically, the bladder mucosa shows acute and chronic inflammation and ulceration and metaplastic changes, including squamous metaplasia and intestinal metaplasia that often persist after surgical closure [25]. The malignant potential of the exstrophied bladder mucosa is well known, with 95% of tumors being adenocarcinomas and 3% to 5% being squamous cell carcinomas. Most (60%) of malignant tumors associated with exstrophy of the bladder occur during the fourth and fifth decades of life. Of the remaining, about 20% each occur after 60 years and before 40 years [31].

Ectopic Prostate Tissue

Ectopic prostate tissue is a rare finding that may occur in the bladder or other genitourinary/extragenitourinary sites or even in females [32]. The microscopic appearance is that of prostatic stroma and glandular epithelium and/or a urothelial cell lining. The prostatic glands are characteristically positive for prostate-specific antigen (PSA) and prostatic acid phosphatase (PSAP) [25, 33]. Reported cases presented as polyps or masses within the bladder [34]. One case presented as prostatic adenocarcinoma arising within ectopic prostate tissue in the bladder dome [32]. The main differential diagnosis is with urachal remnant and prostatic urethral polyp, the latter of which has matching histology to ectopic prostate yet only occurs in the prostatic urethra [25].

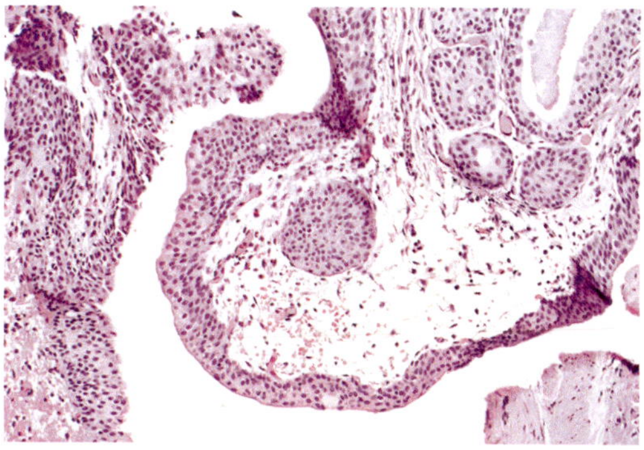

Fig. 2.4 Von Brunn nest. Von Brunn nests are commonly found beneath normal urothelium. They consist of nests of benign urothelial cells with or without a connection to the overlying urothelium. Florid proliferations of Von Brunn nests must be distinguished from nested variants of urothelial carcinoma

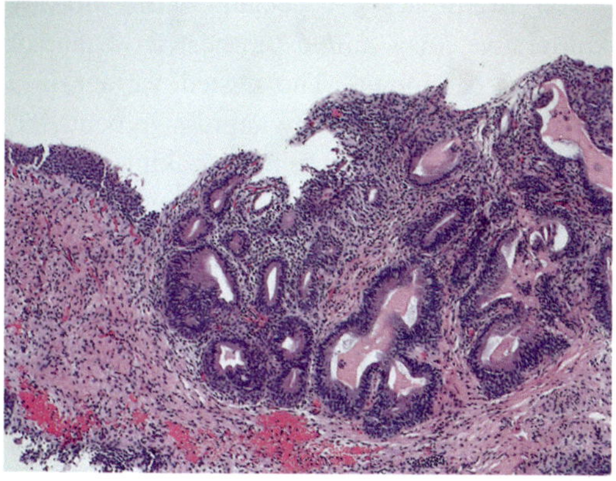

Fig. 2.5 Cystitis glandularis. Von Brunn nests can become cystically dilated and develop a glandular epithelial lining. This is termed cystitis cystica and glandularis (the latter seen here), a potential mimicker of bladder adenocarcinoma

Normal Histologic Variations and Benign Mimickers of Malignancy

von Brunn Nests, Cystitis Cystica, and Cystitis Glandularis

von Brunn nests are benign invaginations of urothelium into the underlying lamina propria and appear as solid nests that may or may not show a connection to the surface (Fig. 2.4). von Brunn nests may become cystic, in which case they are described as cystitis cystica. The epithelial cells lining these cysts are one to several layers thick and are urothelial or cuboidal in shape. The epithelial lining of cystitis cystica may also undergo metaplasia, transforming the lining of the cysts into columnar mucin-secreting cells. This is termed cystitis glandularis (Fig. 2.5). Finally, lining cells of cystitis glandularis can show goblet cell morphology, i.e., intestinal metaplasia [1] (Fig. 2.6). This is known as intestinal-type cystitis glandularis. Von Brunn nests and cystitis cystica are common findings, as 89% and 60% of bladders have these lesions, respectively [35]. These changes are most commonly seen in the bladder neck and trigone [35].

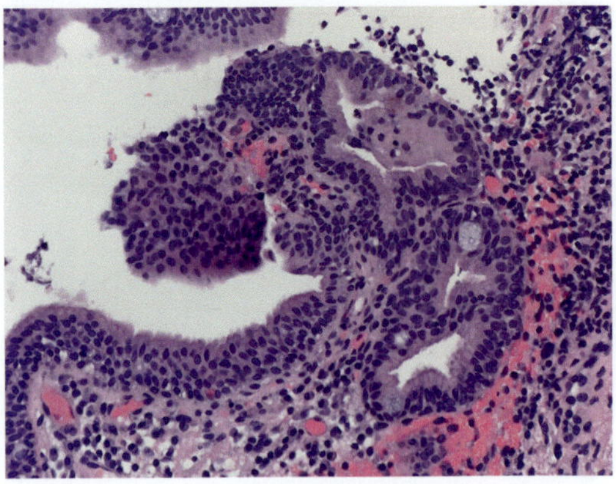

Fig. 2.6 Intestinal metaplasia in cystitis glandularis. Goblet cells are seen in the epithelial lining of cystitis glandularis with intestinal metaplasia. This is a benign finding

von Brunn nests, especially when floridly proliferative, may mimic the nested variant of urothelial carcinoma. The nested variant is a malignancy with generally aggressive behavior, yet frequently bland cytology, making the distinction even more critical. Features that help distinguish this malignancy from von Brunn nests include (1) the variable and smaller size of nests in the nested variant; (2) the more pronounced cyst formation, apical glandular differentiation, and eosinophilic secretions in the nested variant; (3) the complete absence of atypia in von Brunn nests versus occasional atypia in the nested variant; (4) presence of a flat, proliferative base in von Brunn nests versus a more infiltrative pattern in the nested variant; and (5) muscularis propria invasion, which usually indicates malignancy [36].

A recently described variant of nested urothelial carcinoma, the large nested variant, can also appear similar to von Brunn nests. The large size of nests in this variant can even more closely mimic von Brunn nests. However, unlike von Brunn nests, the large nested variant often has a haphazard arrangement of nests within the lamina propria with ample lamina propria in between the nests. Also, although the large nested variant usually shows minimal cytologic atypia, a certain degree of nuclear pleomorphism consisting of small nucleoli, scattered hyperchromatic cells, and mild nuclear pleomorphism is often detectable. Additionally, invasion of the nests into the muscularis propria indicates a malignant process, and the concurrence of usual type urothelial carcinoma can aid in the diagnosis [37]. A recent study has shown that the detection of TERT promoter mutations may help distinguish von Brunn nests from nested and large nested variants of urothelial carcinoma, as this mutation was not detected in any von Brunn nests, whereas it was detected in several cases of malignancy. However, further studies and validation are needed before incorporating TERT molecular testing into routine practice in this setting [38].

Intestinal metaplasia in cystitis glandularis may also mimic adenocarcinoma of the urinary bladder [39, 40]. Both can show mucin extravasation, atypia, and mitoses; however, the extent of these features is more pronounced in adenocarcinoma [39]. Tubular adenomas [41] and dysplasia of cystitis glandularis [42] have also been described. Although it appears that non-dysplastic intestinal metaplasia is not a precursor lesion for adenocarcinoma [43], the presence of dysplasia was associated with adenocarcinoma or urothelial carcinoma in several cases. Therefore, clinical follow-up is recommended whenever dysplasia is present [42].

Squamous Metaplasia

Squamous metaplasia is the transformation of the urothelium into a squamous-lined epithelium. Squamous metaplasia is divided into two types: non-keratinizing and keratinizing. The former, also known as vaginal metaplasia, is a common finding in the bladders of women, especially in the trigone area. Indeed, 72% of bladders removed at autopsy in women dying of non-urinary tract diseases showed this type of metaplasia [44]. Therefore, non-keratinizing squamous metaplasia is considered a normal histologic finding in women.

Keratinizing squamous metaplasia is more insidious and can occur in men and, less commonly, in women. Keratinizing squamous metaplasia is caused by a variety of factors that cause infection and/or irritation to the bladder mucosa,

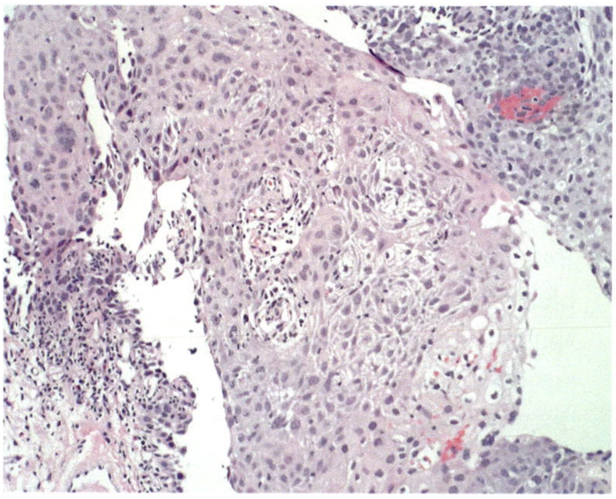

Fig. 2.7 Squamous cell carcinoma. Keratinizing metaplasia is a potential risk factor for the development of primary squamous cell carcinoma of the urinary bladder, which is shown here

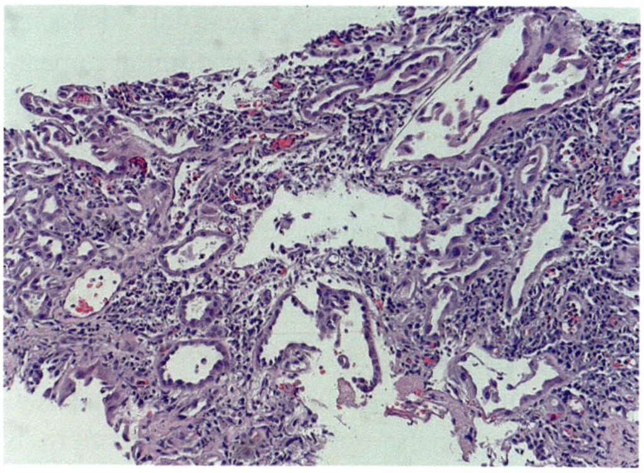

Fig. 2.8 Nephrogenic adenoma (tubular). This case of nephrogenic adenoma shows a tubular growth pattern and single-cell-lined glands with hobnailing of cells within the tubular lumens

including bacterial urinary tract infections, Schistosoma parasite eggs, indwelling catheters, and urinary stones [45]. It is not certain whether keratinizing squamous metaplasia is a precursor to carcinoma; however, it is often found concurrently in patients with pure squamous cell carcinoma of the bladder or urothelial carcinoma with squamous differentiation [45, 46] (Fig. 2.7). Because of this association, surveillance cystoscopy with possible transurethral resections is indicated.

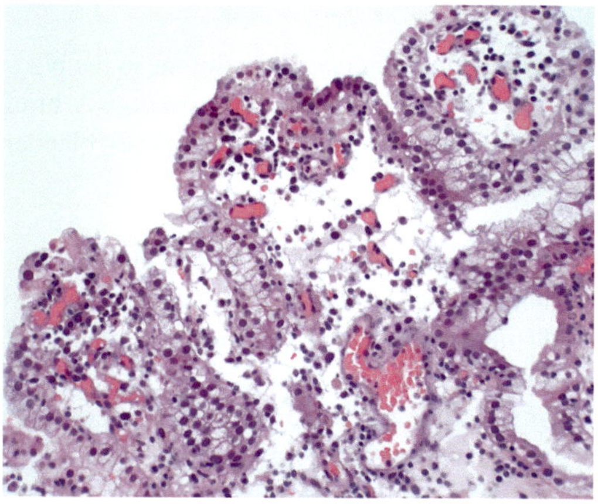

Fig. 2.9 Nephrogenic adenoma (polypoid). Nephrogenic adenoma displaying a single-cell lining of bland cuboidal cells with clear to eosinophilic cytoplasm. This case shows a polypoid configuration

Nephrogenic Adenoma

Nephrogenic adenoma is a benign proliferation that is most commonly encountered in the bladder [47]. It is characterized by a variety of growth patterns, most commonly tubular (Fig. 2.8), cystic, polypoid, and papillary [47, 48]. Additional, less common patterns have been described, including fibromyxoid [49] and flat [50]. The lining cells are distinctively single-layered, are cuboidal to low columnar, and have scant cytoplasm, with occasional cells displaying abundant eosinophilic or clear cytoplasm (Fig. 2.9). A hobnail appearance is also frequently seen. The cells are bland, although they occasionally have prominent nucleoli. Mitoses are usually not seen. The origin of nephrogenic adenoma may be metaplastic or originate from renal tubular cells, as suggested by a recent study of renal transplant patients [51]. Nearly all cases of nephrogenic adenomas occur in patients with a history of prior surgical treatment or inflammatory disease [52].

Several morphologies of nephrogenic adenoma may mimic malignant diagnoses and therefore merit attention from the pathologist. The tubules of nephrogenic adenoma may appear infiltrative and therefore lead to confusion with adenocarcinoma. Small tubules may also contain mucin and be lined by a single cell, mimicking signet ring cell adenocarcinoma [48]. Additionally, a nephrogenic adenoma-like clear cell adenocarcinoma has been described [53]. Similar appearances may confuse nephrogenic adenoma with prostatic adenocarcinoma, particularly when it involves the prostatic urethra or prostate. Staining with alpha-methyl acyl-coenzyme A racemase (AMACR) in this last scenario is potentially risky, as it is positive in both nephrogenic adenoma and prostatic carcinoma. However, PSA is usually negative and PAX8 positive in nephrogenic adenoma, whereas the opposite staining pattern is seen in prostatic adenocarcinoma [48]. Thus, performing PSA and PAX8 staining is preferred over AMACR in this scenario.

Cystitis

A variety of inflammatory conditions in the bladder are grouped under the term cystitis. A brief overview of the different types of urinary bladder cystitis follows [25]:

- *Follicular cystitis*: Cystitis with lymphoid follicles in the lamina propria. It is important to distinguish follicular cystitis from malignant lymphoma.
- *Giant cell cystitis*: Refers to the presence of atypical stromal cells within the lamina propria of the bladder. The cells are nonmalignant and of macrophage origin.
- *Interstitial cystitis*: A diagnosis of exclusion which clinically presents as recurrent discomfort or pain of the bladder and adjacent pelvic region. Mast cells may frequently be seen; however, they are a nonspecific finding. Although usually idiopathic, some cases of interstitial cystitis appeared to be related to IgG4 inflammation [54].
- *Eosinophilic cystitis*: Characterized by infiltrates consisting of abundant eosinophils in the lamina propria and bladder wall. It is usually a nonspecific reaction to injury; however, it may rarely be associated with allergic diseases and parasitic infections.
- *Infectious cystitis*: Cystitis caused by various infectious organisms, including bacteria, fungi, viruses, and parasites.
- *Encrusted cystitis*: Describes the deposition of inorganic salts in injured bladder mucosa due to the presence of urea-splitting bacteria. Calcified and necrotic debris mixed with inflammatory cells and covered with fibrin are present microscopically.
- *Emphysematous* cystitis: Consists of gas-filled blebs that appear microscopically as empty spaces within the lamina propria. The spaces are lined by attenuated cells, and there is frequent foreign-body giant cell reaction.
- *Granulomatous cystitis*: Is seen most commonly following bacille Calmette-Guerin (BCG) therapy for urothelial carcinoma in situ. It consists of noncaseating granulomas in the lamina propria (Fig. 2.10) with possible overlying urothelial reactive atypia or denudation. Granulomas following transurethral resection of bladder tumors (postsurgical granulomas) are another form of granulomatous inflammation and, unlike BCG granulomas, may contain necrosis.
- *Radiation cystitis*: Follows radiation therapy. Acutely, it is characterized by edema and vascular congestion in the lamina propria, mucosal erosion and ulceration, and cytologic atypia that can mimic carcinoma in situ. Some cases may include giant cells and multinucleated cells or pseudocarcinomatous hyperplasia of the epithelium. Extravasated red blood cells, fibrin deposition, inflammation, hemosiderin, mucosal ulceration, atypical fibro-

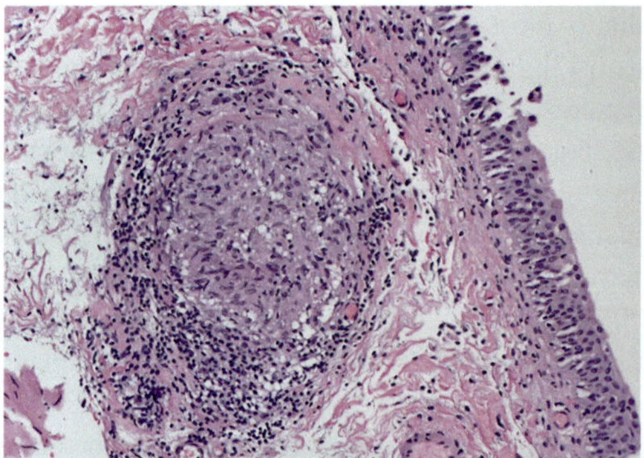

Fig. 2.10 BCG granuloma. Noncaseating granuloma in the lamina propria of a bladder treated with BCG therapy

blasts, hyperplastic or atrophic urothelium, and squamous metaplasia are also features. Chronically, radiation cystitis may lead to collagenization of the lamina propria and muscularis propria and myointimal proliferation or hyalinization of the media of arterioles.

- *Chemotherapy-induced cystitis*: Refers to cystitis caused by systemic or topical chemotherapeutic or immunologic drugs. According to the agent used, cystitis may be (1) hemorrhagic (due to cyclophosphamide), (2) atypical (due to mitomycin C) with degenerative changes and atypia of the urothelial lining, or (3) granulomatous (due to BCG; see granulomatous cystitis above).

Polypoid Cystitis

Polypoid cystitis is a mucosal lesion in the bladder with a polypoid or papillary configuration. Polypoid cystitis arises in the setting of an inflammatory insult to the bladder, such as long-standing indwelling catheterization [55]. The main differential diagnosis is with papillary urothelial carcinoma [56], which is a malignancy, while polypoid cystitis is a benign condition. Microscopically, polypoid cystitis is characterized by broad fibrovascular cores with dilated vessels, edematous stroma, and mixed acute and chronic inflammation in the stroma. Papillae should be simple without complex branching, and the overlying urothelium is normal or with reactive changes or metaplasia but no diagnostic features of malignancy [25, 56].

Malakoplakia

Malakoplakia is an inflammatory process that characteristically appears as multiple yellow or yellow-brown plaques on the bladder mucosal surface. It can occur throughout the genitourinary tract, though the bladder is the most common site. Microscopically, the lesion consists of sheets of macrophages and characteristic Michaelis-Gutmann bodies in the cytoplasm (von Hansemann cells). The Michaelis-Gutmann bodies are 2–10 μm structures that have a targetoid appearance and stain positively for calcium (von Kossa stain) and iron (Perls Prussian blue stain). Malakoplakia is thought to be caused by impaired bactericidal activity of macrophages and is related to chronic immunosuppression and bacterial infections, the most common of which is *Escherichia coli.* Malakoplakia is a benign disease and is usually self-limiting. The main differential diagnosis includes Langerhans cell histiocytosis and xanthogranulomatous inflammation, which also show abundant histiocytic cells within their lesions [57].

Fibroepithelial Polyp

Fibroepithelial polyps are uncommon benign lesions that occur most commonly in pediatric patients but can occur in adults. Histologically, fibroepithelial polyps are usually characterized by a polypoid lesion covered with normal urothelial lining and may display either of three architectural patterns: (1) polypoid with club-like projections, florid cystitis cystica, and cystitis glandularis, (2) papillary with multiple small fibrovascular cores containing dense fibrous tissue, and (3) polypoid with secondary tall finger-like projections. These polyps lack the prominent edema and inflammation of polypoid cystitis [58] (see above section "Polypoid Cystitis").

Mullerian Lesions

Endometriosis can occur in the bladder and is characterized by endometrial glands, stroma, and recent or old hemorrhage. Endocervicosis can also occur and has endocervical-like glands with a haphazard appearance, a columnar mucin-secreting epithelial lining, frequent ciliated cells, and mucin extravasation [25, 59]. When endometriosis, endocervicosis, and endosalpingiosis (fallopian tube-type epithelial inclusions) coexist, the lesion is termed mullerianosis. Although rare, it is important to recognize these Mullerian lesions, as they may mimic primary adenocarcinoma of the bladder [60].

Conclusion

In summary, normal bladder anatomy and histology have direct relevance for bladder pathology and tumors. Basic knowledge of the normal bladder, as well as the benign entities described herein, constitutes an important foundation for genitourinary and general surgical pathologists alike.

References

1. Reuter VE, Al-Ahmadie H, Tickoo SK. Chapter 35: Urinary bladder, ureter, and renal pelvis. In: Mills SE, editor. Histology for pathologists. Philadelphia: Lippincott, Williams and Wilkins; 2012.
2. Amin MB, Edge SB, Greene FL, Schilsky RL, Gaspar LE, Washington M. AJCC cancer staging manual. New York: Springer; 2017.
3. Paner GP, Zhou M, Srigley JR, Amin MB, Allan R, Delahunt B, et al. Protocol for the examination of cystectomy specimens from patients with carcinoma of the urinary bladder: College of American Pathologists; 2019. https://documents.cap.org/protocols/cp-urinary-bladder-resection-20-4020.pdf.
4. Magers MJ, Lopez-Beltran A, Montironi R, Williamson SR, Kaimakliotis HZ, Cheng L. Staging of bladder cancer. Histopathology. 2019;74:112–34. https://doi.org/10.1111/his.13734.
5. Weledji E, Eyongeta D, Ngounou E. The anatomy of urination: what every physician should know: urinary control. Clin Anat. 2018;32 https://doi.org/10.1002/ca.23296.
6. Lopez-Beltran A, Bassi P, Pavone-Macaluso M, Montironi R. Handling and pathology reporting of specimens with carcinoma of the urinary bladder, ureter, and renal pelvis. A joint proposal of the European Society of Uropathology and the Uropathology Working Group. Virchows Arch. 2004;445:103–10. https://doi.org/10.1007/s00428-004-1039-8.
7. Paner GP, Zhou M, Srigley JR, Amin MB, Allan R, Delahunt B, et al. Protocol for the examination of biopsy and transurethral resection of bladder tumor (TURBT) specimens from patients with carcinoma of the urinary bladder: College of American Pathologists; 2019. https://documents.cap.org/protocols/cp-urinary-bladder-biopsy-20-4020.pdf.
8. Lemos MB, Shen SS. Chapter 6: Genitourinary. In: Lemos MB, Okoye E, editors. Atlas of surgical pathology grossing. Cham, Switzerland: Springer; 2019.
9. Renshaw A, Gould E. High-grade urothelial carcinoma on urine cytology resembling umbrella cells. Acta Cytol. 2017;62 https://doi.org/10.1159/000481908.
10. Brimo F, Epstein J. Selected common diagnostic problems in urologic pathology perspectives from a large consult service in genitourinary pathology. Arch Pathol Lab Med. 2012;136:360–71. https://doi.org/10.5858/arpa.2011-0187-RA.
11. Jost SP, Gosling JA, Dixon JS. The morphology of normal human bladder urothelium. J Anat. 1989;167:103–15.
12. Ro J, Ayala A, El-Naggar A. Muscularis mucosa of urinary bladder importance for staging and treatment. Am J Surg Pathol. 1987;11:668–73. https://doi.org/10.1097/00000478-198709000-00002.
13. Dixon J, Gosling J. Histology and fine structure of the muscularis mucosae of the human urinary bladder. J Anat. 1983;136:265–71.
14. Vakar-Lopez F, Shen S, Zhang S, Tamboli P, Ayala A, Ro J. Muscularis mucosae of the urinary bladder revisited with emphasis on its hyperplastic patterns: a study of a large series of cystectomy specimens. Ann Diagn Pathol. 2008;11:395–401. https://doi.org/10.1016/j.anndiagpath.2006.12.014.
15. Paner G, Ro J, Wojcik E, Venkataraman G, Datta M, Amin M. Further characterization of the muscle layers and lamina propria of the urinary bladder by systematic histologic mapping. Am J Surg Pathol. 2007;31:1420–9. https://doi.org/10.1097/PAS.0b013e3180588283.
16. Paner G, Shen S, Lapetino S, Venkataraman G, Barkan G, Quek M, et al. Diagnostic utility of antibody to smoothelin in the distinction of muscularis propria from muscularis mucosae of the urinary bladder. Am J Surg Pathol. 2008;33:91–8.
17. Council L, Hameed O. Differential expression of immunohistochemical markers in bladder smooth muscle and myofibroblasts, and the potential utility of desmin, smoothelin, and vimentin in staging of bladder carcinoma. Mod Pathol. 2009;22:639–50. https://doi.org/10.1038/modpathol.2009.9.
18. Bovio I, Al-Quran S, Rosser C, Algood C, Drew P, Allan R, et al. Smoothelin immunohistochemistry is a useful adjunct for assessing muscularis propria invasion in bladder carcinoma. Histopathology. 2010;56:951–6. https://doi.org/10.1111/j.1365-2559.2010.03575.x.
19. Paner G, Brown J, Lapetino S, Nese N, Gupta R, Shen S, et al. Diagnostic use of antibody to smoothelin in the recognition of muscularis propria in transurethral resection of urinary bladder tumor (TURBT) specimens. Am J Surg Pathol. 2010;34:792–9. https://doi.org/10.1097/PAS.0b013e3181da7650.
20. Miyamoto H, Sharma R, Illei P, Epstein J. Pitfalls in the use of smoothelin to identify muscularis propria invasion by urothelial carcinoma. Am J Surg Pathol. 2010;34:418–22. https://doi.org/10.1097/PAS.0b013e3181ce5066.
21. Elkady N, Abdou A, Kandil M, Ghanem N. Diagnostic value of smoothelin and vimentin in differentiating muscularis propria from muscularis mucosa of bladder carcinoma. Int J Biol Markers. 2017;32(3):e305–12. https://doi.org/10.5301/jbm.5000252.
22. Lindh C, Nilsson R, Lindstrom M, Lundin L, Elmberger G. Detection of smoothelin expression in the urinary bladder is strongly dependent on pretreatment conditions: a critical analysis with pos-

sible consequences for cancer staging. Virchows Arch. 2011;458:665–70. https://doi.org/10.1007/s00428-011-1076-z.
23. Amin MB, Trpkov K, Lopez-Beltran A, Grignon D; Members of the ISUP Immunohistochemistry in Diagnostic Urologic Pathology Group. Best practices recommendations in the application of immunohistochemistry in the bladder lesions: report from the International Society of Urologic Pathology consensus conference. Am J Surg Pathol. 2014;38(8):e20–34. https://doi.org/10.1097/PAS.0000000000000240. PMID: 25029121.
24. Philip A, Amin M, Tamboli P, Lee T, Hill C, Ro J. Intravesical adipose tissue: a quantitative study of its presence and location with implications for therapy and prognosis. Am J Surg Pathol. 2000;24:1286–90.
25. Magi-Galluzzi C, Zhou M. Genitourinary pathology. Philadelphia: Elsevier/Saunders; 2015.
26. Naiditch J, Radhakrishnan J, Chin A. Current diagnosis and management of urachal remnants. J Pediatr Surg. 2013;48:2148–52. https://doi.org/10.1016/j.jpedsurg.2013.02.069.
27. Gopalan A, Sharp D, Fine S, Tickoo S, Herr H, Reuter V, et al. Urachal carcinoma a clinicopathologic analysis of 24 cases with outcome correlation. Am J Surg Pathol. 2009;33(5):659–68.
28. Idrees MT, Alexander RE, Kum JB, Cheng L. The spectrum of histopathologic findings in vesical diverticulum: implications for pathogenesis and staging. Hum Pathol. 2013;44:1223–32.
29. Kong MX, Zhao X, Kheterpal E, Lee P, Taneja S, Lepor H, et al. Histopathologic and clinical features of vesical diverticula. Urology. 2013;82(1):142–7.
30. Siffel C, Correa A, Amar E, Bakker MK, Bermejo-Sanchez E, Bianca S, et al. Bladder exstrophy: an epidemiologic study from the international clearinghouse for birth defects surveillance and research, and an overview of the literature. Am J Med Genet C Semin Med Genet. 2011;0(4):321–32. https://doi.org/10.1002/ajmg.c.30316.
31. Sharma PK, Pandey PK, Vijay MK, Bera MK, Singh JP, Saha K. Squamous cell carcinoma in exstrophy of the bladder. Korean J Urol. 2013;54(8):555–7.
32. Gardner JM, Khurana H, Leach FS, Ayala AG, Zhai J, Ro JY. Adenocarcinoma in ectopic prostate tissue at dome of bladder: a case report of a patient with urothelial carcinoma of the bladder and adenocarcinoma of the prostate. Arch Pathol Lab Med. 2010;134:1271–5.
33. Halat S, Eble JN, Grignon DJ, Lacy S, Montironi R, MacLennan GT, et al. Ectopic prostate tissue: histogenesis and histopathological characteristics. Histopathology. 2011;58:750–8. https://doi.org/10.1111/j.1365-2559.2011.03799.x.
34. Adhya AK, Pradhan MR. Ectopic prostatic tissue presenting as a mucosal tumor in urinary bladder. Indian J Pathol Microbiol. 2018;61:452–3.
35. Wiener D, Koss L, Sablay B, Freed S. The prevalence and significance of Brunn's nests, cystitis cystica and squamous metaplasia in normal bladders. J Urol. 1979;122:317–21. https://doi.org/10.1016/S0022-5347(17)56384-3.
36. Volmar K, Chan T, De Marzo A, Epstein J. Florid von Brunn nests mimicking urothelial carcinoma. Am J Surg Pathol. 2003;27:1243–52. https://doi.org/10.1097/00000478-200309000-00008.
37. Cox R, Epstein J. Large nested variant of urothelial carcinoma: 23 cases mimicking von Brunn nests and inverted growth pattern of noninvasive papillary urothelial carcinoma. Am J Surg Pathol. 2011;35:1337–42. https://doi.org/10.1097/PAS.0b013e318222a653.
38. Tian W, Zhuge J, Zheng X, Huang T, Cai D, Zhang D, et al. Distinguishing nested variants of urothelial carcinoma from benign mimickers by TERT promoter mutation. Am J Surg Pathol. 2014;39 https://doi.org/10.1097/PAS.0000000000000305.
39. Jacobs L, Brooks J, Epstein J. Differentiation of colonic metaplasia from adenocarcinoma of urinary bladder. Hum Pathol. 1997;28:1152–7. https://doi.org/10.1016/S0046-8177(97)90253-7.
40. Young R, Bostwick D. Florid cystitis glandularis of intestinal type with mucin extravasation: a mimic of adenocarcinoma. Am J Surg Pathol. 1997;20:1462–8. https://doi.org/10.1097/00000478-199612000-00005.
41. Kao C-S, Epstein J. Tubular adenoma of the urinary tract: a newly described entity. Hum Pathol. 2013;44 https://doi.org/10.1016/j.humpath.2013.02.017.
42. Gordetsky J, Epstein J. Intestinal metaplasia of the bladder with dysplasia: a risk factor for carcinoma? Histopathology. 2015;67 https://doi.org/10.1111/his.12661.
43. Corica F, Husmann D, Churchill B, Young R, Pacelli A, Lopez-Beltran A, et al. Intestinal metaplasia is not a strong risk factor for bladder cancer: study of 53 cases with long-term follow-up. Urology. 1997;50:427–31. https://doi.org/10.1016/S0090-4295(97)00294-X.
44. Long ED, Shepherd RT. The incidence and significance of vaginal metaplasia of the bladder trigone in adult women. Br J Urol. 1983;55(2):189–94.
45. Ahmad I, Barnetson R, Nalagatla S. Keratinizing squamous metaplasia of the bladder: a review. Urol Int. 2008;81:247–51. https://doi.org/10.1159/000151398.
46. Guo C, Fine S, Epstein J. Noninvasive squamous lesions in the urinary bladder: a clinicopathologic analysis of 29 cases. Am J Surg Pathol. 2006;30:883–91. https://doi.org/10.1097/01.pas.0000213283.20166.5a.
47. Oliva E, Young R. Nephrogenic adenoma of the urinary tract: a review of the microscopic appearance of 80 cases with emphasis on unusual features. Mod Pathol. 1995;8:722–30.
48. Young R. Tumor-like lesions of the urinary bladder. Mod Pathol. 2009;22(Suppl 2):S37–52. https://doi.org/10.1038/modpathol.2008.201.
49. Hansel D, Nadasdy T, Epstein J. Fibromyxoid nephrogenic adenoma: a newly recognized variant mimicking mucinous adenocarcinoma. Am J Surg Pathol. 2007;31:1231–7. https://doi.org/10.1097/PAS.0b013e31802e290d.
50. Piña-Oviedo S, Shen S, Truong L, Ayala A, Ro J. Flat pattern of nephrogenic adenoma: previously unrecognized pattern unveiled using PAX2 and PAX8 immunohistochemistry. Mod Pathol. 2013;26 https://doi.org/10.1038/modpathol.2012.239.

51. Mazal P, Schaufler R, Altenhuber-Müller R, Haitel A, Watschinger B, Kratzik C, et al. Derivation of nephrogenic adenomas from renal tubular cells in kidney-transplant recipients. N Engl J Med. 2002;347:653–9. https://doi.org/10.1056/NEJMoa013413.
52. Porcaro AB, D'Amico A, Ficarra V, Balzarro M, Righetti R, Martignoni G, et al. Nephrogenic adenoma of the urinary bladder: our experience and review of the literature. Urol Int. 2001;66:152–5. https://doi.org/10.1159/000056596.
53. Herawi M, Drew P, Pan C-C, Epstein J. Clear cell adenocarcinoma of the bladder and urethra. Cases diffusely mimicking nephrogenic adenoma. Hum Pathol. 2010;41:594–601. https://doi.org/10.1016/j.humpath.2009.10.011.
54. Crumley S, Ge Y, Zhou H, Shen SS, Ro JY. Interstitial cystitis: another IgG4-related inflammatory disease? Ann Diagn Pathol. 2013;17:403–7.
55. Roh JE, Cho BS, Jeon MH, Kang MH, Lee SY, Song HG. Polypoid cystitis in an adult without history of catheterization. Iran J Radiol. 2011;8(3):173–5. https://doi.org/10.5812/kmp.iranjradiol.17351065.3145.
56. Lane Z, Epstein JI. Polypoid/papillary cystitis: a series of 41 cases misdiagnosed as papillary urothelial neoplasia. Am J Surg Pathol. 2008;32(5):758–64.
57. Cieszczyk K, Puderecki M, Wronecki L, Burdan F, Szumilo J. Malakoplakia of the urinary system. Folia Med Cracov. 2019;59:67–74.
58. Tsuzuki T, Epstein JI. Fibroepithelial polyp of the lower urinary tract in adults. Am J Surg Pathol. 2005;29:460–6.
59. Nazeer T, Ro JY, Tornos C, Ordonez NG, Ayala AG. Endocervical-type glands in urinary bladder: a clinicopathologic study of six cases. Hum Pathol. 1996;27:816–20.
60. Branca G, Barresi V. Mullerianosis of the urinary bladder: a rare tumor-like lesion. Arch Pathol Lab Med. 2014;138:432–6.

3 Flat Urothelial Lesions

Gang Wang

Introduction

There are several clinical scenarios in which flat urothelial lesion needs to be evaluated by surgical pathologists [1]. The first is the random biopsies of the bladder mucosa. Usually, the patients present with urinary symptoms such as hematuria, dysuria, and increased frequency of micturition and do not respond to routine medical treatments. In this setting, cystoscopy is performed, and biopsies are taken to evaluate other causes for the symptoms. Less commonly, the patients have positive urine cytology and positive FISH UroVysion or are at high risk of developing bladder cancer. Under cystoscopy, there is no apparent lesion identified, so random biopsies are taken [2]. The second type of specimens is lesional biopsies, which are taken from the cystoscopy that detected flat urothelial lesions, typically at the mucosa with erythema. In this scenario, the main clinical question is whether they are reactive atypia, dysplasia, or urothelial carcinoma in situ (CIS) [3]. In the specimens of transurethral resection of bladder tumor (TURBT), with the presence of papillary urothelial carcinoma (with or without invasion), the typical pathological question regarding the flat lesion is whether there is concomitant CIS [4]. Another clinical setting is to evaluate the mucosal margins in the surgical resection specimens, typically radical cystectomies. Although invasive carcinoma may rarely be seen in the soft tissue around the ureter or urethra, in most of the time, the main question is to rule out CIS involving the mucosal margins.

Approaches to the Diagnosis of Flat Urothelial Lesions

Pathological diagnosis of flat urothelial lesions should always correlate with the clinical history and gross findings. The previous history of urothelial neoplasm and therapy, the presentation/symptoms, the concurrent urine cytology findings, and the gross appearing of the lesion under cystoscopy will provide beneficial information for correct interpretation of the specimen.

Under the microscope, the general approach to the diagnosis of flat urothelial lesions can be categorized into three aspects: architecture arrangements, cytologic features, and background stroma [1].

The architecture arrangements include the thickness of urothelium, cell polarity, and preservation of surface umbrella cells. The normal urothelium usually has three to seven layers in thickness, depending on the state of distention. Increased number of urothelial layers can be seen

G. Wang (✉)
Department of Pathology and Laboratory Medicine, British Columbia Cancer Vancouver Centre, Vancouver, BC, Canada
e-mail: gang.wang1@bccancer.bc.ca

H. Zhou et al. (eds.), *Urinary Bladder Pathology*, https://doi.org/10.1007/978-3-030-71509-0_3

in the tangential section, benign urothelial hyperplasia, or CIS. Denudation may be seen in reactive conditions (trauma, infection, or instrumentation) or CIS. In the normal urothelium, cells are arranged orderly, composed of compacted basal cells, vertically oriented intermediate cells, and horizontal superficial umbrella cells. The loss of normal polarity and presence of nuclear crowding are often suggestive of a neoplastic process, either urothelial dysplasia or CIS, depending on the degree of cytological atypia. Preservation of surface umbrella cells is a sign of benign lesion and is very helpful to distinguish reactive atypia from CIS.

Cytologic features include cytoplasmic clearing, nucleomegaly, nuclear pleomorphism, nuclear shape and contour, chromatin distribution, number and size of nucleoli, number and location of mitoses, and presence of atypical mitoses. Loss of cytoplasmic clearing (increased eosinophilia), especially enriched eosinophilic cytoplasm in the basal layer of the urothelium, is a sign of dysplasia or CIS. One of the essential diagnostic criteria for CIS is nucleomegaly, which is determined by comparison to the normal urothelium or stromal lymphocytes. Nuclei larger than five times of a normal lymphocyte is a widely accepted cutoff for the diagnosis of CIS, whereas the nuclear size of normal urothelium and dysplastic urothelium is only approximately twice the size of lymphocytes [2]. It should be noted that in some reactive processes, particularly radiation cystitis, the nuclei of reactive urothelium could be markedly enlarged and may even show bizarre nuclei. In such cases, clinical history and other histological features have to be correlated to make a correct diagnosis. Other than nucleomegaly, the cytological features favoring dysplasia or CIS are nuclear pleomorphism, irregular nuclear contour, nuclear hyperchromasia, coarse chromatin distribution, and multiple prominent nucleoli. An increased mitotic index can be seen in a reactive process but should be mainly located in the basal or lower half of the urothelium, while in CIS mitotic figures typically present throughout the full thickness of mucosa. Atypical mitotic figures should be only seen in urothelial CIS.

The background stroma can also provide useful clues for the nature of the flat urothelial lesions. Without a history of previous treatment, neovascularization in the superficial lamina propria suggests the presence of host response to an intraurothelial neoplastic process. The background inflammation could cause urothelial atypia, but if the severity of atypia appears to be out of proportion to the extent of inflammation, urothelial dysplasia or CIS has to be considered.

The diagnostic features for each flat urothelial lesion are summarized in Table 3.1.

Normal Urothelium

The normal bladder wall usually has no or minimal inflammation. Depending on the state of distention, the urothelium arranges between three and seven cell layers and is composed of three cell types: basal, intermediate, and superficial (see Chap. 2, "Normal Anatomy and Histology of the Urinary Bladder with Pathologic Correlates," Fig. 2.1). The basal cells are small (with the nuclear size less than twice of a lymphocyte) and tightly lined or palisaded above the basement membrane. The intermediate cells constitute variable layers of medium-sized urothelium with clear to amphophilic cytoplasm and oval to elongated nuclei typically oriented perpendicularly to the basement membrane. The superficial cells are also called umbrella cells, which are relatively large, with voluminous clear to light eosinophilic cytoplasm and small nucleoli. The umbrella cells are arranged parallel to the basement membrane, spanning or covering the intermediate cells (like an umbrella). It should be noted that due to the tangential or thick sectioning, the apparent layers and polarity may not be appreciable.

Table 3.1 Histologic features of flat urothelial lesions

	Flat hyperplasia	UPUMP	Reactive atypia	UAUS	Dysplasia	CIS
Thickness	>10–12 layers	>10–12 layers	Varies	Varies	Varies	Varies
Polarity	Preserved	Preserved	Usually preserved	May loss	Loss	Loss
Umbrella cells	Preserved	Preserved	May loss	May loss	Loss	Loss
Stroma	No/mild inflammation	No/mild inflammation	Inflamed	Marked inflammation	No/mild inflammation	Variable inflammation, neovascularization
Nuclear size	Same as normal	Same as normal	Enlarged (2–3 lymphocytes)	Enlarged (3–4 lymphocytes)	Enlarged (3–4 lymphocytes)	Enlarged (>5 lymphocytes)
Nuclear shape	Same as normal	Same as normal	Round/oval	Round/polygonal	Round/polygonal	Polygonal
Chromatin	Fine	Fine	Fine	Mild variation	Mild variation	Marked variation
Nucleoli	Absent	Absent	Inconspicuous	Inconspicuous	Inconspicuous	Multiple prominent
Mitotic figures	Absent	Absent	Rare, basal	Occasional	Occasional	Frequent, full thickness
Atypical mitosis	Absent	Absent	Absent	Absent	Usually absent	Present

UPUMP: Urothelial proliferation of uncertain malignant potential
UAUS: Urothelial atypia of unknown significance
CIS: Urothelial carcinoma in situ

Flat Urothelial Hyperplasia

Definition: markedly thickened (more than 10–12 layers) or densified urothelium with no or at most minimal cytologic atypia.

In flat urothelial hyperplasia, the increased number of layers should be the only finding, and these lesions have otherwise the same architecture and cytological features as normal urothelium, such as cell polarity, surface umbrella cells, no or minimal cytological atypia, and occasional mitosis confined to the basal half of the lesion (Fig. 3.1). Flat urothelial hyperplasia is often seen in inflammation (Fig. 3.2) or adjacent to low-grade papillary urothelial lesions. This lesion alone, as a de novo finding, has no clinical significance and no evidence as a premalignant lesion.

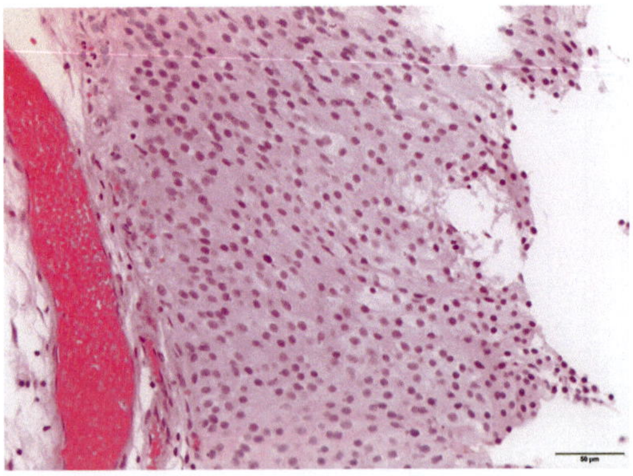

Fig. 3.1 Flat urothelial hyperplasia with markedly thickened urothelium (>12 layers) and no cytological atypia

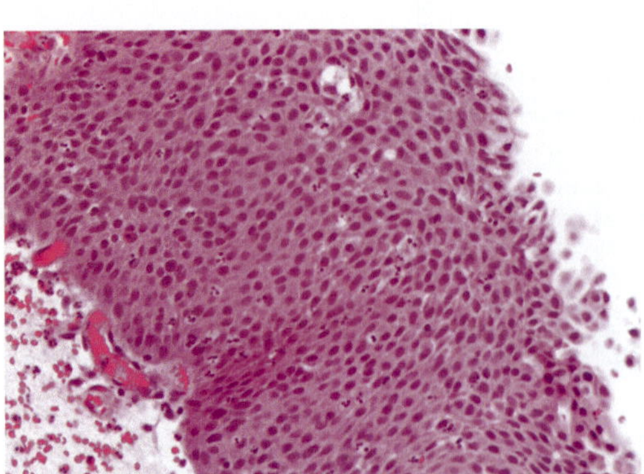

Fig. 3.2 Flat urothelial hyperplasia with acute inflammation and minimal cytological atypia

Urothelial Proliferation of Uncertain Malignant Potential (UPUMP)

Definition: marked thickening of the urothelium with no or minimal cytological atypia and no true papillary formation [3].

UPUMP is most frequently seen in patients with a prior history of papillary urothelial carcinoma or seen adjacent to papillary lesions [4]. Under the cystoscopy, the lesion is typically focal and may be described as bleb-like, papillary, raised, sessile, frondular, or irregular. Microscopically, UPUMP shows a thickened urothelium (usually more than 10–12 layers) arranged into narrow undulating mucosal folds of various heights (Fig. 3.3). In contrast to papillary neoplasms, these lesions lack the well-formed papillary fronds or secondary branching that are diagnostic of a papillary urothelial neoplasm. UPUMP likely represents the lateral extension ("shoulder lesion") of a papillary neoplasm or an early (incipient) manifestation of papillary urothelial neoplasia. This assumption is supported by a high incidence of chromosome 9 deletions and less frequently the FGFR3 abnormalities [5–7]. Like in the flat urothelial hyperplasia, there should be no or minimal cytological atypia in UPUMP. For the lesions with significant cytological atypia, they should be classified as urothelial carcinoma and graded accordingly. In de

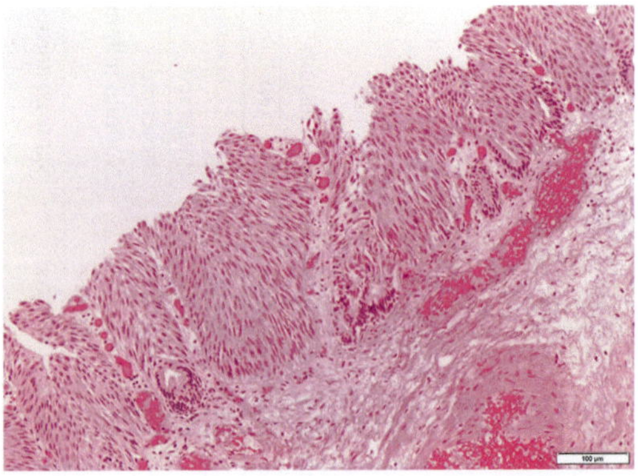

Fig. 3.3 Urothelial proliferation of uncertain malignant potential shows a thickened urothelium arranged into narrow undulating mucosal folds with various heights. Note there are no well-formed papillary fronds or secondary branching and no cytological atypia

novo UPUMP, 15.4% of patients developed subsequent urothelial neoplasia within a mean follow-up of 68.9 months [8].

Reactive Atypia

Definition: benign urothelium with mild cytological atypia secondary to inflammation, therapy, or instrumentation.

Typically the patients have a clinical history of stones, infection, or frequent instrumentation [9]. Microscopically, there is usually prominent background inflammation, particularly intraepithelial inflammatory cell infiltrate, either acute, chronic, or both. Nucleomegaly is the most prominent finding in reactive urothelial atypia, with the size of two to three times of the lymphocyte nucleus, but with no nuclear pleomorphism [10]. The nuclei are usually round or oval, maintaining their polarity perpendicular to the basement membrane, with smooth nuclear contour and evenly distributed vesicular chromatin. The reactive urothelium could have prominent pinpoint nucleoli but should not have macro-nucleoli (Fig. 3.4). There could be increased mitotic activity, but they usually present predominantly in the basal and intermediate layers and should not have atypical mitosis seen. The umbrella cells may or may not be preserved. However, if they are present, they frequently exhibit multinucleation or nucleomegaly, cytoplasmic vacuolation, and a low nuclear to cytoplasmic ratio.

Radiation atypia is defined as benign urothelium with cytological atypia secondary to radiation therapy, also called radiation cystitis. Clinically, the symptoms of radiation cystitis can occur from as early as 4–6 weeks after initiation of the therapy to 10 years later after radiation [11]. The clinical severity and histologic features are both time- and dose-dependent. Microscopically, depending on the stage of the changes, the lamina propria can show marked edema, hyperemia, hemorrhage, fibrin deposition, and fibrosis, often with large atypical fibroblasts. It may be accompanied by desquamation and ulceration of the surface urothelium (Fig. 3.5). The remaining urothelial cells often show significant cytological atypia (Fig. 3.6), demonstrated by prominent and hyperchromatic nuclei, giant cells, and multinucleated cells, which make them look even more bizarre than the cells in CIS [11]. The key diagnostic hints are cytoplasmic and nuclear vacuolation, normal nuclear to cytoplasmic ratio, and lack of mitotic activity. Of course, the clinical history of radiation therapy, typically for prostate, anorectal, or gynecological malignancies, would be very helpful for correct diagnosis.

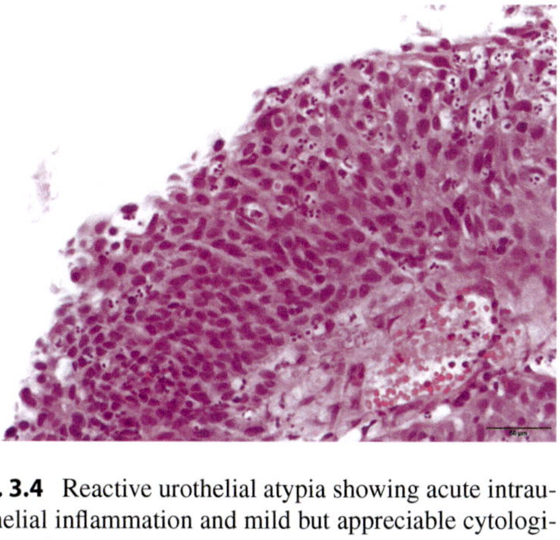

Fig. 3.4 Reactive urothelial atypia showing acute intraurothelial inflammation and mild but appreciable cytological atypia

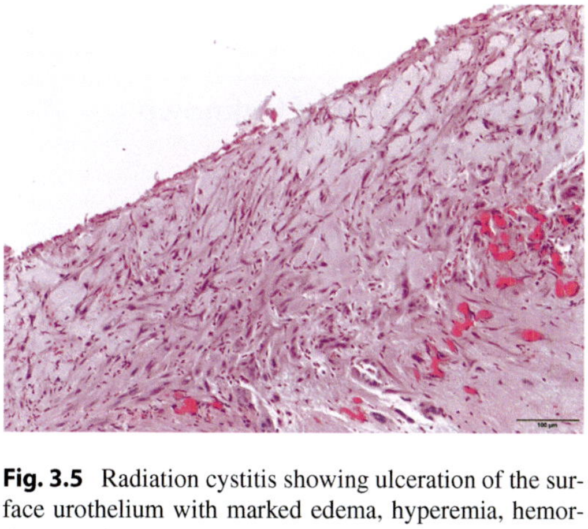

Fig. 3.5 Radiation cystitis showing ulceration of the surface urothelium with marked edema, hyperemia, hemorrhage, and large atypical fibroblasts

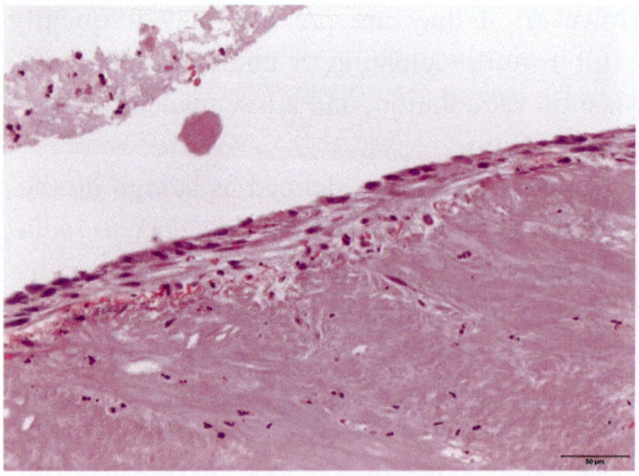

Fig. 3.6 Radiation cystitis showing atypical urothelial cells with fibrinoid stroma and hemosiderin deposition

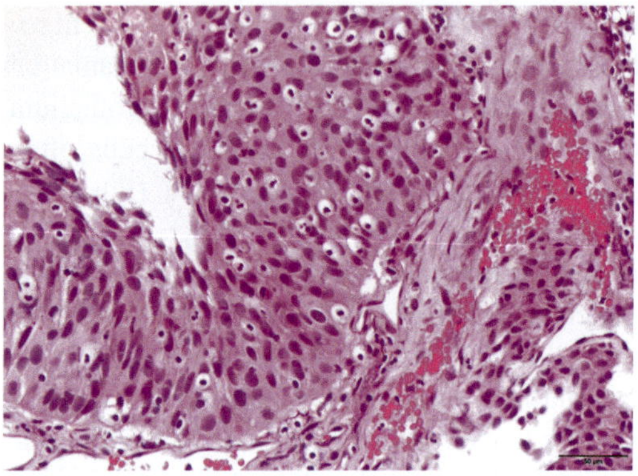

Fig. 3.7 Urothelial atypia of unknown significance showing acute intraurothelial inflammation and apparent cytological atypia which is out of proportion to the extent of inflammation. Note the nucleomegaly of the atypical urothelial cells compared to the benign urothelium in the right lower corner

Urothelial Atypia of Unknown Significance (UAUS)

Definition: flat urothelial lesion with inflammation and cytological atypia where the severity of atypia appears to be out of proportion to the extent of inflammation, such that urothelial dysplasia or CIS cannot be confidently excluded (Figs. 3.7) [12, 13].

Urothelial atypia of unknown significance is not a diagnostic entity. It is merely a descriptive term used for a flat urothelial lesion, in which the atypia cannot be explained by the extent of inflammation but does not meet the criteria of dysplasia or CIS. Clinically, these patients should be followed and reexamined after inflammation subsides.

Urothelial Dysplasia

Definition: flat urothelial lesion, in the background of no or minimal inflammation, with unequivocal cytological atypia but does not meet the diagnostic threshold for urothelial CIS [3]. It is also called low-grade intraurothelial neoplasia.

In urothelial dysplasia, the thickness of the urothelium can vary. The stroma has no or minimal inflammation. The urothelial cells are rounded to polygonal with crowded nuclei and have a loss of polarity (Fig. 3.8). Nuclear atypia is evident, demonstrated by mild nucleomegaly, minimal irregularity of nuclear contours, and altered chromatin distribution, but lacks the nuclear pleomorphism and significant nucleomegaly (nuclear size larger than five lymphocytes) as seen in CIS. Nucleoli can be conspicuous but are not typically present throughout. The mitotic activity is variable but usually not in the upper layers [12–14]. Conceptually, the cytological findings seen in urothelial dysplasia are analogous to those seen in noninvasive low-grade papillary urothelial

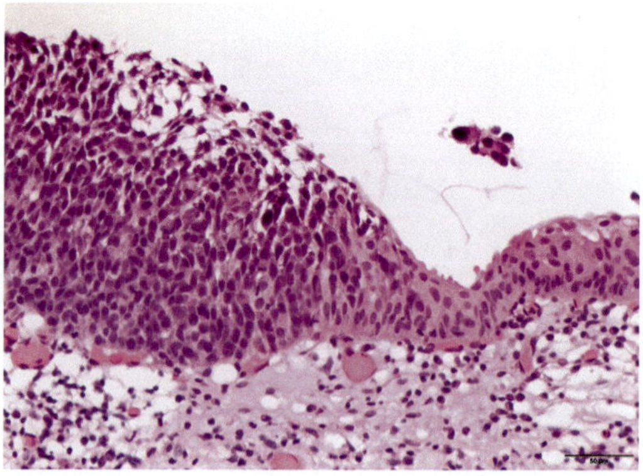

Fig. 3.8 Urothelial dysplasia (left) showing apparent architectural and cytological atypia compared to the benign urothelial (right) but falls short of the diagnostic threshold for CIS. Note the minimal inflammation in the background

carcinoma, while CIS is analogous in its histology to noninvasive high-grade papillary urothelial carcinoma [15]. Nonetheless, the differences between urothelial dysplasia and CIS and between urothelial dysplasia and urothelial atypia of unknown significance are somehow subjective. Therefore, the diagnosis of low-grade urothelial dysplasia is controversial with poor interobserver reproducibility, even among expert genitourinary pathologists [16]. Dysplasia is usually a histologic finding seen most commonly to be associated with other bladder neoplasia, such as papillary urothelial carcinoma, CIS, or invasive urothelial carcinoma. In the absence of prior history or concomitant urothelial neoplasia, the diagnosis of low-grade urothelial dysplasia should be made with great caution. Due to the lack of screening in the general population, there is little known about de novo low-grade dysplasia. Therefore, the diagnosis of low-grade dysplasia should be used with a great precaution when it is de novo presentation. The poor interobserver reproducibility also precludes the accurate evaluation of the nature of low-grade urothelial dysplasia. The few studies published on de novo low-grade dysplasia indicate that 15–19% of the patients progress to urothelial CIS or invasive disease [17, 18]. When the diagnosis of low-grade dysplasia is made, a careful close follow-up is recommended.

Urothelial Carcinoma in Situ (CIS)

Definition: flat urothelial lesion with cytologically malignant cells.

Several molecular changes have been identified in CIS. Next-generation sequencing revealed 92% of CIS harboring at least one potentially actionable genetic alterations, including TP53/cell cycle pathway-related genes (e.g., TP53 and MDM2), genes encoding chromatin-modifying proteins (e.g., ARID1A and KDM6A), DNA damage repair genes (e.g., BRCA2 and ATM), and phosphatidylinositol 3-kinase/mitogen-activated protein kinase pathway genes (e.g., ERBB2 and FGFR1) [19]. The amplification/mutation of the p53 gene, the most frequent genetic change, has been widely applied in ancillary study to facilitate the diagnosis of CIS.

Urothelial CIS is commonly seen to be associated with adjacent high-grade papillary urothelial carcinoma or invasive carcinomas but can also be seen in pure form which accounts for 1–3% of newly diagnosed urothelial neoplasms. The clinical presentation of CIS is not specific, commonly dysuria, urinary frequency or urgency, and microscopic or gross hematuria. Under the cystoscopy, CIS often appears to be mucosal erythema, with occasional erosion. Urothelial CIS is often multifocal and sometimes diffuse. Mapping studies of cystectomy specimens have shown extensive urothelial CIS, with the involvement of the prostatic urethra and of the ureter in as many as 67% and 57% of cases, respectively [20, 21]. There are two proposed theories to explain the frequency of multifocality of CIS. The first is the monoclonal theory suggesting that the multifocal tumors arise from a single transformed cell that proliferates and spreads throughout the urothelium either by intraluminal implantation or by intraepithelial migration. The second theory, the so-called the field cancerization theory, suggests independent transforming genetic alterations at different sites in the urothelial lining caused by chemical carcinogens [22, 23].

The principal histological features of CIS include loss of polarity, marked nuclear crowding, pleomorphism, and frequent mitoses (Fig. 3.9). The lamina propria is frequently

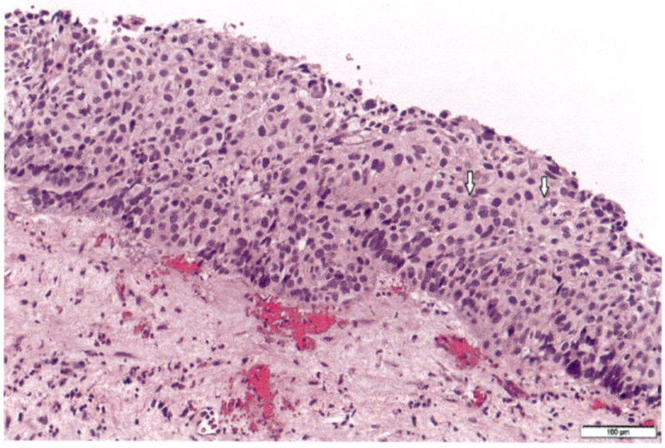

Fig. 3.9 Urothelial carcinoma in situ showing severe architectural, cytological atypia, and frequent mitoses

inflamed and congested with prominent vascularization, reflecting the erythematous appearance under cystoscopy. The thickness of CIS can be variable, ranging from denuded to normal to hyperplastic, depending on the discohesive nature of the neoplastic cells or the procedure artifact. The neoplastic cells may involve either full or partial thickness of the urothelium. The nuclear atypia is generally obvious but may show a spectrum of severity. Generally, there is marked nucleomegaly with the nuclear size larger than five times of quiescent lymphocytes. The chromatin is usually coarse and condensed, with prominent and multiple nucleoli. The number of mitoses can be variable, from occasional to plenty, but typically involving from base to surface. Atypical mitoses are often seen [3].

Additionally, there are varied cytologic and architectural patterns in the histologic presentation of CIS [15, 24]. The most common pattern of CIS is recognized as large cell pleomorphic CIS (Figs. 3.10). The neoplastic cells show considerable loss of polarity with haphazard arrangement and nucleomegaly with marked variation in nuclear shape and size but frequently retain abundant eosinophilic cytoplasm. This pattern usually has abundant mitotic features and atypical mitoses. In some other CIS, the neoplastic cells may not show marked pleomorphism. Instead, they are composed of a more monomorphic population of neoplastic cells. However, they still have a degree of high-grade cytologic features, including nucleomegaly, hyperchromasia, irregular chromatin distribution, and one or a few prominent nucleoli, meeting the diagnostic criteria for CIS. Such lesions are called large cell CIS without pleomorphism (Fig. 3.9). Occasionally, the neoplastic cells of CIS have scant cytoplasm, so they appear smaller than usual CIS cells. Nevertheless, they still have all the nuclear features (markedly enlarged with nuclear chromatin abnormalities) of CIS, therefore called small cell CIS (Fig. 3.11). Small cell CIS is merely a descriptive term; there is no precursor relationship with small cell carcinoma of the bladder, and it does not denote neuroendocrine differentiation. Due to the discohesive nature of CIS cells, it is not uncommon that some or most of the neoplastic cells of CIS lift off, leaving only a few remaining cells attached to the base of mucosa, the so-called clinging-type CIS. Microscopically, this type of CIS is characterized by a partially denuded urothelium with a patchy, usually single layer of residual urothelial cells or even only a few atypical single cells clinging to the base of the mucosa. Although they could be very few, these atypical cells demonstrate all the features of cytological atypia meeting the morphologic criteria for CIS (Figs. 3.12). In the case of complete denudation, the hypervascular

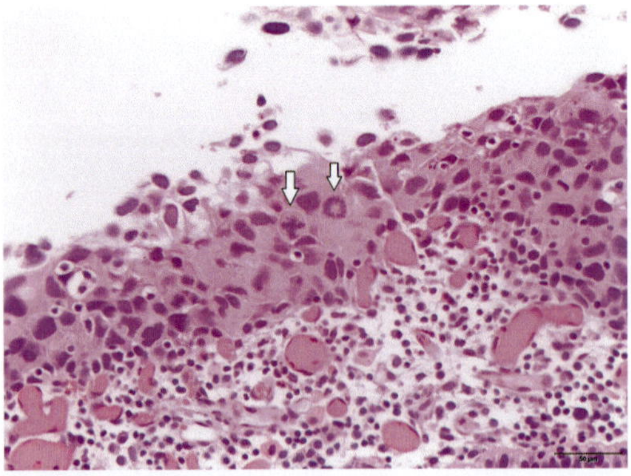

Fig. 3.10 Pleomorphic urothelial carcinoma in situ showing considerable loss of polarity, haphazard arrangement, and nucleomegaly with marked variation in nuclear shape and size and abundant eosinophilic cytoplasm. Note the two atypical mitoses in the center (arrows)

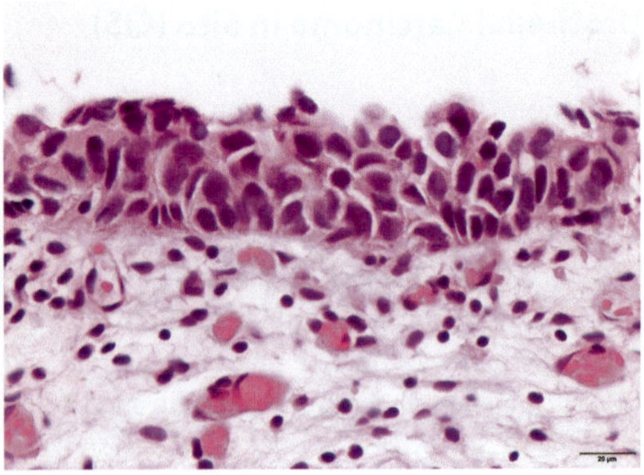

Fig. 3.11 Small cell urothelial carcinoma in situ showing scant cytoplasm, appearing smaller than usual CIS cells. Nevertheless, they still have all the nuclear features (markedly enlarged with nuclear chromatin abnormalities) of CIS

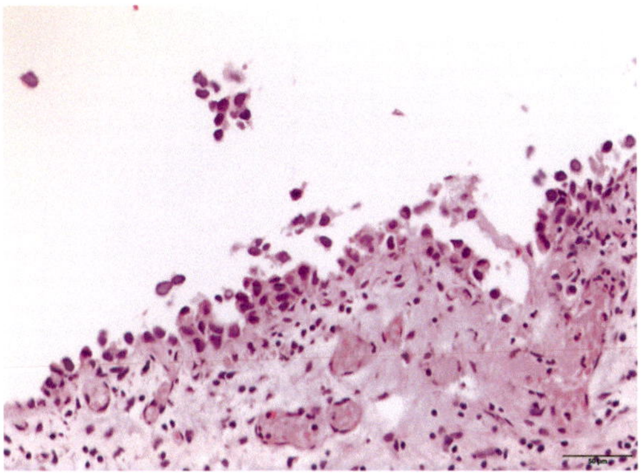

Fig. 3.12 Clinging-type carcinoma in situ characterized by a partially denuded urothelium with a patchy or single layer of residual urothelial cells demonstrating all the features of cytological atypia meeting the morphologic criteria for CIS. Note the floating lifted neoplastic cells

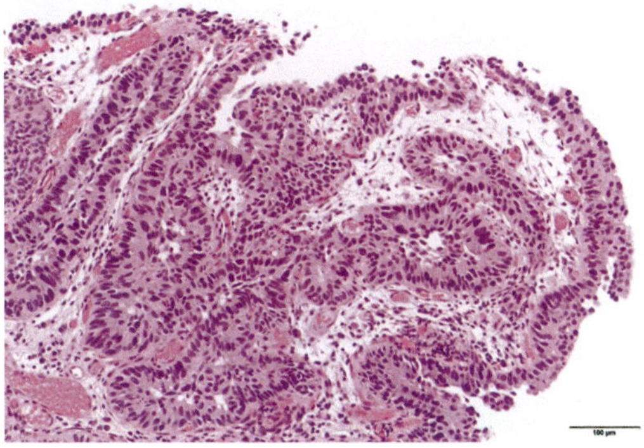

Fig. 3.13 Urothelial carcinoma in situ with glandular differentiation

(neovascularization) and inflamed lamina propria may be the only clue for the overlying abnormal urothelium. In such a case, deeper sections through the block may be extremely helpful to identify or rule out clinging CIS. In cases of completely denuded CIS, cystoscopic urine or bladder wash cytology specimens should be correlated since they may contain a large number of neoplastic cells [25]. Rarely, CIS may demonstrate glandular differentiation (CIS-GL) (Fig. 3.13), but the majority of the cases are associated with concurrent high-grade papillary urothelial carcinoma, conventional CIS, or invasive carcinoma components. CIS-GL has four architectural patterns that can exist alone or in combination: glandular, papillary, cribriform, or flat. The mixture of two patterns, especially glandular and papillary, is commonly seen [3, 26]. The expression of CDX2 would be evidence of glandular differentiation (Fig. 3.14). CIS-GL must be distinguished from florid cystitis cystica, and the later lacks significant cytologic atypia, mitotic figures, and apoptosis seen with CIS-GL. The evidence from the available literature supports that CIS-GL is a variant of CIS as opposed to in situ adenocarcinoma [3, 26]. Some literatures have suggested the association between CIS-GL and small cell carcinoma, but they were based on relatively few cases [26, 27].

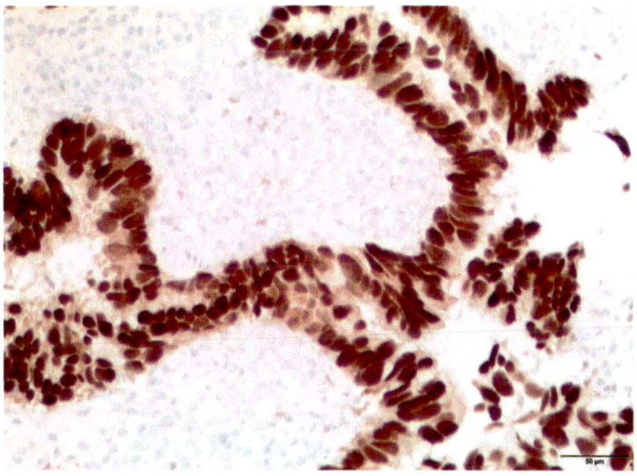

Fig. 3.14 CDX-2 expression in urothelial carcinoma in situ with glandular differentiation

In some cases of CIS, neoplastic cells may only partially involve the normal urothelium, the so-called cancerization. CIS can cancerize non-neoplastic urothelium with two patterns. The first pattern is pagetoid spread, characterized by clusters or isolated single cells with features of CIS within normal urothelium, resembling mammary Paget disease (Fig. 3.15). The pagetoid spread is commonly seen in cases with diffuse and multifocal CIS and could be the only pattern of involvement seen along the upper and lower urinary tract in these patients. The other pattern of cancerization is the undermining of the normal urothelium by adjacent CIS. Sometimes there are only surface benign urothelium left with the underneath extension of the CIS cells (Figs. 3.16).

Very often, CIS can colonize into von Brunn nests, showing variable-sized nests of neoplastic cells within the superficial lamina propria

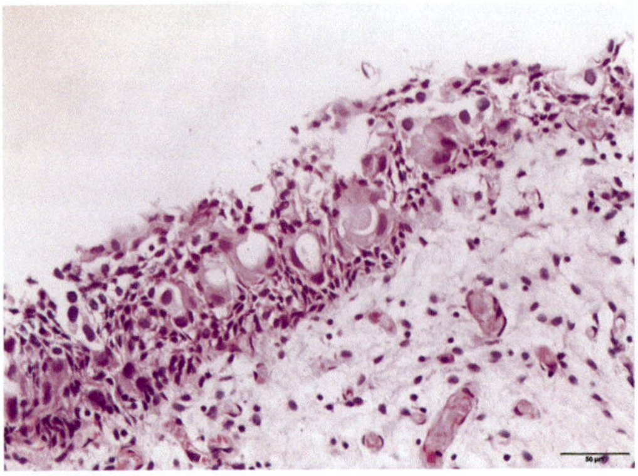

Fig. 3.15 Pagetoid spreading of CIS characterized by clusters or isolated single cells with features of CIS within normal urothelium, resembling mammary Paget disease

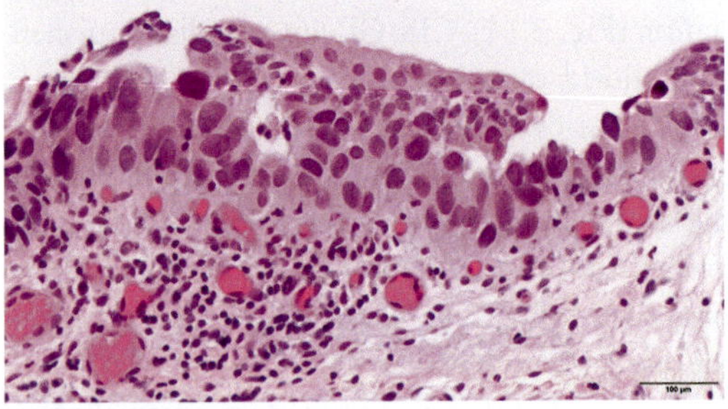

Fig. 3.16 Undermining of the normal urothelium by CIS. Note the superficial umbrella cells left with the underneath extension of the CIS cells

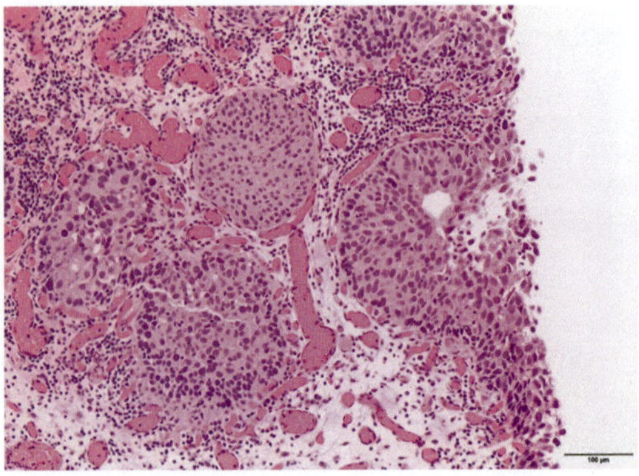

Fig. 3.17 Carcinoma in situ colonizing into von Brunn nests, showing variable-sized nests of neoplastic cells within the superficial lamina propria. Note the comparison between the colonized von Brunn nests and adjacent uninvolved von Brunn nest

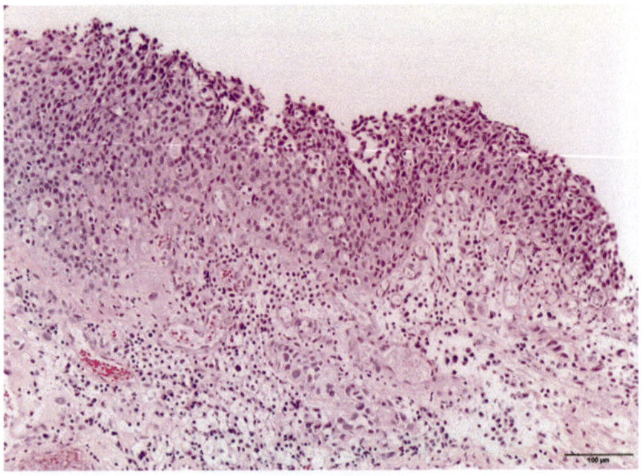

Fig. 3.18 Carcinoma in situ with microinvasion showing the direct extension of single cells or clusters of neoplastic cells into the superficial lamina propria (lower part)

(Fig. 3.17), which may simulate stromal invasion, especially in the presence of inflammation when the basement membrane may be obscured and distorted. The diagnostic hint of CIS colonization of von Brunn nests rather than stromal invasion includes the round contour, sharp border, and lack of retraction artifact or surrounding stromal changes (desmoplasia). On the other hand, stromal microinvasion is the direct extension in cords, single cells, or clusters of neoplastic cells into the superficial lamina propria (Fig. 3.18), often with a retraction artifact that mimics vascular invasion. It might be subtle and easily underdiagnosed histologically; especially if the background is inflamed, microinvasion may be obscured. Desmoplasia or retraction artifact is useful in recognizing invasion, but the stromal response may not always be present [28]. In such cases, immunohistochemical study with cytokeratin would be constructive in identifying single-cell invasion or small clusters of invasion.

The diagnosis of CIS would have a significant impact on the clinical management; therefore, the distinction of CIS from reactive atypia is critical. Most of the time, the diagnosis of CIS is straightforward, based on nuclear characteristics. However, from time to time, the distinction of the neoplastic process from reactive conditions can be difficult. In such cases, ancillary studies should be applied to facilitate the diagnosis.

Several immunohistochemical markers have diagnostic utility for CIS [29, 30]. Among them, the most widely applied markers are CK20 and p53 [10, 31, 32]. In normal urothelium, CK20 only stains the superficial umbrella cells, while nuclear staining of p53 is variably weak and patchy. Urothelium with reactive atypia usually shows CK20 and p53 reactivity patterns identical to those seen in the normal urothelium. In contrast, CIS frequently shows full-thickness, diffuse, and strong cytoplasmic staining for CK20 (Fig. 3.19) and diffuse nuclear reactivity for p53 (Fig. 3.20). It should be noted that the intensity of p53 immunostain varies among different laboratories. The interpretation may be tricky, and the requirement for strong and diffuse nuclear staining must adhere. CD44 is another useful immunomarker for the diagnosis of CIS, but not all the laboratories have this stain. In normal urothelium, CD44 staining is limited to the basal and parabasal urothelial cells. Urothelium with reactive atypia shows increased reactivity for CD44 in all layers of the urothelium, while CD44 reactivity is often absent in CIS [10]. Other immunomarkers with potential value in the diagnosis of CIS include strong membranous staining of HER2 and intense cytoplasmic staining of AMACR and p16, but their utility in routine practice remains in question [33–35]. Ki67 immunohistochemistry for the mitotic index would be useful in distinguishing radiation atypia and CIS. However, the application of Ki67 must be made with great caution, as the reactive urothelium can also have an increased proliferation index, which may overlap with CIS lesions. Ideally, an immune panel consisting of multiple antibodies should be applied because not all cases of CIS consistently exhibit the characteristic immunostaining pattern specified above. Furthermore, the immunohistochemical panel should be only used as an adjunct to morphology. Additionally, there is no immunostain applicable in the distinction of dysplasia from CIS, as this distinction is only based on the diagnostic threshold in histology [15].

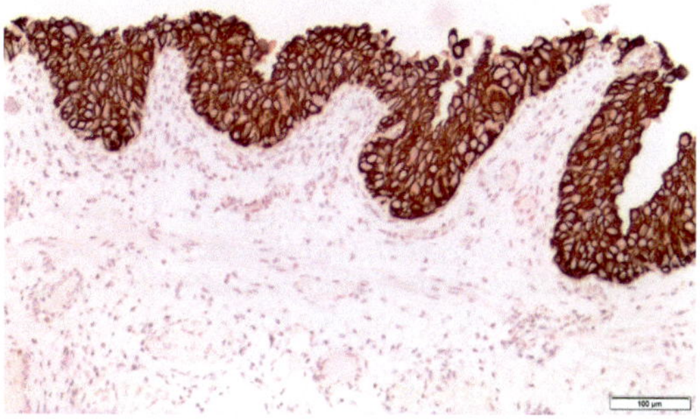

Fig. 3.19 Carcinoma in situ showing full-thickness, diffuse, and strong cytoplasmic staining for CK20

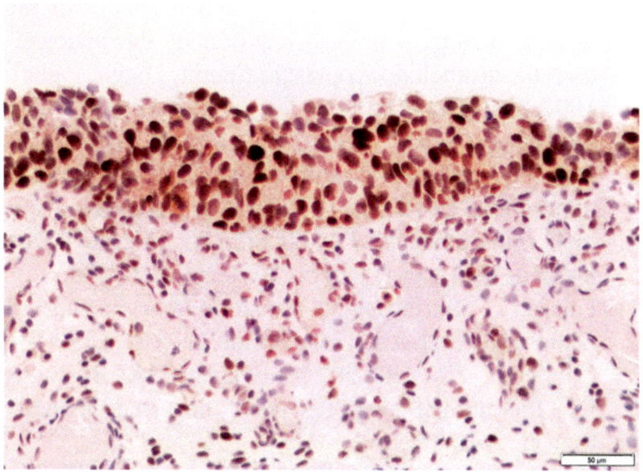

Fig. 3.20 Carcinoma in situ showing full-thickness, diffuse, and strong nuclear staining for p53

Similar to muscle-invasive urothelial carcinoma, CIS can also be subclassified based on its genotype. Using a representative immunohistochemistry panel, a large case series (n = 156) demonstrated that about 85% of CIS express luminal markers (CK20, GATA3, and ER-β), one-third of the CIS overexpress Her2, and only a few cases express basal markers (CK5/CK6) [36]. Interestingly, a phenotypic study in paired CIS and invasive tumors from the same biopsy showed a significant loss of luminal marker expression in the course of progression while an increase of basal marker expression in the invasive compartment, which indicates the luminal type of CIS undergoing a class switch to basal type during progression [36].

Intravesical BCG is currently the standard treatment for CIS [37]. Most patients respond to BCG, but virtually all cases will eventually recur, and as many as 25–50% of the cases are expected to progress to invasive disease [38]. For the refractory CIS, cystectomy may be considered. Actually, in the patients who underwent cystectomy for CIS, 15–25% of the cases harbor microinvasive disease. The prognosis of CIS is variable depending on multiple factors, including the extent of disease (focal, multifocal, or extensive), the involvement of prostatic urethra, and the response to therapy [39]. Multifocal CIS of the bladder is associated with concurrent or subsequent development of CIS in both the upper tract (ureter and renal pelvis) and lower tract (urethra) [40]. Patients with de novo pure CIS are likely to have better disease-free survival (62% vs. 45%) and a lower rate of progression (28% vs. 59%) and death from disease (7% vs. 45%) compared to patients with CIS and concomitant papillary bladder neoplasia [41]. The responsiveness to intravesical therapy is also associated with the prognosis of CIS, and poor response to BCG is an indication for early cystectomy [38].

Summary

In summary, the flat urothelial lesions can be classified into urothelial hyperplasia, UPUMP, reactive atypia, UAUS, urothelial dysplasia, and CIS, based on the architecture and cytological features. The key diagnostic criteria for CIS include nucleomegaly, hyperchromasia, pleomorphism, and mitotic activity in the mid to upper layers of the urothelium. CIS can present with several morphologic patterns, and might not involve the full thickness of the urothelium. Awareness of the morphologic heterogeneity of CIS will facilitate its distinction from its histologic mimics. For difficult cases, immunohistochemical markers, such as CK20 and p53, may be applied to help the diagnosis of CIS. The prognosis of CIS depends on multiple factors, including the extent of disease and response to local therapy.

References

1. Amin MB, McKenney JK. An approach to the diagnosis of flat intraepithelial lesions of the urinary bladder using the World Health Organization/International Society of Urological Pathology consensus classification system. Adv Anat Pathol. 2002;9(4):222–32.
2. Milord RA, Lecksell K, Epstein JI. An objective morphologic parameter to aid in the diagnosis of flat urothelial carcinoma in situ. Hum Pathol. 2001;32(9):997–1002.
3. Moch H, Humphrey PA, Ulbright TM, Reuter V. WHO Classification of Tumours of the Urinary System and Male Genital Organs. Lyon, France: International Agency for Research on Cancer; 2016.
4. Wang G, McKenney JK. Urinary bladder pathology: World Health Organization classification and American Joint Committee on Cancer staging update. Arch Pathol Lab Med. 2019;143(5):571–7.
5. Hartmann A, Moser K, Kriegmair M, Hofstetter A, Hofstaedter F, Knuechel R. Frequent genetic alterations in simple urothelial hyperplasias of the bladder in patients with papillary urothelial carcinoma. Am J Pathol. 1999;154(3):721–7.
6. Obermann EC, Junker K, Stoehr R, Dietmaier W, Zaak D, Schubert J, et al. Frequent genetic alterations in flat urothelial hyperplasias and concomitant papillary bladder cancer as detected by CGH, LOH, and FISH analyses. J Pathol. 2003;199(1):50–7.
7. van Oers JMM, Adam C, Denzinger S, Stoehr R, Bertz S, Zaak D, et al. Chromosome 9 deletions are more frequent than FGFR3 mutations in flat urothelial hyperplasias of the bladder. Int J Cancer. 2006;119(5):1212–5.
8. Lowenthal BM, Sahoo D, Amin MB, Hansel DE. Urothelial proliferation of unknown malignant potential involving the bladder: histopathologic features and risk of progression in de novo cases and cases with prior neoplasia. Arch Pathol Lab Med. 2020;144(7):853–62.
9. Amin MB, Young RH. Intraepithelial lesions of the urinary bladder with a discussion of the histogenesis of urothelial neoplasia. Semin Diagn Pathol. 1997;14(2):84–97.
10. McKenney JK, Desai S, Cohen C, Amin MB. Discriminatory immunohistochemical staining of urothelial carcinoma in situ and non-neoplastic urothelium: an analysis of cytokeratin 20, p53, and CD44 antigens. Am J Surg Pathol. 2001;25(8):1074–8.
11. Fajardo LF, Berthrong M. Radiation injury in surgical pathology. Part I. Am J Surg Pathol. 1978;2(2):159–99.
12. Cheng L, Cheville JC, Neumann RM, Bostwick DG. Flat intraepithelial lesions of the urinary bladder. Cancer. 2000;88(3):625–31.
13. Epstein JI, Amin MB, Reuter VR, Mostofi FK. The World Health Organization/International Society of Urological Pathology consensus classification of urothelial (transitional cell) neoplasms of the urinary bladder. Bladder Consensus Conference Committee. Am J Surg Pathol. 1998;22(12):1435–48.

14. Cheng L, Cheville JC, Neumann RM, Bostwick DG. Natural history of urothelial dysplasia of the bladder. Am J Surg Pathol. 1999;23(4):443–7.
15. Epstein JI, Reuter VE, Amin MB. Biopsy interpretation of the bladder. 3rd ed. Philadelphia: Wolters Kluwer; 2016.
16. Murata S, Iseki M, Kinjo M, Matsuzaki O, Moriuchi A, Ohtani H, et al. Molecular and immunohistologic analyses cannot reliably solve diagnostic variation of flat intraepithelial lesions of the urinary bladder. Am J Clin Pathol. 2010;134(6):862–72.
17. Smith G, Elton RA, Beynon LL, Newsam JE, Chisholm GD, Hargreave TB. Prognostic significance of biopsy results of normal-looking mucosa in cases of superficial bladder cancer. Br J Urol. 1983;55(6):665–9.
18. Zuk RJ, Rogers HS, Martin JE, Baithun SI. Clinicopathological importance of primary dysplasia of bladder. J Clin Pathol. 1988;41(12):1277–80.
19. Garczyk S, Ortiz-Bruchle N, Schneider U, Lurje I, Guricova K, Gaisa NT, et al. Next-generation sequencing reveals potential predictive biomarkers and targets of therapy for urothelial carcinoma in situ of the urinary bladder. Am J Pathol. 2020;190(2):323–32.
20. Moschini M, Soria F, Susani M, Korn S, Briganti A, Roupret M, et al. Impact of the level of urothelial carcinoma involvement of the prostate on survival after radical cystectomy. Bladder Cancer. 2017;3(3):161–9.
21. Nese N, Gupta R, Bui MH, Amin MB. Carcinoma in situ of the urinary bladder: review of clinicopathologic characteristics with an emphasis on aspects related to molecular diagnostic techniques and prognosis. J Natl Compr Canc Netw. 2009;7(1):48–57.
22. Jones TD, Wang M, Eble JN, MacLennan GT, Lopez-Beltran A, Zhang S, et al. Molecular evidence supporting field effect in urothelial carcinogenesis. Clin Cancer Res. 2005;11(18):6512–9.
23. Cheng L, Davidson DD, Maclennan GT, Williamson SR, Zhang S, Koch MO, et al. The origins of urothelial carcinoma. Expert Rev Anticancer Ther. 2010;10(6):865–80.
24. McKenney JK, Gomez JA, Desai S, Lee MW, Amin MB. Morphologic expressions of urothelial carcinoma in situ: a detailed evaluation of its histologic patterns with emphasis on carcinoma in situ with microinvasion. Am J Surg Pathol. 2001;25(3):356–62.
25. Parwani AV, Levi AW, Epstein JI, Ali SZ. Urinary bladder biopsy with denuded mucosa: denuding cystitis-cytopathologic correlates. Diagn Cytopathol. 2004;30(5):297–300.
26. Yang Z, Epstein JI. Urothelial carcinoma in situ of the bladder with glandular differentiation: report of 92 cases. Am J Surg Pathol. 2018;42(7):971–6.
27. Lopez-Beltran A, Jimenez RE, Montironi R, Patriarca C, Blanca A, Menendez CL, et al. Flat urothelial carcinoma in situ of the bladder with glandular differentiation. Hum Pathol. 2011;42(11):1653–9.
28. Amin MB, Gomez JA, Young RH. Urothelial transitional cell carcinoma with endophytic growth patterns: a discussion of patterns of invasion and problems associated with assessment of invasion in 18 cases. Am J Surg Pathol. 1997;21(9):1057–68.
29. Aron M, Luthringer DJ, McKenney JK, Hansel DE, Westfall DE, Parakh R, et al. Utility of a triple antibody cocktail intraurothelial neoplasm-3 (IUN-3-CK20/CD44s/p53) and alpha-methylacyl-CoA racemase (AMACR) in the distinction of urothelial carcinoma in situ (CIS) and reactive urothelial atypia. Am J Surg Pathol. 2013;37(12):1815–23.
30. Amin MB, Trpkov K, Lopez-Beltran A, Grignon D, Epstein JI, Ulbright TM, et al. Best practices recommendations in the application of immunohistochemistry in the bladder lesions report from the International Society of Urologic Pathology Consensus Conference. Am J Surg Pathol. 2014;38(8):E20–34.
31. Harnden P, Eardley I, Joyce AD, Southgate J. Cytokeratin 20 as an objective marker of urothelial dysplasia. Br J Urol. 1996;78(6):870–5.
32. Sarkis AS, Dalbagni G, Cordoncardo C, Zhang ZF, Sheinfeld J, Fair WR, et al. Nuclear overexpression of P53-protein in transitional cell bladder-carcinoma – a marker for disease progression. J Natl Cancer Inst. 1993;85(1):53–9.
33. Alston ELJ, Zynger DL. Does the addition of AMACR to CK20 help to diagnose challenging cases of urothelial carcinoma in situ? Diagn Pathol. 2019;14(1):91.
34. Jung S, Wu C, Eslami Z, Tanguay S, Aprikian A, Kassouf W, et al. The role of immunohistochemistry in the diagnosis of flat urothelial lesions: a study using CK20, CK5/6, P53, Cd138, and Her2/Neu. Ann Diagn Pathol. 2014;18(1):27–32.
35. Yin M, Bastacky S, Parwani AV, McHale T, Dhir R. p16ink4 immunoreactivity is a reliable marker for urothelial carcinoma in situ. Hum Pathol. 2008;39(4):527–35.
36. Barth I, Schneider U, Grimm T, Karl A, Horst D, Gaisa NT, et al. Progression of urothelial carcinoma in situ of the urinary bladder: a switch from luminal to basal phenotype and related therapeutic implications. Virchows Arch. 2018;472(5):749–58.
37. Dalbagni G. The management of superficial bladder cancer. Nat Clin Pract Urol. 2007;4(5):254–60.
38. Gofrit ON, Pode D, Pizov G, Zorn KC, Katz R, Duvdevani M, et al. The natural history of bladder carcinoma in situ after initial response to bacillus Calmette-Guerin immunotherapy. Urol Oncol. 2009;27(3):258–62.
39. Cheng L, Cheville JC, Neumann RM, Leibovich BC, Egan KS, Spotts BE, et al. Survival of patients with carcinoma in situ of the urinary bladder. Cancer. 1999;85(11):2469–74.
40. Nixon RG, Chang SS, Lafleur BJ, Smith JJ, Cookson MS. Carcinoma in situ and tumor multifocality predict the risk of prostatic urethral involvement at radical cystectomy in men with transitional cell carcinoma of the bladder. J Urol. 2002;167(2 Pt 1):502–5.
41. Orozco RE, Martin AA, Murphy WM. Carcinoma in situ of the urinary bladder. Clues to host involvement in human carcinogenesis. Cancer. 1994;74(1):115–22.

Papillary and Inverted Tumors

4

Haijun Zhou, Charles C. Guo, and Jae Y. Ro

Introduction

The architectural growth patterns of noninvasive urothelial neoplasms include flat, papillary, and inverted [1, 2]. Under cystoscopy, flat lesions usually are subtle with erythematous changes. These lesions are discussed in depth in the previous chapter. Papillary urothelial neoplasms are characterized by single or multiple finger-like projections on cystoscopy examination. When papillary neoplasms show endophytic or inverted growth patterns, there may be a dome-shaped, nodular, or flat appearance of the bladder mucosa. These visible lesions are usually biopsied and/or resected during the cystoscopic examination.

When papillary lesions are seen, it is important to determine whether it is true neoplastic condition or reactive, inflammatory condition or tangential section of urothelial mucosa. When the papillary growth is true neoplastic condition, it is important to determine the lining cell is single cell layer or multiple stratified cell layer. Figure 4.1 illustrates diagnostic algorithm of papillary lesions (see Fig. 4.1). In single-layer papillary lesion, it is important to determine whether it is true single cell layer or exfoliated to leave a single layer. The single-layered papillary lesion is papillary nephrogenic adenoma, and multiple-layered or exfoliated papillary lesions are papillary urothelial neoplasm.

The classification and grading systems for papillary urothelial neoplasms have evolved over many years. The current system is the 2016 World Health Organization (WHO), which is largely based on the 2004 WHO/1998 International Society of Urological Pathology (2004 WHO/1998 ISUP) classification system [1]. The 2016 WHO divides papillary urothelial neoplasms into urothelial papilloma, papillary urothelial neoplasm of low malignant potential (PUNLMP), low-grade papillary urothelial carcinoma (LGPUC), and high-grade papillary urothelial carcinoma (HGPUC).

To avoid complexity and confusion, this chapter generally follows the WHO classification system and emphases of pathologic features, differential diagnosis, and diagnostic pitfalls.

H. Zhou (✉) · J. Y. Ro
Department of Pathology and Genomic Medicine, Weill Medical College of Cornell University/Houston Methodist Hospital, Houston, TX, USA
e-mail: hzhou@houstonmethodist.org; JaeRo@houstonmethodist.org

C. C. Guo
Department of Pathology, The University of Texas MD Anderson Cancer Center, Houston, TX, USA
e-mail: ccguo@mdanderson.org

H. Zhou et al. (eds.), *Urinary Bladder Pathology*, https://doi.org/10.1007/978-3-030-71509-0_4

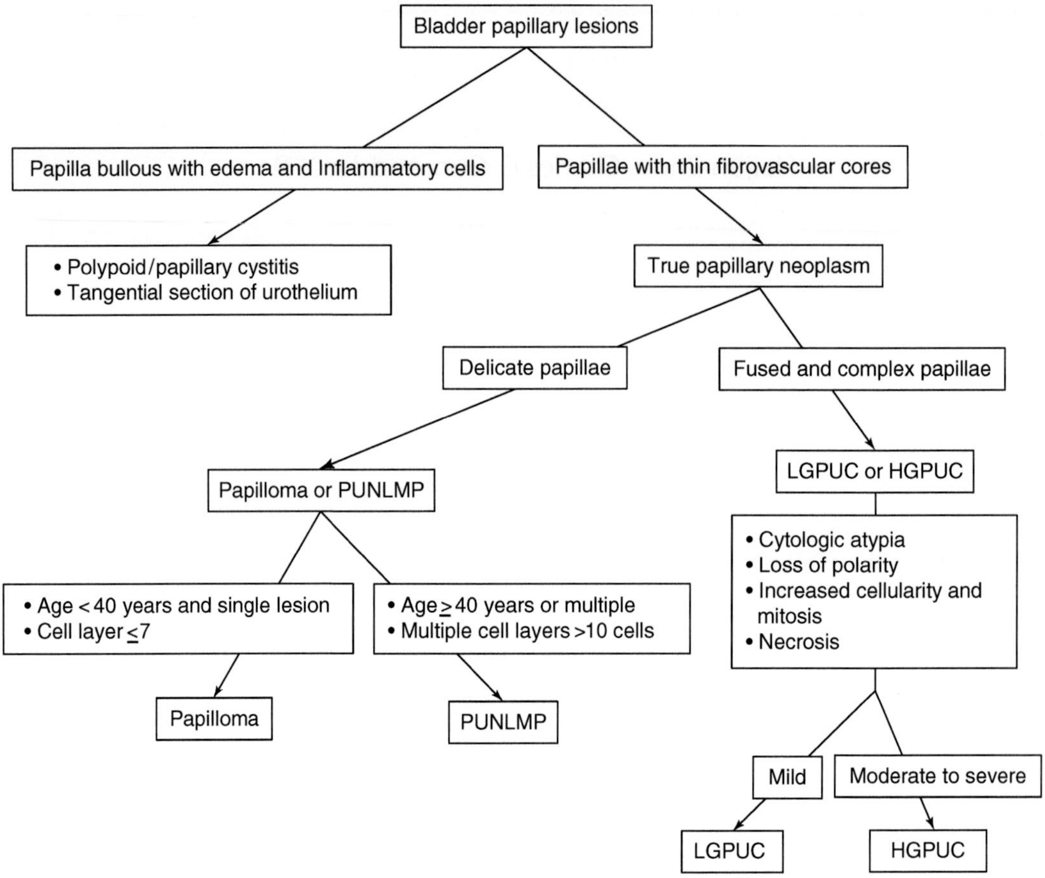

Fig. 4.1 Diagnostic algorithm of bladder papillary lesions. LGPUC, low-grade papillary urothelial carcinoma; HGPUC, high-grade papillary urothelial carcinoma; PUNLMP, papillary urothelial neoplasm of low malignant potential

Benign Neoplastic Papillary Lesions

Urothelial Papilloma

Urothelial papilloma is a benign papillary urothelial neoplasm with delicate fibrovascular cores lined by urothelium of normal appearance and thickness [3].

The diagnostic criteria for urothelial papilloma in the 2016 WHO classification system are identical to those defined in the 1973 WHO classification system [3]. Urothelial papilloma represents less than 4% of noninvasive urothelial neoplasms and typically occurs in patients younger than 50 years of age [4, 5]. The male-to-female ratio of incidence is about 2:1 [4, 6]. The main symptom is hematuria, and most tumors are located in the trigone area of the urinary bladder.

Urothelial papilloma has no fusion of papillae and there is no or minimal branching. The urothelium is cytologically and architecturally normal with no more than seven layers of cells. Umbrella cells are present with or without reactive atypia (Fig. 4.2). Urothelial papilloma has true fibrovascular cores that differentiate it from papillary hyperplasia and papillary cystitis. PUNLMP shares similar urothelial cytologic features with urothelial papilloma; however, PUNLMP exhibits a thickened urothelium, and papillae fusion and branching may occur but rare in PUMLMP.

Molecular studies show frequent mutations in fibroblast growth factor receptor 3 (FGFR3) and

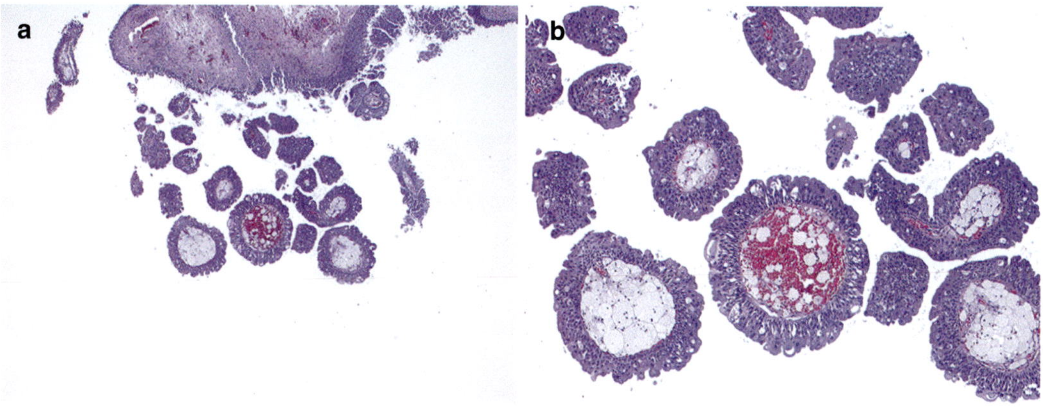

Fig. 4.2 Urothelial papilloma has delicate papillary fronds without branching or fusion. The overlying urothelium is normal without thickening or atypia (**a**, 4X, and **b**, 10X). Of note, there is a collection of macrophage in the fibrovascular core in this case

the promoter of telomerase reverse transcriptase (TERT) [7, 8]. Cytokeratin (CK) 20 expression is confined to superficial umbrella cells [9]. Urothelial papilloma can recur, but recurrent papilloma usually does not progress [4–6, 10]. The treatment of choice is complete transurethral resection.

Inverted Urothelial Papilloma

Inverted urothelial papilloma is a urothelial neoplasm with a complex, anastomosing inverted growth pattern and no to minimal cytological atypia [3].

Inverted urothelial papilloma occurs in a wide range of ages, but it is usually found in the sixth or seventh decade of life with a male-to-female ratio of incidence of 7:1 [11, 12]. The common symptoms are hematuria and urinary obstruction [12]. Inverted papilloma occurs frequently in the urinary bladder trigone area and ureteric orifices. A significant number of patients have a history of smoking [11].

Inverted urothelial papilloma appears as polypoid growth with a smooth overlying surface in the bladder mucosa under cystoscopy. Histologically, inverted papilloma shows an endophytic growth pattern, usually with thin, anastomosing cords and trabeculae of normal-appearing urothelial cells with intervening stromal tissue. The inverted urothelium has multiple connections to the overlying mucosal surface and usually does not grow into the muscularis propria. The intact inverted feature may not be preserved when disrupted during resection. The fragments of inverted papilloma may show a partially exophytic appearance.

The urothelial cells at the edge of the trabeculae can show peripheral palisading. The cells in the center of the trabeculae may exhibit mild spindling and streaming or even cuboidal and columnar changes with a gland-like appearance. Cytologically, the cells preserve polarity and may show mild atypia without significant nuclear pleomorphism. The stroma has no desmoplastic changes.

Recent molecular studies have demonstrated that inverted papilloma does not harbor the key genetic abnormalities that predispose it to develop urothelial carcinoma, such as LOH, TP53 mutations, telomere shortening, and FGFR3 mutations [12–15]. The recurrence of inverted papilloma is low [16], and transurethral resection of inverted papilloma is adequate treatment [11].

Squamous Papillary Lesions

Squamous papilloma is a rare benign neoplasm that is unrelated to HPV infection [17, 18]. It usually occurs in elderly women. Other exophytic squamous lesions, such as verrucous squamous hyperplasia and condyloma acuminatum, are also reported in the bladder [18].

Urothelial Proliferation of Uncertain Malignant Potential/Papillary Urothelial Hyperplasia

Papillary urothelial hyperplasia is an old term to describe small papillary urothelial lesions with thickened but normal-appearing urothelium and without true fibrovascular core formation. There is no cytologic atypia in the urothelium. The 2016 WHO classification of tumors of the urinary tract recommended that urothelial proliferation of uncertain malignant potential (UPUMP) should be used for the lesions previously known as papillary urothelial hyperplasia and flat urothelial hyperplasia [3]. Flat lesions are discussed in the previous chapter.

UPUMP is found most commonly on follow-up cystoscopy in patients with either a prior or concurrent low-grade papillary urothelial neoplasia, and it may be a precursor lesion to urothelial papillary tumor [19]. On cystoscopic examination, the lesion exhibits focally elevated bleb-like papillary structure or a raised, sessile, frondular appearance. Histologically, UPUMP lesions show undulating folds of thickened urothelium without fibrovascular cores [19, 20]. Cytologically, the cells in UPUMP have no atypia and maintain nuclear polarity (Fig. 4.3). The base of the papillary folds may have increased vascularity in the stroma. The finding of these lesions may indicate the presence of adjacent low-grade papillary urothelial neoplasm with lateral extension. Therefore, a comment in the pathology report suggesting clinical follow-up is warranted.

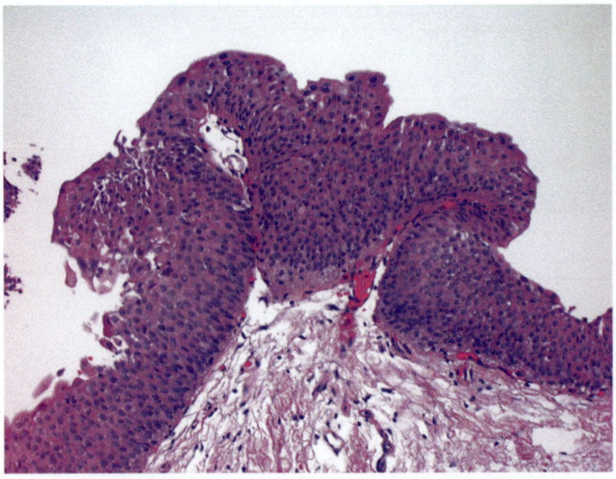

Fig. 4.3 Urothelial proliferation of uncertain malignant potential (UPUMP) showing undulating folds of thickened urothelium without true fibrovascular cores. The base of the papillary folds has increased vascularity in the stroma. The urothelial cells have no atypia and maintain nuclear polarity

Papillary Urothelial Neoplasm of Low Malignant Potential (PUNLMP)

PUNLMP is a papillary urothelial neoplasm that resembles urothelial papilloma with its delicate papillae, but with increased cellular proliferation exceeding the thickness of normal-appearing urothelium. The urothelium is usually more than seven cells thick with no to minimal nuclear atypia.

PUNLMP defines a group of lesions that have features beyond the criteria of urothelial papilloma, but without the overly malignant features to warrant diagnosis as carcinoma. PUNLMP has a low incidence of recurrence and progression [21–29], and it was previously classified as grade 1 transitional cell carcinoma (TCC) by the 1973 WHO grading system. PUNLMP is more often seen in male patients (male-to-female ratio of incidence is about 3:1), with a mean age of 65 years [30]. Gross or microscopic hematuria is the most common clinical presentation.

These lesions are typically located on the lateral wall of the bladder or near the ureteral orifices and may exhibit a “seaweed in the ocean” appearance on cystoscopy [30]. The urothelial cells surrounding the fibrovascular cores have no or minimal cytologic atypia, and architectural abnormalities are minimal with preserved cellular polarity. Mitotic figures are usually not seen. Molecular abnormalities can be detected, and a study reports that TERT promoter mutations are present in 43% of PUNLMP cases [8].

Of note, PUNLMP is not a benign neoplasm, and because of its risk for tumor recurrence and disease progression, long-term clinical follow-up is recommended for patients [22, 23].

Low-Grade Papillary Urothelial Carcinoma (LGPUC)

LGPUC has thin papillary fronds that show frequent branching, minimal fusion, and mild variation in architecture. There is mild nuclear atypia including variation in nuclear polarity, enlarged nuclei with irregular shapes, vesicular chromatin, and noticeable nucleoli. Mitotic figures can be seen in low-grade papillary urothelial carcinoma [31, 32] (Fig. 4.4). Molecular studies have shown that aneuploidy, FGFR3 mutations, and altered expression of CK20, CD44, p53, and p63 are frequently seen in LGPUC [33, 34].

LGPUC was previously classified as grade 1 or 2 TCC in the 1973 WHO classification scheme. The male-to-female ratio of incidence is about 3:1, and the mean age of patients is 70 years [29, 35, 36]. Patients with LGUC usually present with hematuria. Most patients have a single tumor located in the posterior or lateral bladder wall. However, multiple low-grade papillary urothelial carcinomas may be seen in 22% of patients [37].

LGPUC has a higher recurrence rate (about 50%) than PUNLMP, and the grade or stage progression rate is about 10% [25]. Stage progression has been reported to be as high as 13% [25]. A large study has placed the tumor-related mortality rate at approximately 2% [29]. Invasive LGPUC is also reported with a subset of patients progressing to high-grade invasive urothelial carcinoma and even metastatic disease [38, 39]. Treatment for LGPUC is complete resection with close clinical follow-up, and certain patients with increased risk may require intravesical therapy [40].

A major challenge in the diagnosis of low-grade papillary urothelium neoplasms is interobserver variability and reproducibility. From the introduction of the 1973 WHO system to the adoption of the most recent 2004/2016 WHO system with its defined and detailed histologic criteria for each diagnostic category, the improvement in intraobserver and interobserver variability has been limited [22, 23, 41–43]. Therefore, review with patient's previous materials is highly recommended to reduce intraobserver and interobserver variability.

High-Grade Papillary Urothelial Carcinoma (HGPUC)

HGPUC is characterized by papillary fronds lined by urothelial cells with obvious disordered arrangement and cytologic atypia. Both architectural and cytologic abnormalities are easily recognizable at a low magnification [25]. The papillae frequently show fusion and branching, and the thickness of the urothelium varies. The cells lose polarity with pleomorphic nuclei and prominent nucleoli, and mitotic figures are easily detectable (Fig. 4.5). Carcinoma in situ is frequently identified in the adjacent urothelial mucosa.

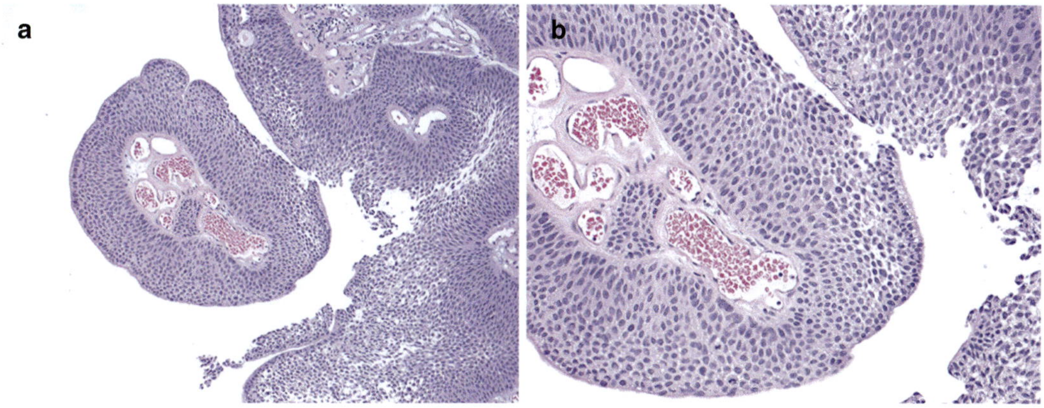

Fig. 4.4 Low-grade papillary urothelial carcinoma (LGPUC) has thin papillary fronds with frequent branching, minimal fusion, and mild variation in architecture. Mild nuclear atypia including variation in nuclear polarity, nuclei enlargement with irregularity, and inconspicuous nucleoli. Mitotic figures can be seen (**a**, 10 X, and **b**, 20 X)

Patients with HGPUC commonly have hematuria. On cystoscopy, HGPUC can appear as single or multiple papillary, nodular, or solid lesions. All grade 3 tumors and some grade 2 TCCs assigned in the 1973 WHO scheme are now classified as high-grade carcinomas in the 2004/2016 WHO classification. Molecularly, HGPUC resembles invasive tumors. Deletions at 2q, 5q, 10q, and 18q and gains at 5p and 20q are commonly detected in HGPUC [44]. Biomarker changes such as the overexpression of p53, HER2, or EGFR and loss of p21 or p27 are frequently present in HGPUC [45].

HGPUC has a high risk of recurrence and progression to invasive disease. Stage progression is observed in as many as 65% of patients, and the tumor-related mortality rate is approximately 22% [29]. The treatment for HGPUC is complete resection followed by intravesical therapy [40].

Grade heterogeneity is a common feature seen in papillary neoplasms, many of which show morphology of mixed grades within the same lesion [1, 46–51] (Fig. 4.6). The 2004 WHO/ISUP system recommends classifying according to the highest-grade present when lesions have mixed grades [1]. Studies have shown that lesions with mixed grades typically have lower staging than purely high-grade lesions [46, 47, 49, 50]. However, additional studies are needed to define to what extent a tumor can be classified as mixed grade tumor. Practically, pathologists may provide a comment in the report to indicate which grade is predominant for a mixed grade tumor, for example, HGPUC (10%) is seen in the background of LGPUC.

There are several basic features to differentiate papillary lesions. The urothelial papilloma has a delicate fibrovascular core with benign urothelial lining. PUNLMP has thickened benign-appearing urothelium compared to papilloma. UPUMP shares a similar urothelium with PUNLMP but lacks its fibrovascular core. LGPUC starts to have mild papillae fusion and mild cytologic atypia compared to PUNLMP. HGPUC has severe architectural and cytologic atypia that is easily recognizable at a low power.

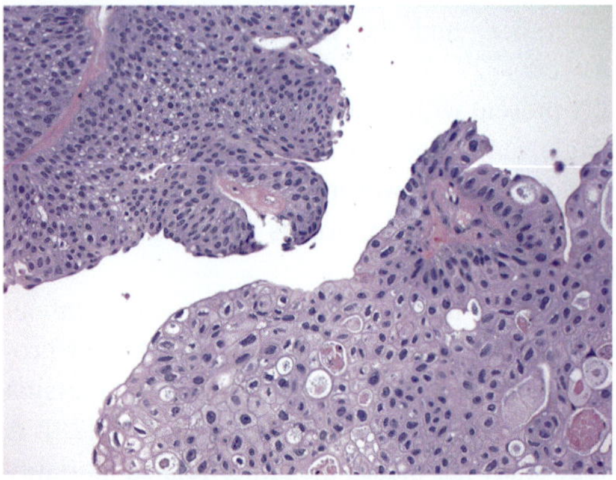

Fig. 4.6 A case of mixed low-grade (left upper) and high-grade (right lower) papillary urothelial carcinomas

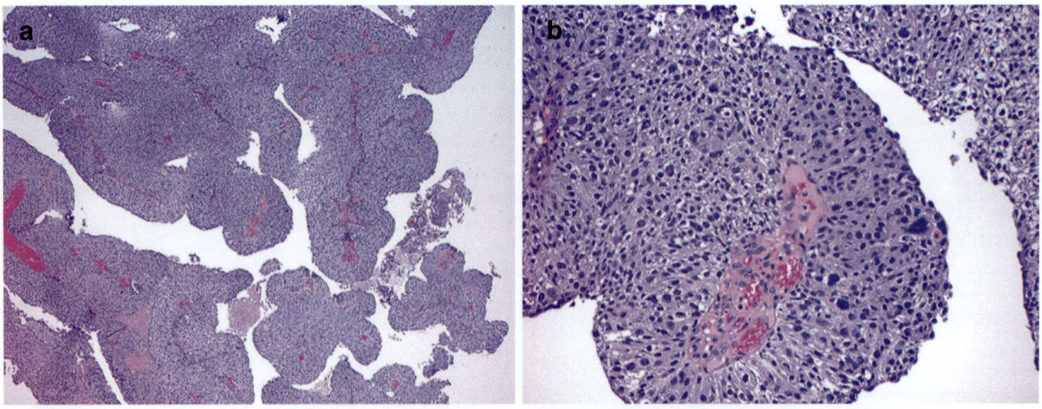

Fig. 4.5 High-grade papillary urothelial carcinoma (HGPUC) has architectural and cytologic abnormalities which are easily recognizable at scanning magnification. The papillae frequently show fusion and branching, and the thickness of the urothelium varies. Urothelial cells have obvious disordered arrangement and cytologic atypia, including pleomorphic nuclei, prominent nucleoli, and frequent mitotic figures (**a**, 4 X, and **b**, 20 X)

Urothelial Carcinoma with Inverted Growth Pattern

UPUMP, PUNLMP, LGPUC, and HGPUC may show inverted growth, which is characterized by large nests or nodules in the lamina propria with a pushing border (Fig. 4.7). Although they share the same endophytic growth pattern with inverted papilloma, anastomosing cords, central streaming, and peripheral palisading in the trabeculae are usually not present in inverted UPUMP, PUNLMP, LGPUC, and HGPUC [52–55].

The inverted variant of urothelial carcinoma is often associated with an exophytic high-grade papillary or invasive component [52, 56]. The inverted component demonstrates nuclear pleomorphism, architectural abnormality, and mitotic activity similar to those in its exophytic high-grade counterpart (Fig. 4.8). The presence of irregular neoplastic nests and single cells in the lamina propria with desmoplastic reaction and inflammation often indicates stroma invasion.

Immunohistochemical studies can be helpful in difficult cases. Urothelial carcinomas with an inverted growth pattern frequently express Ki67, p53, and/or CK20. It often demonstrates genetic alterations that are commonly seen in bladder cancer [52]. Telomere shortening and TERT promoter mutations are more frequently seen in inverted pattern urothelial carcinomas than in inverted papillomas (70% versus 9% and 58% versus 15%, respectively) [13, 57].

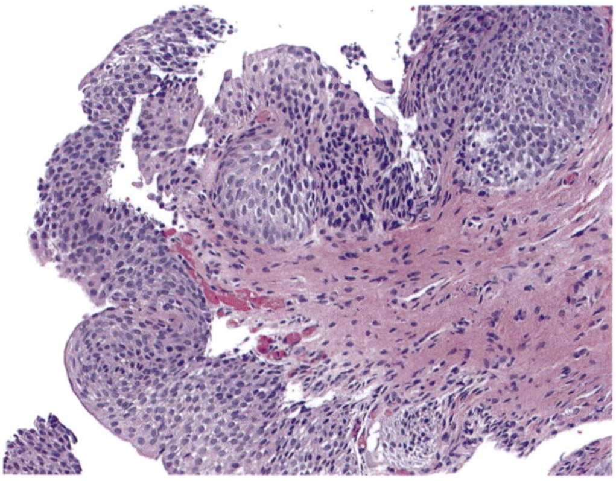

Fig. 4.7 The surface urothelial proliferation meets the diagnosis of urothelial proliferation of uncertain malignant potential (UPUMP). The underneath inverted nests have pushing borders and share the similar cytologic features with the surface urothelium

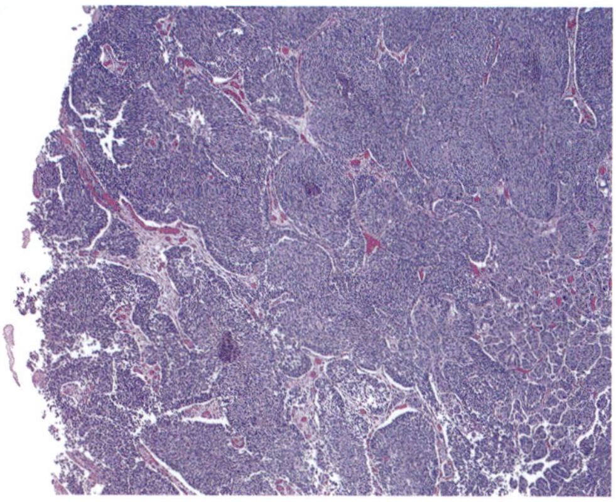

Fig. 4.8 The inverted variant of high-grade papillary urothelial carcinoma demonstrates nuclear pleomorphism, architectural abnormality, and frequent mitotic activity. The irregular neoplastic nests and single cells in the lamina propria indicate stromal invasion

Nonneoplastic Papillary Lesions

Papillary lesions seen in the urinary bladder are not all neoplastic. Commonly encountered reactive papillary lesions include polypoid/papillary cystitis, papillary nephrogenic adenoma, and fibroepithelial polyps.

Polypoid/papillary cystitis is a secondary mucosa reaction to chronic inflammation in the bladder, which is commonly seen in patients with indwelling catheter and vesical fistula [58–60]. On cystoscopy, these papillary or polypoid lesions are often located in the dome or on the posterior wall of the urinary bladder. Tissue biopsy is usually performed to rule out papillary urothelial carcinoma [61, 62].

Microscopically, papillary cystitis has finger-like papillae lined by a reactive urothelium, and polypoid cystitis has a broad-based edematous lamina propria (Fig. 4.9). Chronic inflammation in the lamina propria and dilated blood vessels are prominent in both papillary and polypoid cystitis. Metaplastic changes may be present in the epithelium covering or adjacent to the lesion.

Papillary and polypoid cystitis may be distinguished from papillary urothelial carcinoma by the following features: the broader fronds of polypoid

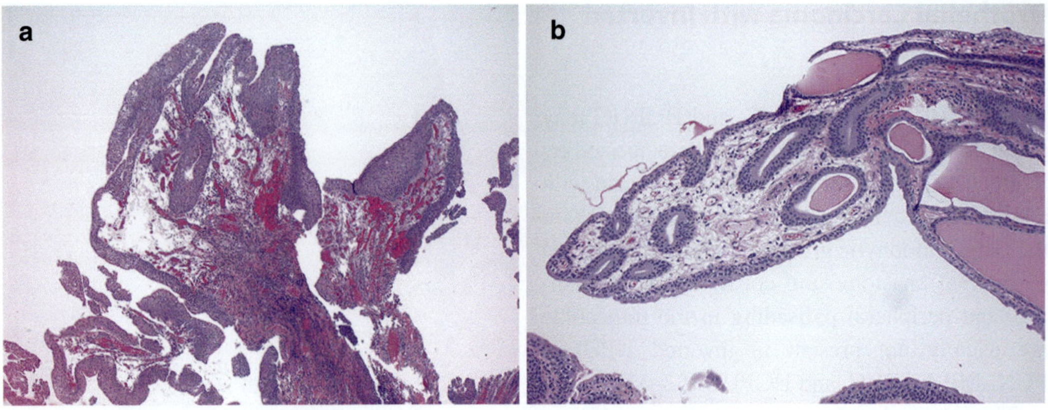

Fig. 4.9 Polypoid/papillary cystitis has finger-like papillae lined by a reactive urothelium with/without broad-based edematous lamina propria (**a**). Cystitis glandularis is present with the polypoid/papillary cystitis (**b**)

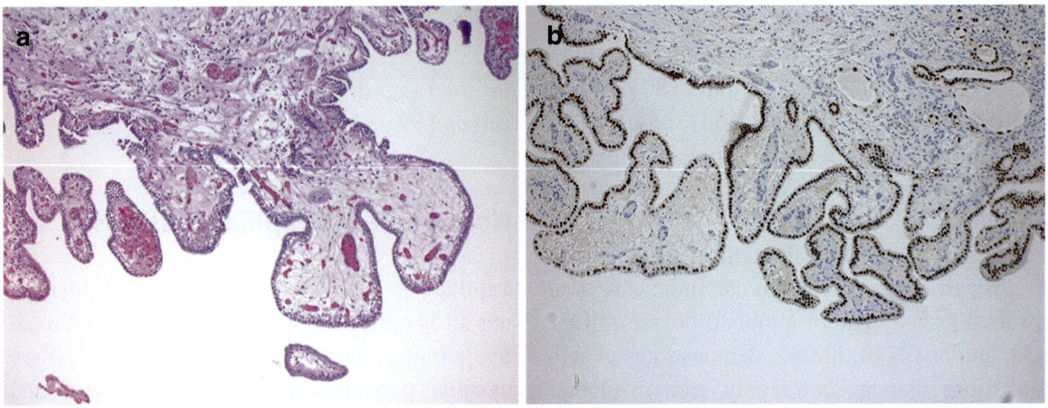

Fig. 4.10 Papillary nephrogenic adenoma has a single layer of cuboidal cell lining on the surface of the papillae (**a**). The lining cells are positive for Pax-8 (**b**)

cystitis, the less branching papillae of papillary cystitis, the lesser hyperplasia in the epithelium of papillary cystitis, and the more frequently present umbrella cells of papillary cystitis.

Nephrogenic adenoma can present with multiple growth patterns (see Chap. 2 for further discussion). Papillary nephrogenic adenoma has a cuboidal single cell lining on the surface of the papillae. It may be differentiated from papillary urothelial carcinoma by its denuded surface. Immunohistochemical studies show that nephrogenic adenomas are positive for Pax-8 and negative for p63 and GATA3 [63, 64] (Fig. 4.10).

Fibroepithelial polyps are most commonly seen in children but may occur at all ages. Fibroepithelial polyps contain broader stalks with dense fibrous stroma as compared to the thin delicate fibrovascular cores seen in urothelial papilloma [65].

References

1. Epstein JI, Amin MB, Reuter VR, Mostofi FK. The World Health Organization/International Society of Urological Pathology consensus classification of urothelial (transitional cell) neoplasms of the urinary bladder. Bladder Consensus Conference Committee. Am J Surg Pathol. 1998; 22(12):1435–48.
2. Montironi R, Mazzucchelli R, Scarpelli M, Lopez-Beltran A, Cheng L. Morphological diagnosis of urothelial neoplasms. J Clin Pathol. 2008;61(1):3–10.
3. Moch H. HPA, Ulbright T.M., Reuter V.E. WHO Classification of Tumours of the Urinary Stem and Male Genital Organs. Lyon, France: International Agency for Research on Cancer (IARC) 2016.
4. Cheng L, Darson M, Cheville JC, Neumann RM, Zincke H, Nehra A, et al. Urothelial papilloma of the bladder. Clinical and biologic implications. Cancer. 1999;86(10):2098–101.
5. McKenney JK, Amin MB, Young RH. Urothelial (transitional cell) papilloma of the urinary bladder:

a clinicopathologic study of 26 cases. Mod Pathol. 2003;16(7):623–9.
6. Magi-Galluzzi C, Epstein JI. Urothelial papilloma of the bladder: a review of 34 de novo cases. Am J Surg Pathol. 2004;28(12):1615–20.
7. van Rhijn BW, Montironi R, Zwarthoff EC, Jöbsis AC, van der Kwast TH. Frequent FGFR3 mutations in urothelial papilloma. J Pathol. 2002;198(2):245–51.
8. Cheng L, Montironi R, Lopez-Beltran A. TERT Promoter Mutations Occur Frequently in Urothelial Papilloma and Papillary Urothelial Neoplasm of Low Malignant Potential. Eur Urol. 2017;71(3):497–8.
9. Harnden P, Mahmood N, Southgate J. Expression of cytokeratin 20 redefines urothelial papillomas of the bladder. Lancet. 1999;353(9157):974–7.
10. Al Bashir S, Yilmaz A, Gotto G, Trpkov K. Long term outcome of primary urothelial papilloma: a single institution cohort. Pathology. 2014;46(1):37–40.
11. Sung MT, Maclennan GT, Lopez-Beltran A, Montironi R, Cheng L. Natural history of urothelial inverted papilloma. Cancer. 2006;107(11):2622–7.
12. Hodges KB, Lopez-Beltran A, Maclennan GT, Montironi R, Cheng L. Urothelial lesions with inverted growth patterns: histogenesis, molecular genetic findings, differential diagnosis and clinical management. BJU Int. 2011;107(4):532–7.
13. Williamson SR, Zhang S, Lopez-Beltran A, Montironi R, Wang M, Cheng L. Telomere shortening distinguishes inverted urothelial neoplasms. Histopathology. 2013;62(4):595–601.
14. Montironi R, Cheng L, Lopez-Beltran A, Scarpelli M, Mazzucchelli R, Mikuz G, et al. Inverted (endophytic) noninvasive lesions and neoplasms of the urothelium: the Cinderella group has yet to be fully exploited. Eur Urol. 2011;59(2):225–30.
15. Lott S, Wang M, Zhang S, MacLennan GT, Lopez-Beltran A, Montironi R, et al. FGFR3 and TP53 mutation analysis in inverted urothelial papilloma: incidence and etiological considerations. Mod Pathol. 2009;22(5):627–32.
16. Cheng CW, Chan LW, Chan CK, Ng CF, Cheung HY, Chan SY, et al. Is surveillance necessary for inverted papilloma in the urinary bladder and urethra? ANZ J Surg. 2005;75(4):213–7.
17. Cheng L, Leibovich BC, Cheville JC, Ramnani DM, Sebo TJ, Nehra A, et al. Squamous papilloma of the urinary tract is unrelated to condyloma acuminata. Cancer. 2000;88(7):1679–86.
18. Guo CC, Fine SW, Epstein JI. Noninvasive squamous lesions in the urinary bladder: a clinicopathologic analysis of 29 cases. Am J Surg Pathol. 2006;30(7):883–91.
19. Taylor DC, Bhagavan BS, Larsen MP, Cox JA, Epstein JI. Papillary urothelial hyperplasia. A precursor to papillary neoplasms. Am J Surg Pathol. 1996;20(12):1481–8.
20. Cheng L, Bostwick DG. Overdiagnosis of bladder carcinoma. Anal Quant Cytol Histol. 2008;30(5):261–4.
21. Cheng L, MacLennan GT, Zhang S, Wang M, Pan CX, Koch MO. Laser capture microdissection analysis reveals frequent allelic losses in papillary urothelial neoplasm of low malignant potential of the urinary bladder. Cancer. 2004;101(1):183–8.
22. MacLennan GT, Kirkali Z, Cheng L. Histologic grading of noninvasive papillary urothelial neoplasms. Eur Urol. 2007;51(4):889-97; discussion 897–8.
23. Jones TD, Cheng L. Papillary urothelial neoplasm of low malignant potential: evolving terminology and concepts. J Urol. 2006;175(6):1995–2003.
24. Montironi R, Lopez-Beltran A, Mazzucchelli R, Bostwick DG. Classification and grading of the non-invasive urothelial neoplasms: recent advances and controversies. J Clin Pathol. 2003;56(2):91–5.
25. Lopez-Beltran A, Montironi R. Non-invasive urothelial neoplasms: according to the most recent WHO classification. Eur Urol. 2004;46(2):170–6.
26. Alsheikh A, Mohamedali Z, Jones E, Masterson J, Gilks CB. Comparison of the WHO/ISUP classification and cytokeratin 20 expression in predicting the behavior of low-grade papillary urothelial tumors. World/Health Organization/Internattional Society of Urologic Pathology. Mod Pathol. 2001;14(4):267–72.
27. Montironi R, Lopez-Beltran A, Scarpelli M, Mazzucchelli R, Cheng L. Morphological classification and definition of benign, preneoplastic and non-invasive neoplastic lesions of the urinary bladder. Histopathology. 2008;53(6):621–33.
28. Montironi R, Cheng L, Scarpelli M, Mazzucchelli R, Lopez-Beltran A. How much do you know about benign, preneoplastic, non-invasive and invasive neoplastic lesions of the urinary bladder classified according to the 2004 WHO scheme? Diagn Pathol. 2011;6:31.
29. Pan CC, Chang YH, Chen KK, Yu HJ, Sun CH, Ho DM. Prognostic significance of the 2004 WHO/ISUP classification for prediction of recurrence, progression, and cancer-specific mortality of non-muscle-invasive urothelial tumors of the urinary bladder: a clinicopathologic study of 1,515 cases. Am J Clin Pathol. 2010;133(5):788–95.
30. Cheng L, Neumann RM, Bostwick DG. Papillary urothelial neoplasms of low malignant potential. Clinical and biologic implications. Cancer. 1999;86(10):2102–8.
31. Carbin BE, Ekman P, Gustafson H, Christensen NJ, Sandstedt B, Silfverswärd C. Grading of human urothelial carcinoma based on nuclear atypia and mitotic frequency. I. Histological description. J Urol. 1991;145(5):968–71.
32. Miyamoto H, Brimo F, Schultz L, Ye H, Miller JS, Fajardo DA, et al. Low-grade papillary urothelial carcinoma of the urinary bladder: a clinicopathologic analysis of a post-World Health Organization/International Society of Urological Pathology classification cohort from a single academic center. Arch Pathol Lab Med. 2010;134(8):1160–3.
33. Cheng L, Zhang S, MacLennan GT, Williamson SR, Lopez-Beltran A, Montironi R. Bladder cancer: translating molecular genetic insights into clinical practice. Hum Pathol. 2011;42(4):455–81.
34. van Oers JM, Wild PJ, Burger M, Denzinger S, Stoehr R, Rosskopf E, et al. FGFR3 mutations and a normal CK20 staining pattern define low-grade noninvasive urothelial bladder tumours. Eur Urol. 2007;52(3):760–8.
35. Oosterhuis JW, Schapers RF, Janssen-Heijnen ML, Pauwels RP, Newling DW, ten Kate F. Histological grading of papillary urothelial carcinoma of the blad-

der: prognostic value of the 1998 WHO/ISUP classification system and comparison with conventional grading systems. J Clin Pathol. 2002;55(12):900–5.
36. Holmäng S, Hedelin H, Anderström C, Holmberg E, Busch C, Johansson SL. Recurrence and progression in low grade papillary urothelial tumors. J Urol. 1999;162(3 Pt 1):702–7.
37. Holmäng S, Hedelin H, Anderström C, Holmberg E, Johansson SL. Prospective registration of all patients in a geographical region with newly diagnosed bladder carcinomas during a two-year period. Scand J Urol Nephrol. 2000;34(2):95–101.
38. Watts KE, Montironi R, Mazzucchelli R, van der Kwast T, Osunkoya AO, Stephenson AJ, et al. Clinicopathologic characteristics of 23 cases of invasive low-grade papillary urothelial carcinoma. Urology. 2012;80(2):361–6.
39. Toll AD, Epstein JI. Invasive low-grade papillary urothelial carcinoma: a clinicopathologic analysis of 41 cases. Am J Surg Pathol. 2012;36(7):1081–6.
40. Brausi M, Witjes JA, Lamm D, Persad R, Palou J, Colombel M, et al. A review of current guidelines and best practice recommendations for the management of nonmuscle invasive bladder cancer by the International Bladder Cancer Group. J Urol. 2011;186(6):2158–67.
41. Murphy WM, Takezawa K, Maruniak NA. Interobserver discrepancy using the 1998 World Health Organization/International Society of Urologic Pathology classification of urothelial neoplasms: practical choices for patient care. J Urol. 2002;168(3):968–72.
42. Yorukoglu K, Tuna B, Dikicioglu E, Duzcan E, Isisag A, Sen S, et al. Reproducibility of the 1998 World Health Organization/International Society of Urologic Pathology classification of papillary urothelial neoplasms of the urinary bladder. Virchows Arch. 2003;443(6):734–40.
43. Bol MG, Baak JP, Buhr-Wildhagen S, Kruse AJ, Kjellevold KH, Janssen EA, et al. Reproducibility and prognostic variability of grade and lamina propria invasion in stages Ta, T1 urothelial carcinoma of the bladder. J Urol. 2003;169(4):1291–4.
44. Habuchi T, Ogawa O, Kakehi Y, Ogura K, Koshiba M, Hamazaki S, et al. Accumulated allelic losses in the development of invasive urothelial cancer. Int J Cancer. 1993;53(4):579–84.
45. Eble J.N. SG, Epstein J.I., et al. World Health Organization Classification of Tumours: Pathology and Genetics of Tumours of the Urinary System and Male Genital Organs. Lyon, France: IARC Press 2004.
46. Billis A, Carvalho RB, Mattos AC, Negretti F, Nogueira CR, Oliveira MC, et al. Tumor grade heterogeneity in urothelial bladder carcinoma--proposal of a system using combined numbers. Scand J Urol Nephrol. 2001;35(4):275–9.
47. Cheng L, Neumann RM, Nehra A, Spotts BE, Weaver AL, Bostwick DG. Cancer heterogeneity and its biologic implications in the grading of urothelial carcinoma. Cancer. 2000;88(7):1663–70.
48. Bostwick DG, Mikuz G. Urothelial papillary (exophytic) neoplasms. Virchows Arch. 2002;441(2):109–16.
49. Bircan S, Candir O, Serel TA. Comparison of WHO 1973, WHO/ISUP 1998, WHO 1999 grade and combined scoring systems in evaluation of bladder carcinoma. Urol Int. 2004;73(3):201–8.
50. Krüger S, Thorns C, Böhle A, Feller AC. Prognostic significance of a grading system considering tumor heterogeneity in muscle-invasive urothelial carcinoma of the urinary bladder. Int Urol Nephrol. 2003;35(2):169–73.
51. May M, Brookman-Amissah S, Roigas J, Hartmann A, Störkel S, Kristiansen G, et al. Prognostic accuracy of individual uropathologists in noninvasive urinary bladder carcinoma: a multicentre study comparing the 1973 and 2004 World Health Organisation classifications. Eur Urol. 2010;57(5):850–8.
52. Jones TD, Zhang S, Lopez-Beltran A, Eble JN, Sung MT, MacLennan GT, et al. Urothelial carcinoma with an inverted growth pattern can be distinguished from inverted papilloma by fluorescence in situ hybridization, immunohistochemistry, and morphologic analysis. Am J Surg Pathol. 2007;31(12):1861–7.
53. Lopez-Beltran A, Cheng L. Histologic variants of urothelial carcinoma: differential diagnosis and clinical implications. Hum Pathol. 2006;37(11):1371–88.
54. Amin MB, Gómez JA, Young RH. Urothelial transitional cell carcinoma with endophytic growth patterns: a discussion of patterns of invasion and problems associated with assessment of invasion in 18 cases. Am J Surg Pathol. 1997;21(9):1057-68.
55. Sudo T, Irie A, Ishii D, Satoh E, Mitomi H, Baba S. Histopathologic and biologic characteristics of a transitional cell carcinoma with inverted papilloma-like endophytic growth pattern. Urology. 2003;61(4):837.
56. Terai A, Tamaki M, Hayashida H, Tomoyosh T, Takeuchi H, Yoshida O. Bulky transitional cell carcinoma of bladder with inverted proliferation. Int J Urol. 1996;3(4):316–9.
57. Cheng L, Davidson DD, Wang M, Lopez-Beltran A, Montironi R, Wang L, et al. Telomerase reverse transcriptase (TERT) promoter mutation analysis of benign, malignant and reactive urothelial lesions reveals a subpopulation of inverted papilloma with immortalizing genetic change. Histopathology. 2016;69(1):107–13.
58. Young RH. Papillary and polypoid cystitis. A report of eight cases. Am J Surg Pathol. 1988;12(7):542–6.
59. Milles G. Catheter-induced hemorrhagic pseudopolyps of the urinary bladder. Jama. 1965;193:968–9.
60. Ekelund P, Anderström C, Johansson SL, Larsson P. The reversibility of catheter-associated polypoid cystitis. J Urol. 1983;130(3):456–9.
61. Lane Z, Epstein JI. Polypoid/papillary cystitis: a series of 41 cases misdiagnosed as papillary urothelial neoplasia. Am J Surg Pathol. 2008;32(5):758–64.
62. Buck EG. Polypoid cystitis mimicking transitional cell carcinoma. J Urol. 1984;131(5):963.
63. Fromont G, Barcat L, Gaudin J, Irani J. Revisiting the immunophenotype of nephrogenic adenoma. Am J Surg Pathol. 2009;33(11):1654–8.
64. Rahemtullah A, Oliva E. Nephrogenic adenoma: an update on an innocuous but troublesome entity. Adv Anat Pathol. 2006;13(5):247–55.
65. Tsuzuki T, Epstein JI. Fibroepithelial polyp of the lower urinary tract in adults. Am J Surg Pathol. 2005;29(4):460–6.

Invasive Urothelial Carcinoma with Molecular Types

5

Charles C. Guo, Jae Y. Ro, and Bogdan Czerniak

Approximately 30% of bladder cancers are composed of invasive urothelial carcinoma (UC), which is characterized by infiltrating growth through the urothelial basement membrane into the stromal tissue in the bladder wall [1–3]. Unlike noninvasive UC, invasive UC is a highly aggressive disease associated with rapid progression and metastasis, requiring significantly different treatment modality from that of indolent noninvasive UC [1, 4–6]. Cancer stage based on the depth of cancer invasion in the bladder wall is the most important prognostic factor in invasive UC [1, 2, 7]. The muscularis propria (MP) is the major landmark in bladder cancer stage (see Chap. 12), which divides invasive UC into superficially and deeply invasive diseases. The superficial disease compromises bladder cancers that invade only the lamina propria (LP) (pT1), and the deep disease includes bladder cancers that invade into the MP (pT2), perivesical tissue (pT3), and adjacent organs (pT4). Superficially and deeply invasive UC are treated differently – the former usually undergoes local treatment, including transurethral resection of bladder tumor (TURBT) and intravesical therapy, while the latter requires radical surgeries (cystectomy and cystoprostatectomy) with and without systemic chemotherapy and radiation therapy [1, 4–6]. Therefore, it is critical to recognize the morphologic features associated with cancer invasion as well as to determine the depth of cancer invasion. Recent genomic analyses of muscle-invasive bladder cancer (MIBC) have revealed several different molecular subtypes, which demonstrate not only specific molecular signatures but also distinct clinicopathologic features [8–11]. Another remarkable feature of invasive UC is a high propensity for divergent differentiation [2, 12, 13], leading to a number of distinct UC histologic variants, which are detailed in Chap. 6.

C. C. Guo (✉) · B. Czerniak
Department of Pathology, The University of Texas MD Anderson Cancer Center, Houston, TX, USA
e-mail: ccguo@mdanderson.org; bczernia@mdanderson.org

J. Y. Ro
Department of Pathology and Genomic Medicine, Weill Medical College of Cornell University/Houston Methodist Hospital, Houston, TX, USA
e-mail: JaeRo@houstonmethodist.org

Diagnosis of Cancer Invasion

Bladder cancer infiltrates through the basement membrane at the urothelial mucosa, initiating the cancer invasion process. Grossly, invasive UC may present as a sessile, polypoid, ulcerated, or infiltrative lesion. It is often associated with noninvasive papillary UC or erythematous areas of UC in situ (UCIS). Microscopically, invasive UC demonstrates a constellation of morphologic features that are distinct from those in noninvasive

H. Zhou et al. (eds.), *Urinary Bladder Pathology*, https://doi.org/10.1007/978-3-030-71509-0_5

Table 5.1 Diagnostic criteria for invasive urothelial carcinoma

Usually high grade, although not exclusively
Common growth patterns include irregularly shaped nests, sheets, cords, trabeculae, and infiltrating single cells
Absent or disrupted basement membrane
Invasive carcinoma cells may develop "paradoxical differentiation" with higher nuclear grade and more abundant eosinophilic cytoplasm than the adjacent noninvasive carcinoma cells
Often induces reactive changes in the stroma, such as desmoplasia, inflammation, retraction artifact, and myxoid changes
Immunohistochemistry with cytokeratin and deeper sections may be helpful in difficult cases

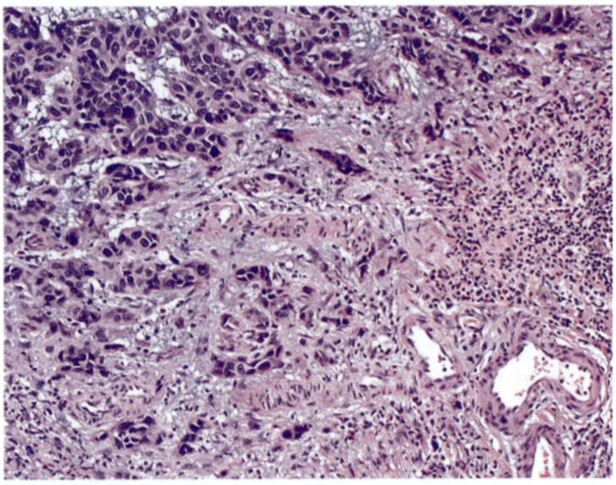

Fig. 5.1 Urothelial carcinoma shows small nests, cords, and single cells with high-grade nuclear atypia. It invades the lamina propria

papillary UC or UCIS (Table 5.1). Invasive UC shows a variety of growth patterns, including nests, sheets, cords, trabeculae, small clusters, and single cells infiltrating the bladder wall (Fig. 5.1). Tumor nests are often irregularly shaped and variably sized, and the basement membrane around tumor nests is often absent or disrupted.

Sometimes tumor shows a diffuse, sheet-like pattern, but focal areas of nests and clusters are generally present, if it is carefully examined. Tumor often displays a mixture of several growth patterns. Infiltrating cords and single cell growth patterns may be associated with worse prognosis than other patterns [14, 15].

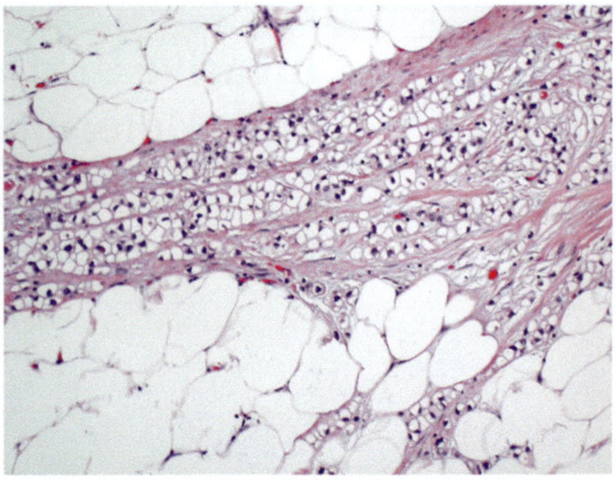

Fig. 5.2 Urothelial carcinoma shows low-grade nuclear atypia and clear cytoplasm. It invades the perivesical adipose tissue

Invasive UC cells have a relatively nondescript morphology with various amounts of pale to eosinophilic cytoplasm, which cannot be easily differentiated from poorly differentiated carcinoma of other types. More than 90% of pT1 UC are high grade characterized by nuclear enlargement, pleomorphism, and increased mitotic activity (Fig. 5.1). However, invasive UC can also be found in a small subset of low-grade UC (Fig. 5.2). The prognostic difference between low-grade and high-grade invasive UC remains uncertain [16–18]. Nonetheless, it is recommended that tumor grade should be reported for invasive UC, particularly pT1 tumors [2]. UC cells may contain abundant glycogen, leading to a clear cell appearance after formalin fixation (Fig. 5.2) [19]. Although cytoplasmic mucin is not easily recognizable on routine hematoxylin and eosin (H&E) stain, it can be detected in up to 60% of high-grade UC on mucin-specific histochemical stains, such as periodic acid-Schiff (PAS) and mucicarmine stains [20]. The presence of cytoplasmic mucin on histochemical stain by itself is insufficient for an indication of glandular differentiation. Sometimes, invasive UC may develop "paradoxical differentiation" or "reverse maturation," a phenomenon in which invasive UC cells show a higher degree of nuclear atypia with abundant eosinophilic cytoplasm than the adjacent noninvasive cells (Fig. 5.3). UC frequently shows divergent differentiation, such as

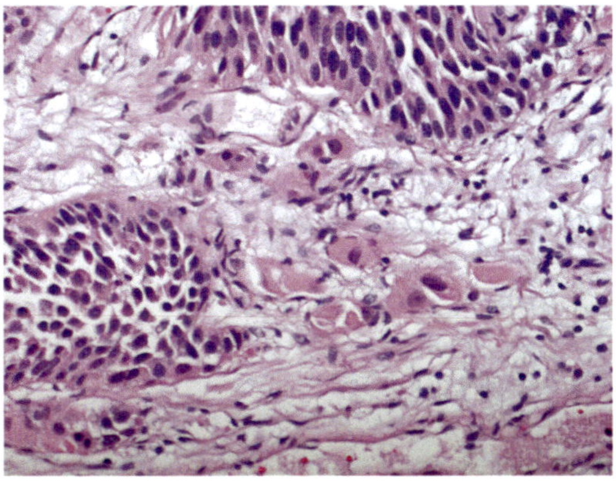

Fig. 5.3 Minimally invasive urothelial carcinoma shows a few tumor cells with abundant eosinophilic cytoplasm ("paradoxical differentiation") in the stroma

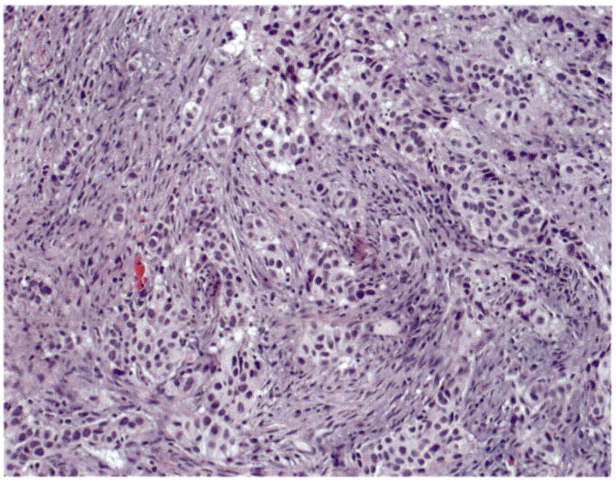

Fig. 5.4 Invasive urothelial carcinoma induces exuberant fibrosis in the stroma

squamous and glandular differentiation, and develops a number of distinct histologic variants [12, 13] (see Chap. 6). The presence of divergent differentiation in a poorly differentiated carcinoma at a metastatic site should raise a possibility of UC. In general, the diagnosis of squamous cell carcinoma or adenocarcinoma in the bladder is only reserved for those that demonstrate pure or almost pure morphology of squamous or glandular differentiation [2] (see Chap. 7).

Invasive UC induces a wide range of reactive changes in the adjacent stroma, which may aid the recognition of cancer invasion. The stroma often becomes desmoplastic or fibrotic with proliferation of fibroblasts/myofibroblasts and accumulation of collagen (Fig. 5.4). Sometimes, the proliferation of spindle fibroblasts and myofibroblasts is exuberant with conspicuous nuclear atypia, mimicking sarcomatoid UC or sarcoma. However, the proliferation is usually non-expansile, and the atypia often has a degenerative appearance. Inflammation is another common reaction associated with cancer invasion (Fig. 5.5). Sometimes the inflammation is intense and diffuse, particularly in lymphoepithelioma-like UC variant, which makes it difficult to recognize single-cell or small-nest cancer invasion. Retraction artifact is another common sign of stromal invasion (Fig. 5.6), which is particularly prominent in micropapillary UC variant.

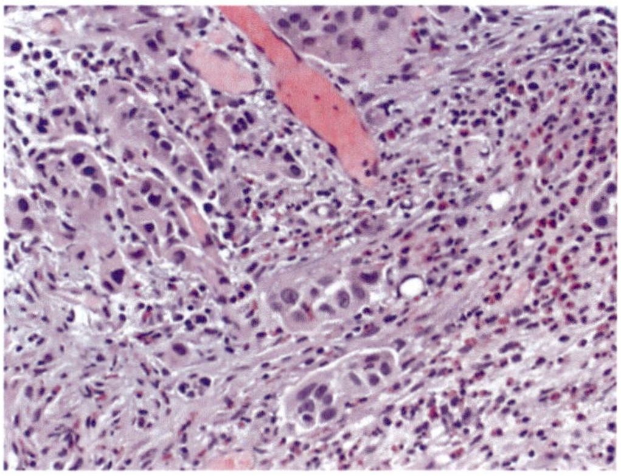

Fig. 5.5 Invasive urothelial carcinoma induces inflammatory reaction in the stroma

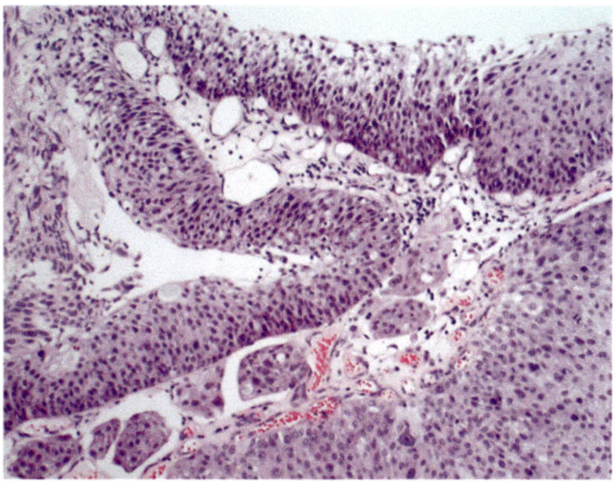

Fig. 5.6 High-grade papillary urothelial carcinoma shows small, irregular nests with retraction artifact. It invades the papillary cores

Although retraction artifact mimics lymphovascular invasion, it lacks an endothelial lining. Sometimes, the stroma may become myxoid with loose and hypocellular stroma. The myxoid stroma is usually positive for PAS with diastase, Alcian blue, and mucicarmine mucin stains [21].

Lamina Propria Invasion

Recognition of cancer invasion is generally not difficult, but it may be challenging in a small subset of TURBT specimens with minimal, superficial invasion into the LP. At the early phase, stromal invasion is usually seen at the base of the papillary UC (Fig. 5.7). Sometimes, UC may invade into the stalks of papillary tumor (Fig. 5.6), which can be difficult to differentiate from tangential section of noninvasive papillary UC.

Interobserver variability is substantial in diagnosing an early-phase, minimal invasion into the LP. In one study, 35% of bladder UC initially diagnosed as stage pT1 were downstaged to pTa, and 3% were upstaged as pT2–4, when they were reviewed by a genitourinary pathologist [22]. In another study, 57% of bladder UC initially diagnosed as stage pT1 were downstaged to pTa, and 13% were upstaged to pT2–3, after when they were reviewed by a panel of genitourinary pathologists [23]. The high interobserver variation of minimal LP invasion is caused by several inherent factors in TURBT specimens: (1) TURBT samples are usually small and fragmented with a poor orientation. (2) Cauterization and crush artifacts are common in TURBT specimens, which severely distort the tumor morphology. (3) Invasive UC frequently induces exuberant inflammation in the adjacent stroma, which may obscure isolated cells or small clusters of invasive cancer cells. (4) UCIS involves von Brunn nests with isolated nests of high-grade cells in the stroma, resembling LP invasion. (5) Noninvasive papillary UC may display an inverted growth pattern characterized by large, smooth, and round nests of tumor cells with regular contour in the LP, mimicking stromal invasion (see Chap. 4); however, the nests in invasive UC are often small and jagged with irregular contours. Deeper levels and cytokeratin immunostaining may be useful in identifying invasive UC (Fig. 5.8), when the presence of minimal LP invasion is uncertain in difficult cases.

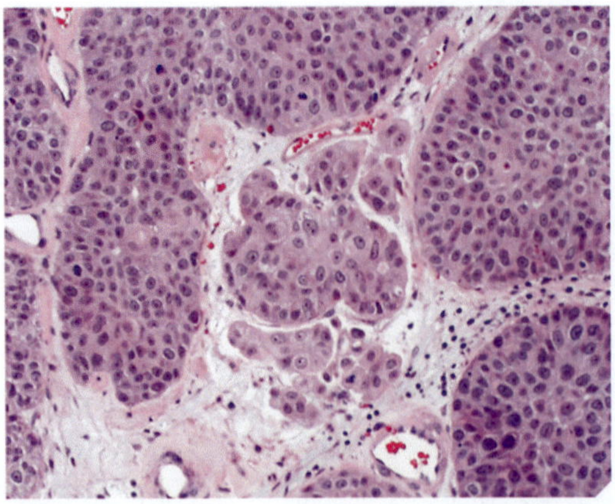

Fig. 5.7 High-grade papillary urothelial carcinoma shows small, irregular nests with retraction artifact. It invades the base of papillary tumor

Interobserver variability in recognizing the minimal LP invasion may lead to the lack of prognostic difference between pTa and pT1 tumors [24]. It is suggested that the report of stromal invasion by a pathologist who is not experienced in TURBT specimens may not be sufficient to justify radical cystectomy treatment [25–27]. The slides should be reviewed by a genitourinary or experienced pathologist to minimize errors before a patient undergoes any forms of radical treatment. Although urologists often combine UCIS, pTa, and pT1 tumors together as the superficial bladder tumors, pathologists should avoid the term "superficial tumor" in their report. Recent studies have demonstrated clear prognostic difference between UCIS, pTa, and pT1 bladder cancers, when TURBT specimens are evaluated by experienced or dedicated genitourinary pathologists [25, 26].

Bladder cancer staging requires histologic examination of radical or partial cystectomy specimens, but TURBT is critical in evaluating the extent of disease. To accurately evaluate the extent of cancer invasion, TURBT should be attempted to obtain adequate tissue sampling, which needs to resect all the visible tumors as well as to sample the underlying MP to determine

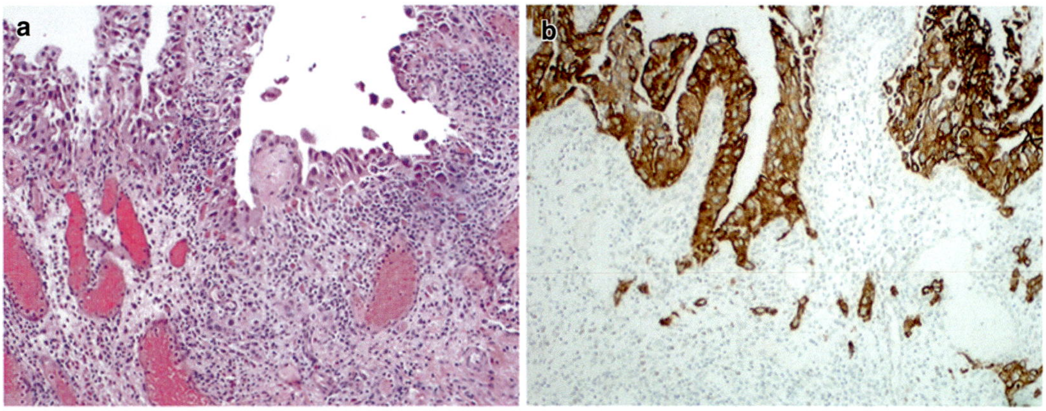

Fig. 5.8 Immunohistochemistry aids the recognition of minimal stromal invasion. (**a**) Scanty tumor cells invade the superficial lamina propria, which is difficult to differentiate from the intense inflammatory reaction. (**b**) Immunostain for cytokeratins highlights invasive carcinoma cells in the stroma

whether the tumor involves the MP. The absence of MP in a TURBT specimen indicates inadequate sampling, which is associated with a high risk of cancer understaging in patients with pT1 bladder cancer [28, 29]. Our previous study demonstrated that 41% of patients without MP in TURBT specimens showed cancer upstaging in the immediately subsequent specimens, whereas the upstaging rate was only 22% in patients with MP in TURBT specimens [28]. Therefore, patients, particularly those with pT1 bladder cancer, should undergo immediate restaging TURBT, when the MP tissue is absent in the initial TURBT specimens. The repeat TURBT can improve cancer staging accuracy and facilitate the selection of optimal treatment. Furthermore, several studies have demonstrated that repeat TURBT also carries therapeutic value, improving the recurrence-free survival rate, progression-free survival rate, and response to BCG therapy [30–33].

A substantial number of patients (30–50%) with pT1 bladder cancer will progress to muscle-invasive disease or develop metastasis. It is important to identify these patients with a high potential for disease progression so that they could benefit from frequent follow-up and aggressive therapy. Several methods have been proposed to substage pT1 bladder cancer. The most common method is to assess the depth of invasion using the muscularis mucosae (MM) as an anatomic landmark: T1a, tumor invades above the MM; T1b, tumor invades into MM or beyond [34–37]. This method is relatively quick and can be performed on small tumors, but it is highly dependent on orientation to the surface urothelium. Furthermore, MM is not always visible in TUBRT specimens because of its discontinuous distribution or displacement by tumor. Sometimes, large vessel plexus in the LP may be used as a substitute for the MM [38]. Others have used % of specimen with invasive tumor, diameter of invasive tumor, number of invasive tumor foci, and depth of invasion in millimeters from the basement membrane, but these methods are time-consuming [39–43]. Some pathologists use focal or extensive disease to substage pT1 disease, and focal invasion (or microinvasion) may be defined by invasive tumor <1 high power field, greatest tumor diameter < 1 mm, the depth of invasion from the basement <2 mm, or pT1a tumor [7]. A number of studies have demonstrated that pT1 substaging using these methods can identify a subset of pT1 bladder cancer with a more adverse prognosis [44–47]. The current World Health Organization (WHO) classification and the eighth edition of the American Joint Committee on Cancer (AJCC) staging manual both recommend that an attempt to substage pT1 disease may be made by the pathologist, although a specific method is not explicitly endorsed [7, 48].

Muscularis Propria Invasion

Invasion of the MP or detrusor muscle in the bladder wall by UC is a crucial factor in the management of bladder cancer [1]. Bladder cancer invading the MP or beyond represents a deeply invasive, advanced diseases [2, 7] (see Chap. 19). Bladder cancer at pT2 invades into but not through the MP (Fig. 5.9), which can be further divided into pT2a (invading the inner half of MP) and pT2b (invading the outer half). Bladder cancer at pT3 is characterized by cancer invasion through the MP into the perivesical soft tissue (Fig. 5.2), which can be further divided into pT3a (microscopic invasion) and pT3b (macroscopic or grossly appreciable invasion). It may be difficult to differentiate between pT2b and pT3a, as the border between the MP and perivesical soft tissue is not well demarcated. To help the distinction, an artificial line may be drawn to delineate the boundary between the MP and perivesical tissue in the bladder wall [49]. However, the presence of tumor in adipose tissue does not necessarily equate to pT3 invading the perivesical fat, as adipose tissue can be found in any layer of the bladder wall including the LP as well as MP. In general, superficial and deeply invasive disease can be differentiated in most TURBT specimens, but further distinction between T2a, T2b, T3, and T4 can be performed only in cystectomy specimens but not TURBT specimens, as the latter lack the appropriate orientation to allow further substaging [2, 7].

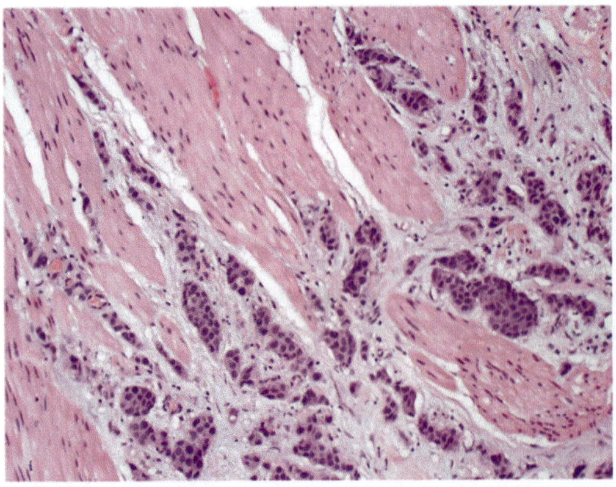

Fig. 5.9 Urothelial carcinoma invades the muscularis propria, which is characterized by thick, compact bundles of smooth muscle fibers

Bladder cancers that invade the MP or beyond are a highly aggressive disease, which generally requires multimodality treatment, including surgery, chemotherapy, radiation therapy, and novel targeted therapy [1] (Chaps. 16 and 17). In general, radical cystectomy or cystoprostatectomy coupled with en bloc pelvic lymphadenectomy is the standard surgical approach to muscle-invasive bladder cancers. Approximately 3–7% of patients treated with radical surgery will have lymph node metastases, and the clinical outcome varies considerably. To augment the impact of surgical treatment, patients with metastatic disease and other adverse risk factors, such as variant histology and lymphovascular invasion, may undergo radiation or chemotherapy singly or in combination as neoadjuvant or adjuvant therapy.

Differentiating Muscularis Mucosae Invasion from Muscularis Propria Invasion

It has to be emphasized that not all bladder cancers that involve the smooth muscle tissue represent an advanced disease with MP invasion, as there are two different types of smooth muscle tissue in the bladder wall, i.e., MP and MM [38, 50] . The smooth muscle tissue in MP invasion is characterized by large, thick, compact bundles (Fig. 5.9), whereas that in the MM invasion is composed of small, thin, loose bundles located at the lamina propria (Fig. 5.10). However, it may be challenging to determine the type of smooth muscle tissue involved by bladder cancer in a small subset of TURBT specimens (Fig. 5.11) [28, 51]. This diagnostic challenge may be caused by the following inherent factors in TURBT: (1) In patients with multiple TURBT procedures, the MM may be displaced and become hyperplastic, mimicking the MP (Fig. 5.11a). (2) Bladder cancer may show extensive growth and disperse the muscle bundles of the MP, causing it to resemble

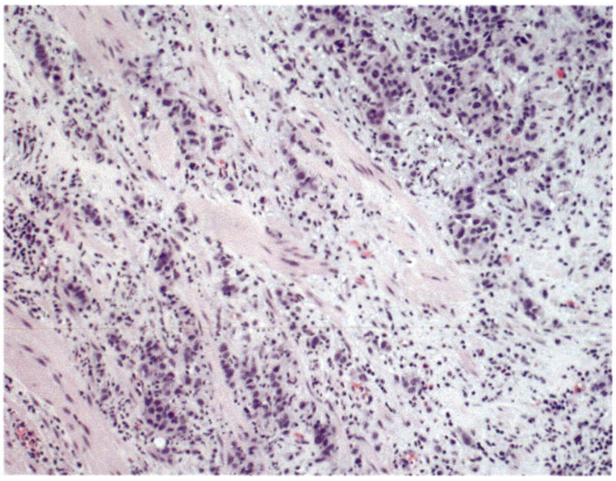

Fig. 5.10 Urothelial carcinoma invades the muscularis mucosae, which is characterized by thin, loose bundles of smooth muscle fibers

the MM (Fig. 5.11b). (3) Invasive UC often induces exuberant fibrosis, which resembles the smooth muscle bundles (Fig. 5.11c). (4) Finally, distortion of TURBT specimens by cautery and crushing artifacts also increases the difficulty in determining the type of smooth muscle involved by bladder cancer (Fig. 5.11d).

Immunohistochemistry has been used to differentiate MM from MP in TURBT speccimens [52]. Desmin stains smooth muscle tissue, which can help distinguish smooth muscle bundles from desmoplasia [53]. It may also aid to differentiate MM and MP in the appropriate setting, where the staining signal is too extensive for the MM and therefore represents the MP. Vimentin is usually

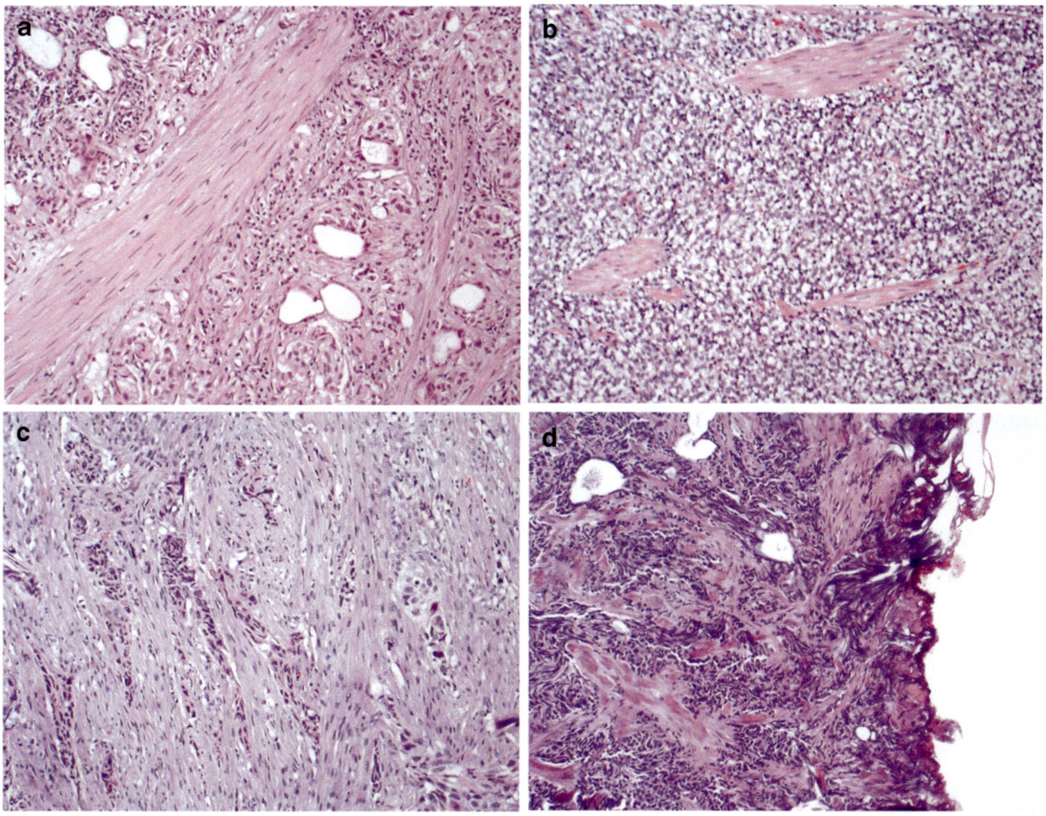

Fig. 5.11 Urothelial carcinoma involves smooth muscle of indeterminate type. (**a**) The muscularis mucosae become hyperplastic due to repeated resections, mimicking the muscularis propria. (**b**) Invasive urothelial carcinoma shows extensive growth and disperses smooth muscle bundles. (**c**) Invasive urothelial carcinoma induces exuberant fibrosis, resembling smooth muscle bundles. (**d**) Transurethral resection causes severe distortion and cautery artifacts in the smooth muscle bundles involved by urothelial carcinoma

expressed in MM but rarely in MP [53]. Smoothelin, a contractile cytoskeleton protein in smooth muscle cells, is another useful marker [54, 55]. Immunohistochemical staining of smoothelin usually shows diffuse strong staining in the MP but negative or focal weak staining in the MM (Fig. 5.12). However, subsequent studies demonstrated a significant overlap of smoothelin staining patterns between the MM and MP in TURBT specimens, which has limited the use of this marker in differentiating MM from MP in routine clinical practice, especially when uninvolved MM and MP are not present as internal reference [56].

Smooth muscle of indeterminate type (SMIT) may be applied, when pathologists are uncertain whether the smooth muscle tissue involved by bladder cancer represents the MM or MP [28, 51] (Fig. 5.11). Bladder cancer with SMIT invasion in TURBT specimens demonstrates a significantly higher rate of cancer upstaging in the subsequent specimens than that invading the MM [28]. Furthermore, patients with SMIT invasion show a significantly worse clinical outcomes than those with MM invasion, which highlights the necessity for restaging TUR, particularly when the MP is not present in TURBT specimens. The subsequent restaging specimens can improve the accuracy of cancer staging, which aid the stratification of these patients into different therapeutic and prognostic groups [28, 51].

Involvement of the Prostate

UC involves the prostate at a variable frequency, ranging from 12% to 48% [57–59] . Several recent series with a large number of cases evaluated by whole-mount section of the prostate demonstrate a more consistent rate of 30–35% [58, 60]. Tumor multifocality and presence of UCIS are associated with a higher probability of prostatic involvement by UC [58, 61]. UC involves the prostate in several patterns: (1) UCIS arises from the prostatic urethra (pTis pu) and then spreads into prostatic ducts (pTis pd) and acini without stromal invasion (Fig. 5.13). (2) UC involves the prostatic urethra and invades through

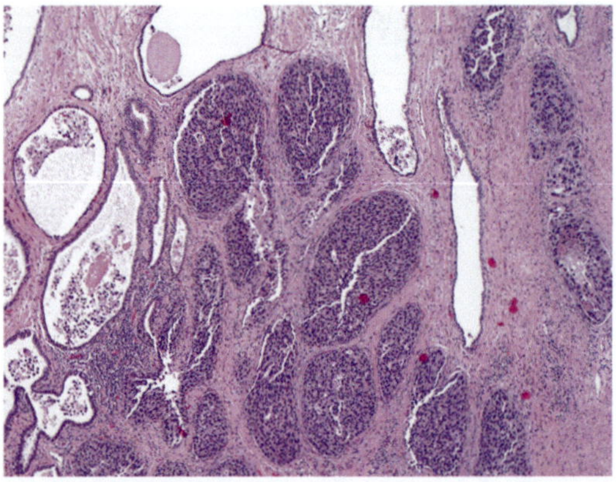

Fig. 5.13 Urothelial carcinoma in situ spreads into the prostatic ducts and large acini

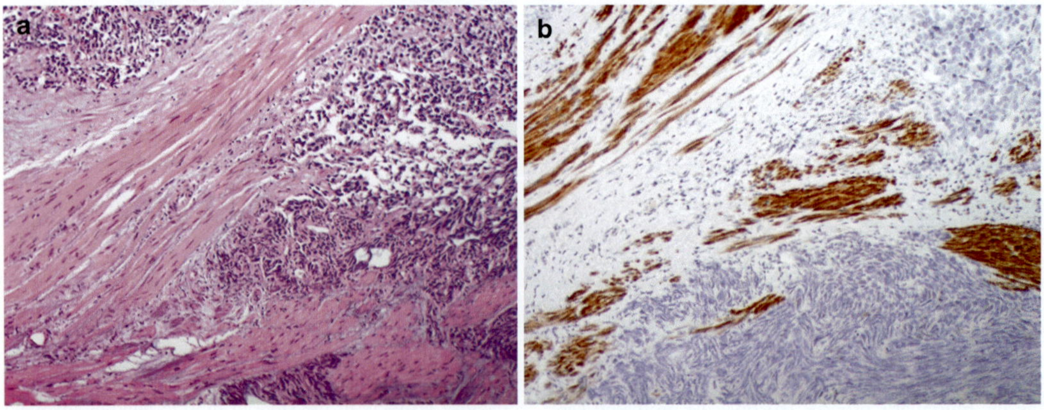

Fig. 5.12 Immunohistochemistry aids the recognition of muscularis propria invasion. (**a**) Urothelial carcinoma involves thick bundles of smooth muscle fibers. (**b**) Immunostain shows strong and diffuse staining for smoothelin, supporting the muscularis propria invasion

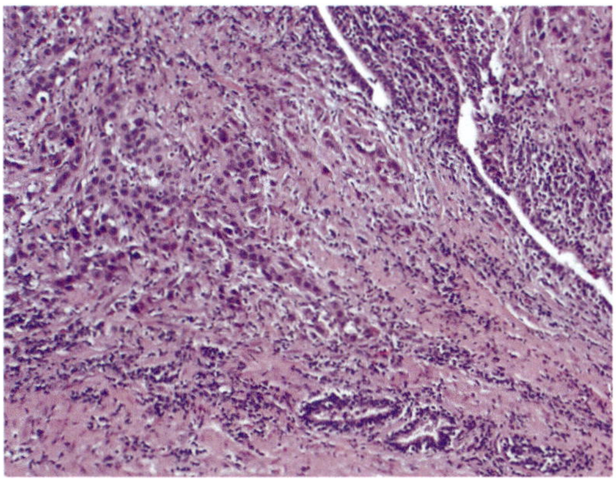

Fig. 5.14 Urothelial carcinoma invades the prostatic stroma

the subepithelial tissue into prostatic stroma. (3) Bladder UC invades through the entire bladder wall into prostatic stroma (Fig. 5.14). It has been well recognized that prostatic involvement by UCIS has a significantly more favorable outcome than that of prostatic stromal invasion [58, 61]. Furthermore, several studies have demonstrated that invasion of the prostatic stroma by bladder UC is associated with a substantially worse prognosis compared to stromal invasion by prostatic urethral UC [58, 61]. Therefore, the prostatic stroma involvement by UC should be staged according to the cancer origin [46, 58]. If the prostatic stroma is involved contiguously by invasive bladder UC, it should be staged as pT4a bladder cancer. However, if the prostatic stroma is invaded by UC arising from the prostatic urethra and not in direct contact with bladder UC, it should be staged as pT2 prostatic urethral cancer. This proposal has been accepted by the current WHO classification system and the eighth edition AJCC staging manual [7, 48].

Lymphovascular Invasion

Lymphovascular invasion (LVI), the presence of tumor thrombi in lymphatic and blood vessels, can be seen in a small subset of invasive bladder UC. In patients with pT1 disease, the presence of LVI in TURBT or biopsy specimens is associated with a high risk of cancer recurrence and progression [62, 63]. A meta-analysis including data from more than 3900 patients demonstrated a significant association between the presence of LVI in TURBT specimens and cancer upstaging in the radical cystectomy specimens, suggesting that early radical cystectomy may be beneficial for some patients with pT1 disease and LVI [64]. In patients with pT2 or above, the presence of LVI in TURBT or biopsy specimens is associated with non-organ-confined disease (pT3–pT4 tumor or lymph node metastases) in the subsequent radical cystectomy specimens [65]. Furthermore, patients with LVI in pT2 disease may benefit from neoadjuvant chemotherapy before radical surgery [66]. Several studies have demonstrated that LVI can independently predict recurrence-free survival, cancer-specific survival, and overall survival in patients with muscle-invasive UC and lymph node-negative disease, but its relevance in patients with lymph node-positive disease remains unclear [67–69].

Although LVI is an important prognostic factor in bladder cancer, it may be challenging to assess LVI in TURBT specimens. Invasive UC, particularly micropapillary variant, frequently exhibits retraction artifacts, which mimic LVI. Carryover artifact can also lead to the false presence of tumor cells in lymphovascular spaces. Several studies have reported that the reproducibility of reporting LVI varies significantly among pathologists [68, 70, 71]. To improve the diagnostic accuracy of LVI, a set of morphologic criteria should be applied strictly: (1) Tumor thrombus conforms to the shape of a vessel (Fig. 5.15). (2) Tumor thrombus is attached to the vascular wall. (3) The lymphovascular space should have an unequivocal endothelial lining. In uncertain cases, immunohistochemical stain for endothelial markers, such as ERG, CD31, and CD34, may be used to confirm the presence of endothelial lining (Fig. 5.16). (4) Blood constituents (red blood cells, white blood cells, or blood thrombus) are present. (5) LVI is preferred at a peritumoral location (at least one high power distance from the tumor advancing edge) over an intratumoral location. (6) It is located in a vascular route adjacent to the artery and vein. The diagnosis of LVI should be based on a constellation of these morphologic features but not solely on any single feature, but it is not recommended to use immunostains routinely for the detection of LVI.

Intrinsic Molecular Subtypes of Invasive Bladder Cancer

A number of contemporary studies have analyzed the genomic profile of invasive bladder cancer on multiple molecular platforms, including somatic DNA mutations, copy number variations, DNA methylation, mRNA expressions, microRNA expressions, microbe analysis, and proteomic analysis [8–11, 72]. These comprehensive analyses demonstrated a remarkable molecular diversity in bladder cancer, which may underlie a wide spectrum of clinical behaviors as well as varied responses to conventional and targeted therapies. The MD Anderson Cancer Center group analyzed the whole-genome mRNA expressions of muscle-invasive bladder cancer (MIBC), which revealed two distinct intrinsic molecular subtypes, basal and luminal (Fig. 5.17) [8]. The molecular subtypes generally reflect the gene expression signature of normal basal (such as CK5/CK6, CK14, p63, and others) and luminal (such as uroplakins, CK18, CK20, GATA3, and others) urothelial cells. Furthermore, the molecular subtypes also demonstrate different clinicopathologic features. Basal UC is typically enriched with squamous features and often present at an advanced stage. Although it is intrinsically aggressive, basal UC is highly sensitive to cisplatin-based chemotherapy. Luminal UC is enriched with papillary morphology and demonstrates *FGFR3* mutations and activation of the peroxisome proliferator activator receptor γ (PPARγ) pathway. Luminal UC is not as aggressive as basal UC, but a subset of luminal UC may be resistant to chemotherapy and may represent a therapeutic challenge.

The Cancer Genome Atlas (TCGA) group recently performed a comprehensive analysis of

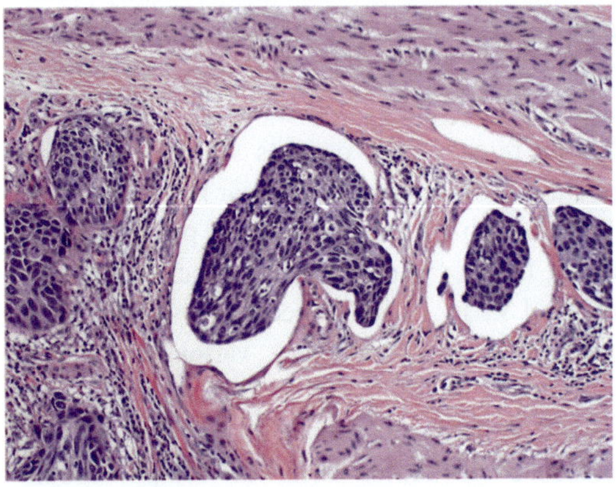

Fig. 5.15 Lymphovascular invasion shows tumor thrombus conforming the shape of vascular space and focally attaching to the vascular wall

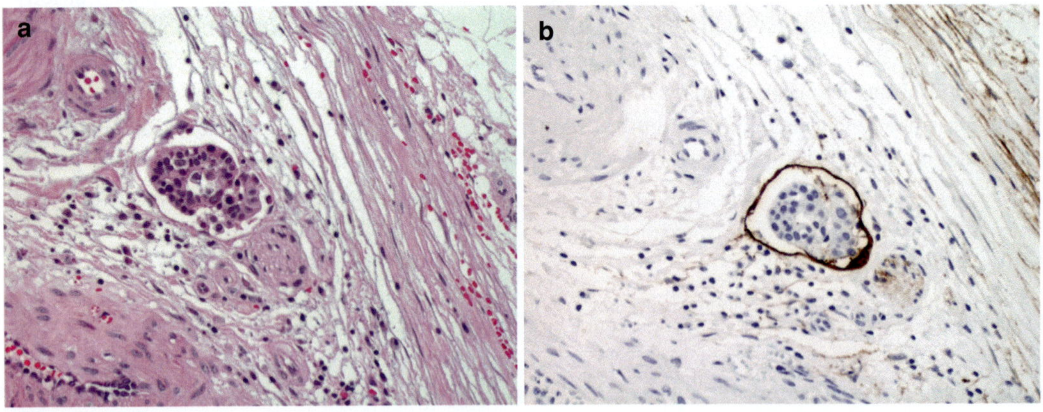

Fig. 5.16 Immunohistochemistry aids the diagnosis of lymphovascular invasion. (**a**) A small tumor thrombus in vascular space resembles retraction artifact. (**b**) Immunostain for CD31 highlights the presence of endothelial lining of the vascular space

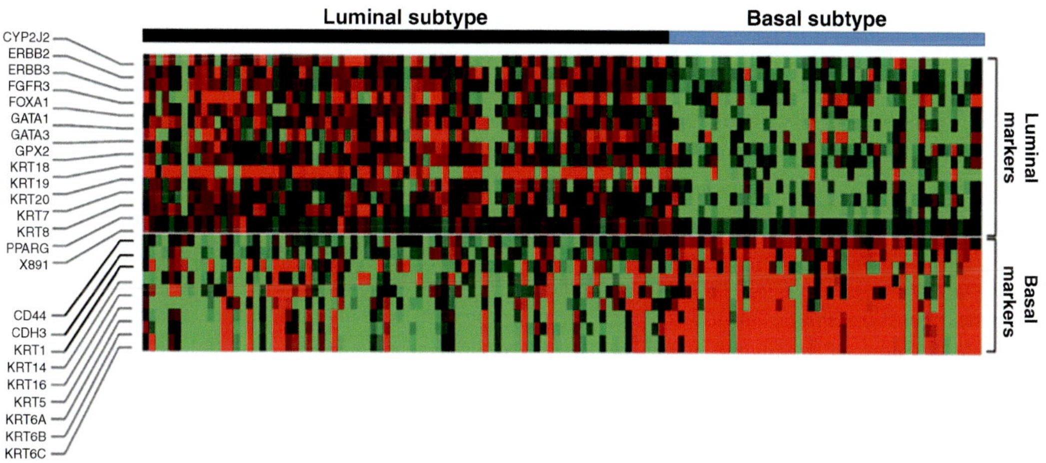

Fig. 5.17 Molecular classification of muscle-invasive bladder cancer by the MD Anderson Cancer Center group. Luminal and basal molecular subtypes show distinct patterns of gene expressions. (Modified and reproduced from Choi et al. Cancer Cell. 2014;25(2):152–165, with permission from Elsevier)

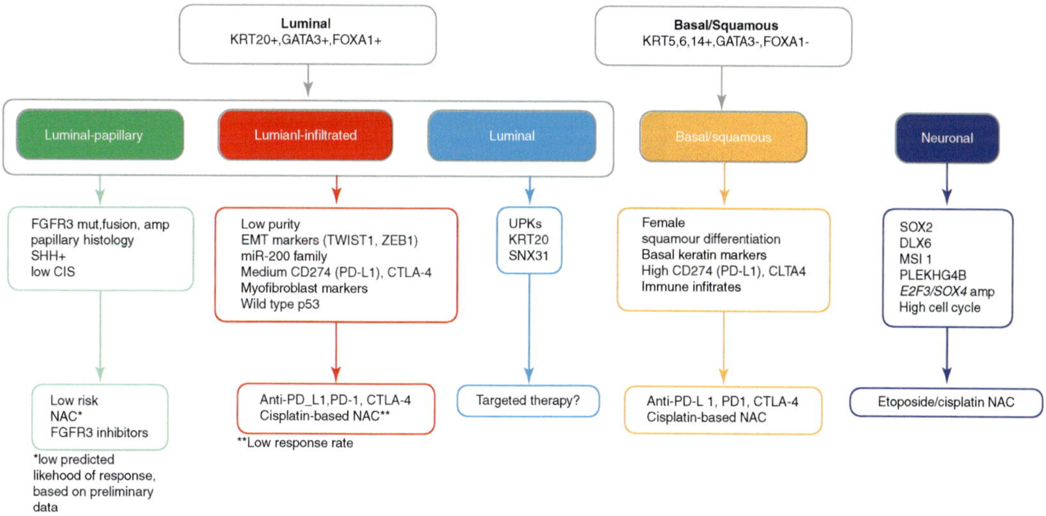

Fig. 5.18 Molecular classification of muscle-invasive bladder cancer by The Cancer Atlas Genome group. It provides a framework for prospective hypothesis testing in clinical trials. (Modified and reproduced from Robertson et al. Cell. 2017;171(3):540–556, with permission from Elsevier)

MIBC on multiple molecular platforms, which demonstrated five distinct molecular subtypes, including luminal-papillary, luminal-infiltrated, luminal, basal-squamous, and neuronal subtypes (Fig. 5.18) [9]. The luminal-papillary subtype is associated with a low risk for cancer progression, but it responds poorly to cisplatin-based chemotherapy. As it shows a high prevalence of FGFR3 gene mutations and overexpression, the luminal-papillary may respond favorably to FGFR3 tyrosine kinase inhibitors. The luminal-infiltrated subtype shows elevated expressions of immune checkpoint markers, including PD-L1, PD-1, and CTLA4, indicating that immune checkpoint therapy may be effective for this subtype. The luminal subtype expresses high levels of uroplakin genes and other genes associated with the terminally differentiated umbrella cells. The basal-squamous subtype shows high expressions of basal markers (CK5, CK6A, CK14) as well as squamous differentiation markers (TGM1, DSC3, PI3). This subtype is likely to respond to cisplatin-based chemotherapy as well as immune checkpoint therapy, because it also shows high expressions of PD-L1 and CTLA4 immune markers. The neuronal subtype is characterized by robust expressions of neuroendocrine and neuronal genes, but it does not exhibit the typical morphologic features of small cell neuroendocrine carcinoma. It shows a high cell-cycle signature with frequent mutations in TP53 and RB1 genes. Although the neuronal type is associated with the worst survival among all the molecular subtypes, it may respond to etoposide-cisplatin chemotherapy, like small cell lung carcinoma. Therefore, the comprehensive molecular analyses of MIBC provide an insightful framework to understand this complex disease, which can facilitate the development of novel therapeutic approaches.

Several other groups also analyzed the genomic expressions of MIUC and proposed different molecular classification systems [8–11, 73–75]. Although the names and numbers of subtypes are somewhat different in these classification systems, there are strong evidences to support that the top-level separation occurs at the basal and luminal differentiation checkpoint (Fig. 5.19). Recently, an international meta-analyses of 1750 MIBC transcriptomic profiles from 18 published datasets proposed a consensus

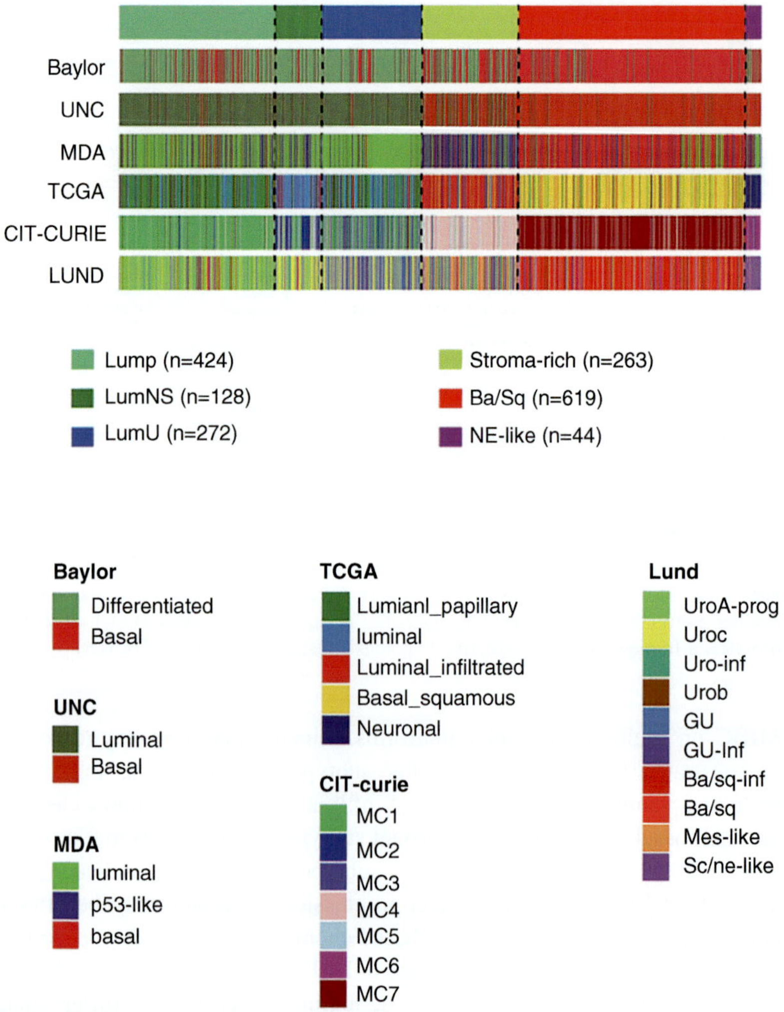

Fig. 5.19 International consensus molecular classification of muscle-invasive bladder cancers. It proposes six distinct molecular subtypes based on a meta-analysis of six independent classification systems. Ba/Sq, basal/squamous; LumNS, luminal nonspecified; LumP, luminal-papillary; LumU, luminal unstable; MDA, MD Anderson Cancer Center; NE-like, neuroendocrine-like; TCGA, The Cancer Genome Atlas; UNC, University of North Carolina. (Modified and reproduced from Kamoun et al. Eur Urol. 2020;77(4):420–433, with permission from Elsevier)

set of six distinct molecular subtypes: luminal-papillary (24%), luminal nonspecified (8%), luminal unstable (15%), stroma-rich (15%), basal/squamous (35%), and neuroendocrine-like (3%) [76]. The luminal UC appears to evolve through the papillary track, while the basal UC develops via the nonpapillary track. Although papillary UC are almost exclusively luminal subtype, invasive bladder UC can be luminal or basal subtype. The invasive UC that show a luminal expression signature likely evolve from the preexisting papillary tumor and represent a progression of superficial papillary tumors. Further studies revealed that various UC histologic variants are associated with characteristic molecular subtypes. For examples, micropapillary variant is almost exclusively composed of the luminal subtype [77], while sarcomatoid variant often shows the basal-type molecular signature [78]. It is evident from these investigations that bladder cancer is a molecularly heterogeneous disease [72].

Although the molecular classification of bladder cancer based on the genomic mRNA expression profiling provides valuable insights into its biological behavior, it cannot be easily applied to the routine clinical practice, because the analytical method is technologically complex and costly. Recent studies have found that immunohistochemistry may be used to aid the molecular classification of bladder UC [79, 80]. Parallel analyses of genomic mRNA expressions and immunohistochemical protein expressions found that a small set of luminal (GATA3, CK20, and uroplakin II) and basal (CK5/CK6, CK14, and p63) markers can be successfully used to classify bladder cancer into different molecular subtypes [79]. Furthermore, the immunohistochemical expression levels of just two signature markers, GATA3 and CK5/CK6, are sufficient to classify bladder cancers into luminal and basal categories with over 80% accuracy (Fig. 5.20). The molecular classification by immunohistochemistry can be performed not only on fresh-frozen tumor specimens but also on formalin-fixed and paraffin-embedded archival samples. However, the performance of this classifier remains to be validated on larger independent cohorts.

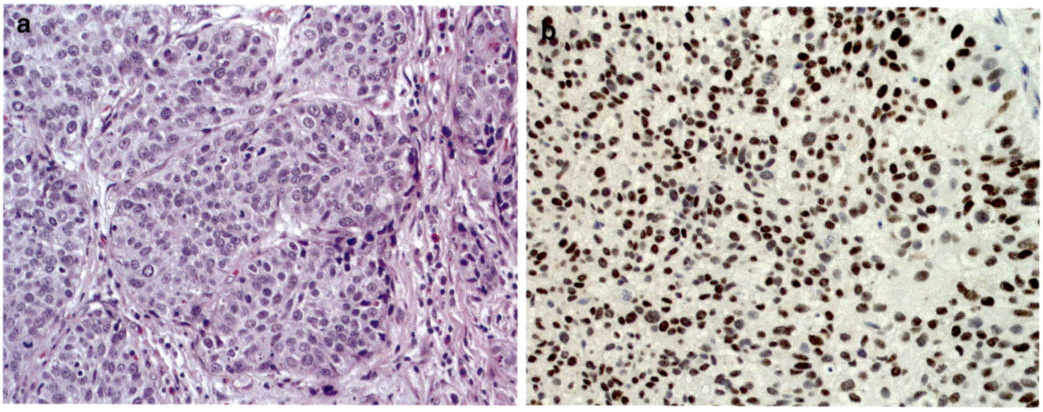

Fig. 5.20 Immunohistochemistry aids the molecular classification of invasive urothelial carcinoma. Luminal subtype tumor (**a**) expresses GATA3 (**b**) but not CK5/CK6 (**c**). Basal subtype tumor (**d**) expresses CK5/CK6 (**e**) but not GATA3 (**f**)

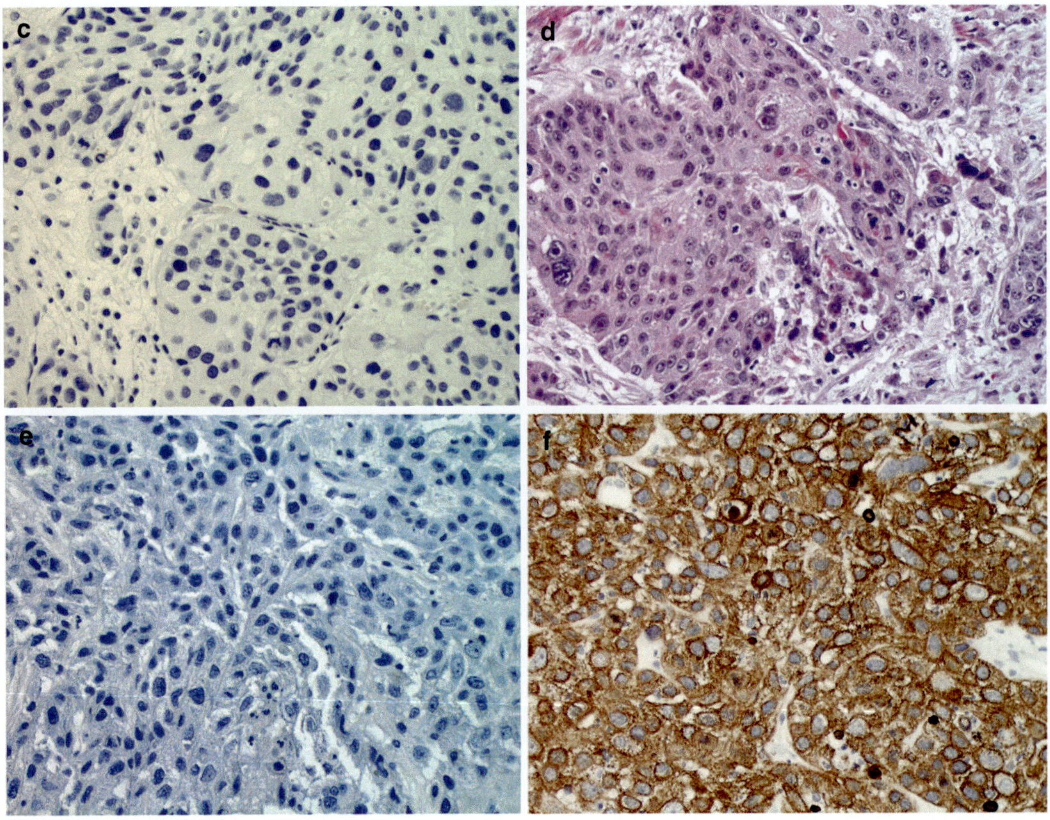

Fig. 5.20 (continued)

References

1. Kamat AM, Hahn NM, Efstathiou JA, Lerner SP, Malmstrom PU, Choi W, et al. Bladder cancer. Lancet. 2016;388(10061):2796–810.
2. Grignon DJ, Al-Ahmadie H, Algaba F, Amin MB, Comperat E, Dyrskjot L, Epstein JI, Hansel DE, Knochel R, Lloreta J, Lopez-Beltran A, McKenney JK, Netto GJ, Paner G, Reuter VE, Shen SS, Van der Kwast T. Tumors of the urinary tract. In: Moch H, Humphrey PA, Ulbright TM, Retuer VE, editors. WHO Classification of Tumours of the Urinary System and Male organs. 4th ed (pp.77–135). Lyon: IARC Press; 2016.
3. Antoni S, Ferlay J, Soerjomataram I, Znaor A, Jemal A, Bray F. Bladder cancer incidence and mortality: a global overview and recent trends. Eur Urol. 2017;71(1):96–108.
4. Chang SS, Boorjian SA, Chou R, Clark PE, Daneshmand S, Konety BR, et al. Diagnosis and treatment of non-muscle invasive bladder cancer: AUA/SUO guideline. J Urol. 2016;196(4):1021–9.
5. Leow JJ, Bedke J, Chamie K, Collins JW, Daneshmand S, Grivas P, et al. SIU-ICUD consultation on bladder cancer: treatment of muscle-invasive bladder cancer. World J Urol. 2019;37(1):61–83.
6. Lobo N, Mount C, Omar K, Nair R, Thurairaja R, Khan MS. Landmarks in the treatment of muscle-invasive bladder cancer. Nat Rev Urol. 2017;14(9):565–74.
7. Bochner BH, Hansel D, Efstathiou JA, Konety B, Lee CT, McKiernan JM, Plimack ER, Reuter VE, Srdhar S, Vikram R, Stadler WM. Urinary bladder. In: Amin MB, editor. AJCC Cancer Staging Manual, 8th ed (pp.757–765). New York: Springer; 2017.
8. Choi W, Porten S, Kim S, Willis D, Plimack ER, Hoffman-Censits J, et al. Identification of distinct basal and luminal subtypes of muscle-invasive bladder cancer with different sensitivities to frontline chemotherapy. Cancer Cell. 2014;25(2):152–65.
9. Robertson AG, Kim J, Al-Ahmadie H, Bellmunt J, Guo G, Cherniack AD, et al. Comprehensive molecular characterization of muscle-invasive bladder cancer. Cell. 2017;171(3):540–56.e25.
10. Damrauer JS, Hoadley KA, Chism DD, Fan C, Tiganelli CJ, Wobker SE, et al. Intrinsic subtypes of high-grade bladder cancer reflect the hallmarks of breast cancer biology. Proc Natl Acad Sci U S A. 2014;111(8):3110–5.
11. Cancer Genome Atlas Research Network. Comprehensive molecular characterization of uro-

thelial bladder carcinoma. Nature. 2014;507(7492):315–22.
12. Amin MB. Histological variants of urothelial carcinoma: diagnostic, therapeutic and prognostic implications. Mod Pathol. 2009;22(Suppl 2):S96–S118.
13. Lopez-Beltran A, Henriques V, Montironi R, Cimadamore A, Raspollini MR, Cheng L. Variants and new entities of bladder cancer. Histopathology. 2019;74(1):77–96.
14. Denzinger S, Burger M, Fritsche HM, Bertz S, Hofstädter F, Wieland WF, et al. Prognostic value of histopathological tumour growth patterns at the invasion front of T1G3 urothelial carcinoma of the bladder. Scand J Urol Nephrol. 2009;43(4):282–7.
15. Jimenez RE, Gheiler E, Oskanian P, Tiguert R, Sakr W, Wood DP Jr, et al. Grading the invasive component of urothelial carcinoma of the bladder and its relationship with progression-free survival. Am J Surg Pathol. 2000;24(7):980–7.
16. Jimenez-Marin A, Collado-Romero M, Ramirez-Boo M, Arce C, Garrido JJ. Biological pathway analysis by ArrayUnlock and Ingenuity Pathway Analysis. BMC Proc. 2009;3(Suppl 4):S6.
17. Nishiyama N, Kitamura H, Maeda T, Takahashi S, Masumori N, Hasegawa T, et al. Clinicopathological analysis of patients with non-muscle-invasive bladder cancer: prognostic value and clinical reliability of the 2004 WHO classification system. Jpn J Clin Oncol. 2013;43(11):1124–31.
18. Pellucchi F, Freschi M, Moschini M, Rocchini L, Maccagnano C, Nazareno S, et al. Oncological predictive value of the 2004 World Health Organisation grading classification in primary T1 non-muscle-invasive bladder cancer. A step forward or back? BJU Int. 2015;115(2):267–73.
19. Mai KT, Bateman J, Djordjevic B, Flood TA, Belanger EC. Clear cell urothelial carcinoma. Int J Surg Pathol. 2017;25(1):18–25.
20. Donhuijsen K, Schmidt U, Richter HJ, Leder LD. Mucoid cytoplasmic inclusions in urothelial carcinomas. Hum Pathol. 1992;23(8):860–4.
21. Tavora F, Epstein JI. Urothelial carcinoma with abundant myxoid stroma. Hum Pathol. 2009;40(10):1391–8.
22. Tosoni I, Wagner U, Sauter G, Egloff M, Knönagel H, Alund G, et al. Clinical significance of interobserver differences in the staging and grading of superficial bladder cancer. BJU Int. 2000;85(1):48–53.
23. Bol MG, Baak JP, Buhr-Wildhagen S, Kruse AJ, Kjellevold KH, Janssen EA, et al. Reproducibility and prognostic variability of grade and lamina propria invasion in stages Ta, T1 urothelial carcinoma of the bladder. J Urol. 2003;169(4):1291–4.
24. Flamm J, Havelec L. Factors affecting survival in primary superficial bladder cancer. Eur Urol. 1990;17(2):113–8.
25. Amin MB, McKenney JK, Paner GP, Hansel DE, Grignon DJ, Montironi R, et al. ICUD-EAU international consultation on bladder cancer 2012: pathology. Eur Urol. 2013;63(1):16–35.
26. van Rhijn BW, van der Kwast TH, Kakiashvili DM, Fleshner NE, van der Aa MN, Alkhateeb S, et al. Pathological stage review is indicated in primary pT1 bladder cancer. BJU Int. 2010;106(2):206–11.
27. Compérat E, Egevad L, Lopez-Beltran A, Camparo P, Algaba F, Amin M, et al. An interobserver reproducibility study on invasiveness of bladder cancer using virtual microscopy and heatmaps. Histopathology. 2013;63(6):756–66.
28. Hwang MJ, Kamat AM, Dinney CP, Czerniak B, Guo CC. Bladder cancer involving smooth muscle of indeterminate type or muscularis mucosae in transurethral biopsy specimens. Am J Clin Pathol. 2020;154(2):208–14.
29. Herr HW, Donat SM. Quality control in transurethral resection of bladder tumours. BJU Int. 2008;102(9 Pt B):1242–6.
30. Shariat SF, Palapattu GS, Karakiewicz PI, Rogers CG, Vazina A, Bastian PJ, et al. Concomitant carcinoma in situ is a feature of aggressive disease in patients with organ-confined TCC at radical cystectomy. Eur Urol. 2007;51(1):152–60.
31. Divrik RT, Sahin AF, Yildirim U, Altok M, Zorlu F. Impact of routine second transurethral resection on the long-term outcome of patients with newly diagnosed pT1 urothelial carcinoma with respect to recurrence, progression rate, and disease-specific survival: a prospective randomised clinical trial. Eur Urol. 2010;58(2):185–90.
32. Sfakianos JP, Kim PH, Hakimi AA, Herr HW. The effect of restaging transurethral resection on recurrence and progression rates in patients with nonmuscle invasive bladder cancer treated with intravesical bacillus Calmette-Guérin. J Urol. 2014;191(2):341–5.
33. Herr HW. Restaging transurethral resection of high risk superficial bladder cancer improves the initial response to bacillus Calmette-Guerin therapy. J Urol. 2005;174(6):2134–7.
34. Angulo JC, Lopez JI, Grignon DJ, Sanchez-Chapado M. Muscularis mucosa differentiates two populations with different prognosis in stage T1 bladder cancer. Urology. 1995;45(1):47–53.
35. Younes M, Sussman J, True LD. The usefulness of the level of the muscularis mucosae in the staging of invasive transitional cell carcinoma of the urinary bladder. Cancer. 1990;66(3):543–8.
36. Jimenez RE, Keane TE, Hardy HT, Amin MB. pT1 urothelial carcinoma of the bladder: criteria for diagnosis, pitfalls, and clinical implications. Adv Anat Pathol. 2000;7(1):13–25.
37. Rouprêt M, Seisen T, Compérat E, Larré S, Mazerolles C, Gobet F, et al. Prognostic interest in discriminating muscularis mucosa invasion (T1a vs T1b) in nonmuscle invasive bladder carcinoma: French national multicenter study with central pathology review. J Urol. 2013;189(6):2069–76.
38. Paner GP, Ro JY, Wojcik EM, Venkataraman G, Datta MW, Amin MB. Further characterization of the muscle layers and lamina propria of the urinary bladder by systematic histologic mapping: implications for

pathologic staging of invasive urothelial carcinoma. Am J Surg Pathol. 2007;31(9):1420–9.
39. Cheng L, Neumann RM, Weaver AL, Spotts BE, Bostwick DG. Predicting cancer progression in patients with stage T1 bladder carcinoma. J Clin Oncol Off J Am Soc Clin Oncol. 1999;17(10):3182–7.
40. Cheng L, Weaver AL, Neumann RM, Scherer BG, Bostwick DG. Substaging of T1 bladder carcinoma based on the depth of invasion as measured by micrometer: a new proposal. Cancer. 1999;86(6):1035–43.
41. Brimo F, Wu C, Zeizafoun N, Tanguay S, Aprikian A, Mansure JJ, et al. Prognostic factors in T1 bladder urothelial carcinoma: the value of recording millimetric depth of invasion, diameter of invasive carcinoma, and muscularis mucosa invasion. Hum Pathol. 2013;44(1):95–102.
42. Hu Z, Mudaliar K, Quek ML, Paner GP, Barkan GA. Measuring the dimension of invasive component in pT1 urothelial carcinoma in transurethral resection specimens can predict time to recurrence. Ann Diagn Pathol. 2014;18(2):49–52.
43. van Rhijn BW, van der Kwast TH, Alkhateeb SS, Fleshner NE, van Leenders GJ, Bostrom PJ, et al. A new and highly prognostic system to discern T1 bladder cancer substage. Eur Urol. 2012;61(2):378–84.
44. Babjuk M, Burger M, Compérat EM, Gontero P, Mostafid AH, Palou J, et al. European Association of Urology guidelines on non-muscle-invasive bladder cancer (TaT1 and carcinoma in situ) – 2019 update. Eur Urol. 2019;76(5):639–57.
45. Fransen van de Putte EE, Behrendt MA, Pigot GL, van der Kwast TH, van Rhijn BW. Prognostic significance of substage and WHO classification systems in T1 urothelial carcinoma of the bladder. Curr Opin Urol. 2015;25(5):427–35.
46. Paner GP, Montironi R, Amin MB. Challenges in pathologic staging of bladder cancer: proposals for fresh approaches of assessing pathologic stage in light of recent studies and observations pertaining to bladder histoanatomic variances. Adv Anat Pathol. 2017;24(3):113–27.
47. Paner GP, Stadler WM, Hansel DE, Montironi R, Lin DW, Amin MB. Updates in the Eighth Edition of the Tumor-Node-Metastasis Staging Classification for Urologic Cancers. Eur Urol. 2018;73:560–69.
48. Grignon DJAAH, Algaba F, Amin MB, Comperat E, Dyrskjot L, Epstein JI, Hansel DE, Knochel R, Lloreta J, Lopez-Beltran A, McKenney JK, Netto GJ, Paner G, Reuter VE, Shen SS, Van der Kwast T. In: Moch H, Humphrey PA, Ulbright TM, Retuer VE, editors. Tumors of the urinary tract. 4th ed. Lyon: IARC Press; 2016.
49. Ananthanarayanan V, Pan Y, Tretiakova M, Amin MB, Cheng L, Epstein JI, et al. Influence of histologic criteria and confounding factors in staging equivocal cases for microscopic perivesical tissue invasion (pT3a): an interobserver study among genitourinary pathologists. Am J Surg Pathol. 2014;38(2):167–75.
50. Ro JY, Ayala AG, El-Naggar A. Muscularis mucosa of urinary bladder. Importance for staging and treatment. Am J Surg Pathol. 1987;11(9):668–73.
51. Miyamoto H, Epstein JI. Transurethral resection specimens of the bladder: outcome of invasive urothelial cancer involving muscle bundles indeterminate between muscularis mucosae and muscularis propria. Urology. 2010;76(3):600–2.
52. Amin MB, Trpkov K, Lopez-Beltran A, Grignon D. Best practices recommendations in the application of immunohistochemistry in the bladder lesions: report from the International Society of Urologic Pathology consensus conference. Am J Surg Pathol. 2014;38(8):e20–34.
53. Council L, Hameed O. Differential expression of immunohistochemical markers in bladder smooth muscle and myofibroblasts, and the potential utility of desmin, smoothelin, and vimentin in staging of bladder carcinoma. Mod Pathol. 2009;22(5):639–50.
54. Paner GP, Shen SS, Lapetino S, Venkataraman G, Barkan GA, Quek ML, et al. Diagnostic utility of antibody to smoothelin in the distinction of muscularis propria from muscularis mucosae of the urinary bladder: a potential ancillary tool in the pathologic staging of invasive urothelial carcinoma. Am J Surg Pathol. 2009;33(1):91–8.
55. Paner GP, Brown JG, Lapetino S, Nese N, Gupta R, Shen SS, et al. Diagnostic use of antibody to smoothelin in the recognition of muscularis propria in transurethral resection of urinary bladder tumor (TURBT) specimens. Am J Surg Pathol. 2010;34(6):792–9.
56. Miyamoto H, Sharma RB, Illei PB, Epstein JI. Pitfalls in the use of smoothelin to identify muscularis propria invasion by urothelial carcinoma. Am J Surg Pathol. 2010;34(3):418–22.
57. Esrig D, Freeman JA, Elmajian DA, Stein JP, Chen SC, Groshen S, et al. Transitional cell carcinoma involving the prostate with a proposed staging classification for stromal invasion. J Urol. 1996;156(3):1071–6.
58. Shen SS, Lerner SP, Muezzinoglu B, Truong LD, Amiel G, Wheeler TM. Prostatic involvement by transitional cell carcinoma in patients with bladder cancer and its prognostic significance. Hum Pathol. 2006;37(6):726–34.
59. Schellhammer PF, Bean MA, Whitmore WF Jr. Prostatic involvement by transitional cell carcinoma: pathogenesis, patterns and prognosis. J Urol. 1977;118(3):399–403.
60. Revelo MP, Cookson MS, Chang SS, Shook MF, Smith JA Jr, Shappell SB. Incidence and location of prostate and urothelial carcinoma in prostates from cystoprostatectomies: implications for possible apical sparing surgery. J Urol. 2004;171(2 Pt 1):646–51.
61. Moschini M, Soria F, Susani M, Korn S, Briganti A, Roupret M, et al. Impact of the level of urothelial carcinoma involvement of the prostate on survival after radical cystectomy. Bladder Cancer (Amsterdam, Netherlands). 2017;3(3):161–9.
62. Shariat SF, Khoddami SM, Saboorian H, Koeneman KS, Sagalowsky AI, Cadeddu JA, et al.

Lymphovascular invasion is a pathological feature of biologically aggressive disease in patients treated with radical prostatectomy. J Urol. 2004;171(3):1122–7.
63. Mathieu R, Lucca I, Rouprêt M, Briganti A, Shariat SF. The prognostic role of lymphovascular invasion in urothelial carcinoma of the bladder. Nat Rev Urol. 2016;13(8):471–9.
64. Kim HS, Kim M, Jeong CW, Kwak C, Kim HH, Ku JH. Presence of lymphovascular invasion in urothelial bladder cancer specimens after transurethral resections correlates with risk of upstaging and survival: a systematic review and meta-analysis. Urol Oncol. 2014;32(8):1191–9.
65. Green DA, Rink M, Hansen J, Cha EK, Robinson B, Tian Z, et al. Accurate preoperative prediction of non-organ-confined bladder urothelial carcinoma at cystectomy. BJU Int. 2013;111(3):404–11.
66. Matulay JT, Kamat AM. Advances in risk stratification of bladder cancer to guide personalized medicine. F1000Res. 2018;7:F1000 Faculty Rev–1137.
67. Mari A, Kimura S, Foerster B, Abufaraj M, D'Andrea D, Gust KM, et al. A systematic review and meta-analysis of lymphovascular invasion in patients treated with radical cystectomy for bladder cancer. Urol Oncol. 2018;36(6):293–305.
68. Berman DM, Kawashima A, Peng Y, Mackillop WJ, Siemens DR, Booth CM. Reporting trends and prognostic significance of lymphovascular invasion in muscle-invasive urothelial carcinoma: a population-based study. Int J Urol. 2015;22(2):163–70.
69. Sonpavde G, Khan MM, Svatek RS, Lee R, Novara G, Tilki D, et al. Prognostic risk stratification of pathological stage T2N0 bladder cancer after radical cystectomy. BJU Int. 2011;108(5):687–92.
70. Mazzucchelli R, Cheng L, Lopez-Beltran A, Scarpelli M, Montironi R. Clinicopathological significance of lymphovascular invasion in urothelial carcinoma. Anal Quant Cytol Histol. 2012;34(4):173–9.
71. Larsen MP, Steinberg GD, Brendler CB, Epstein JI. Use of Ulex europaeus agglutinin I (UEAI) to distinguish vascular and "pseudovascular" invasion in transitional cell carcinoma of bladder with lamina propria invasion. Mod Pathol. 1990;3(1):83–8.
72. Guo CC, Czerniak B. Bladder cancer in the genomic era. Arch Pathol Lab Med. 2019;143(6):695–704.
73. Rebouissou S, Bernard-Pierrot I, de Reyniès A, Lepage M-L, Krucker C, Chapeaublanc E, et al. EGFR as a potential therapeutic target for a subset of muscle-invasive bladder cancers presenting a basal-like phenotype. Sci Transl Med. 2014;6(244):244ra91.
74. Marzouka N-A-D, Eriksson P, Rovira C, Liedberg F, Sjödahl G, Höglund M. A validation and extended description of the Lund taxonomy for urothelial carcinoma using the TCGA cohort. Sci Rep. 2018;8(1):3737.
75. Mo Q, Nikolos F, Chen F, Tramel Z, Lee Y-C, Hayashi K, et al. Prognostic power of a tumor differentiation gene signature for bladder urothelial carcinomas. J Natl Cancer Inst. 2018;110(5):448–59.
76. Kamoun A, de Reynies A, Allory Y, Sjodahl G, Robertson AG, Seiler R, et al. A consensus molecular classification of muscle-invasive bladder cancer. Eur Urol. 2020;77(4):420–33.
77. Guo CC, Dadhania V, Zhang L, Majewski T, Bondaruk J, Sykulski M, et al. Gene expression profile of the clinically aggressive micropapillary variant of bladder cancer. Eur Urol. 2016;70(4):611–20.
78. Guo CC, Majewski T, Zhang L, Yao H, Bondaruk J, Wang Y, et al. Dysregulation of EMT drives the progression to clinically aggressive sarcomatoid bladder cancer. Cell Rep. 2019;27(6):1781–93.e4.
79. Dadhania V, Zhang M, Zhang L, Bondaruk J, Majewski T, Siefker-Radtke A, et al. Meta-analysis of the luminal and basal subtypes of bladder cancer and the identification of signature immunohistochemical markers for clinical use. EBioMedicine. 2016;12:105–17.
80. Sjodahl G. Molecular subtype profiling of urothelial carcinoma using a subtype-specific immunohistochemistry panel. Methods Mol Biol (Clifton, NJ). 2018;1655:53–64.

6 Morphological Variants of Invasive Urothelial Carcinoma

Kyung En Park, Qihui "Jim" Zhai, and Fang-Ming Deng

Invasive urothelial carcinoma (UC) displays many histological variants; some variants are associated with different outcomes compared to conventional UC. Based on the WHO classification system 2016 [1], the variants of infiltrating UC are listed in Table 6.1. In this chapter, the morphological features, diagnostic pitfalls, differential diagnoses, immunoprofile, molecular alterations, and clinical relevance for the common variants will be reviewed.

UC has a high propensity for divergent differentiation. The apparent rise in the incidence of variant histology is largely due to the increased awareness, recognition, and improved reporting by pathologists. The rationales to recognize the variants are for diagnostic, therapeutic, as well as prognostic significance. Some variants may mimic other malignancies or even benign lesions, potentially leading to misdiagnosis. Some variants are correlated with different clinical outcomes from conventional invasive UC. Therefore, familiarity with the diverse morphology of invasive UC is more than just an academic exercise; it directly determines if we can provide the optimal care for patients affected by this disease [2–4].

Most of the time, we can handle these cases with confidence based on hematoxylin and eosin (H&E)-stained sections alone; however, in difficult cases, immunohistochemistry (IHC) and molecular profiling in special situations may play an important role aiding us in reaching an accurate diagnosis in our daily practice.

Table 6.1 Histological variants of infiltrating urothelial carcinoma according to WHO 2016 classification of tumors of the urinary tract

Urothelial carcinoma
With divergent differentiation
With squamous cell differentiation
With glandular differentiation
With trophoblastic differentiation
Others (including small cell and Müllerian differentiation)
Nested urothelial carcinoma (including large nested)
Microcystic urothelial carcinoma
Micropapillary urothelial carcinoma
Lymphoepithelioma-like urothelial carcinoma
Plasmacytoid/signet ring cell/diffuse urothelial carcinoma
Sarcomatoid urothelial carcinoma
Giant cell urothelial carcinoma
Lipid-rich urothelial carcinoma
Clear cell (glycogen-rich) urothelial carcinoma
Poorly differentiated urothelial tumors (including those with osteoclast-like giant cells)

K. E. Park · F.-M. Deng (✉)
Department of Pathology, New York University Langone Health, New York, NY, USA
e-mail: kyung.park@nyulangone.org; fang-ming.deng@nyumc.org

Q. "J." Zhai
Lab Medicine and Pathology, Mayo Clinic Florida, Jacksonville, FL, USA
e-mail: Zhai.Qihui@mayo.edu

H. Zhou et al. (eds.), *Urinary Bladder Pathology*, https://doi.org/10.1007/978-3-030-71509-0_6

Infiltrating Urothelial Carcinoma with Divergent Differentiation

The most common UC variant is UC with divergent differentiation, which includes squamous, glandular, trophoblastic, small cell, and other rare variations of differentiation occurring in a background of conventional UC.

Infiltrating Urothelial Carcinoma with Squamous Differentiation

The presence of squamous differentiation within a conventional invasive UC occurs in up to 40% of bladder UC [5]. The incidence increases with tumor grade and stage. Morphological evidence of squamous differentiation shares the similar histological features of the typical squamous cell carcinoma, including polygonal cells that frequently display dyskeratosis, individual keratinization or keratin pearl formation, and occasional intercellular bridges (Fig. 6.1). It is well documented that normal and neoplastic urothelium can undergo squamous differentiation, such as seen in well-differentiated, noninvasive papillary tumors. Areas of squamous differentiation may have basaloid or clear cell features, and the urothelial component may consist only of UC in situ. The term squamoid should be avoided, because clinicians interpret UC with squamoid differentiation as the same as squamous differentiation, and this may impact the treatment decision.

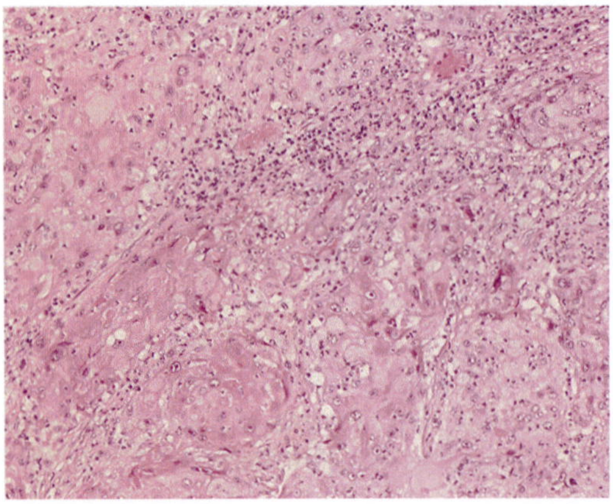

Fig. 6.1 Urothelial carcinoma with squamous differentiation

Pure squamous cell carcinoma is the primary differential diagnosis for this variant; the main difference is that the pure squamous cell carcinoma does not contain any conventional UC and not have surface urothelial dysplasia or UC in situ. No specific markers exist to help with the distinction of squamous differentiation in urothelial carcinoma from pure squamous cell carcinoma, and the diagnosis relies on the clinical history and the absence of a clear-cut conventional UC and/or UC in situ component upon histological analysis. However, UC with squamous differentiation may express urothelial markers (S100P, GATA3, uroplakins). Positivity of these markers in tumor cells strongly favors urothelial differentiation over squamous differentiation [6].

Squamous cell carcinomas are associated with some major risk factors, such as smoking, schistosomiasis, stones, or repetitive trauma. The presence of associated keratin production and squamous dysplasia or squamous carcinoma in situ is more typical of primary squamous cell carcinoma, and these conditions do not appear to be involved in the pathogenesis of UC with squamous differentiation. Although human papillomavirus has been identified in a subset of these cases, it is generally not considered to be causative to the development of this variant of UC [7].

Patients with UCs containing abundant squamous differentiation may have a worse prognosis, possibly because they are typically associated with a higher-grade UC [8]. In the pathology report, the percentage of the squamous component should be estimated and documented, since some data have shown that tumors with squamous differentiation may be more resistant to systemic chemotherapy and radiation treatment [8–10]. However, there are no large studies examining the clinical significance of squamous differentiation or its response to standard therapy to validate these findings. Recently gene sequencing studies have identified the so-called basal/squamous-like type which, having squamous or squamoid morphology, has been linked to poor responsiveness to chemotherapy and decreased cancer-specific survival [11, 12].

Infiltrating Urothelial Carcinoma with Glandular Differentiation

This variant is defined by the presence of true glandular spaces associated with a conventional UC. Glandular differentiation within urothelial carcinoma has an estimated prevalence of up to 18% among cases of UC of the bladder, making it one of the more common variants, though not as common as squamous differentiation [13]. Glandular differentiation can be found in UCs of all stages and grades, with predilection for high-grade and high-stage tumors. The importance of recognizing this pattern of UC and making the distinction is twofold: [1] UC with a predominant glandular pattern may have a worse prognosis than tumors with only focal or limited differentiation, though currently there is limited data to validate this suspicion [13, 14], and [2] UC with glandular differentiation is managed differently from metastatic adenocarcinoma. Furthermore, documenting the proportion of glandular differentiation and following the clinical behavior of these lesions may further clarify the prognostic significance of this variant, if any.

These glandular structures consist of tubular- or enteric-type glands, often associated with variable mucin production. The glands are lined by a single layer of low to high columnar epithelium within nests of conventional invasive UC (Fig. 6.2). Mucin production may be so dominant that occasional tumor cells, especially signet ring cells, may be floating within the mucinous material (so-called colloid pattern). The presence of cytoplasmic mucin (so-called pseudoglandular changes) is not uncommon and is estimated in up to 63% of cases of UC, but this feature alone is not sufficient to make the diagnosis of glandular differentiation. Necrotic debris within tumor nests should not be confused with glandular lumens.

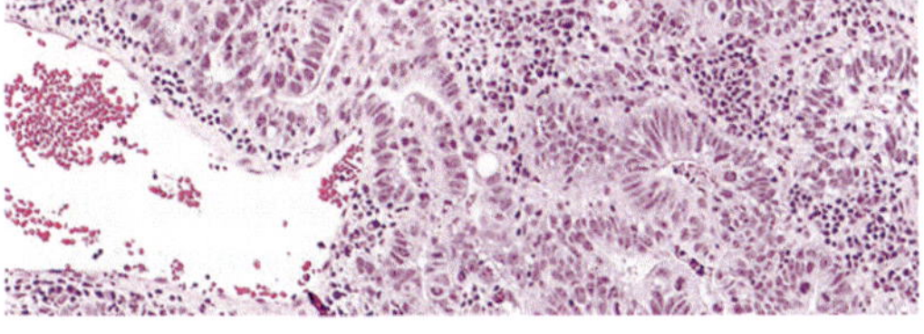

Fig. 6.2 Urothelial carcinoma with glandular differentiation

The major differential diagnoses should include adenocarcinoma of the urinary bladder (both urachal and nonurachal), cystitis glandularis, cystitis cystica, von Brunn nests, microcystic and nested variants of UC, and metastatic adenocarcinoma. The presence of both conventional UC and areas of glandular differentiation with malignant cytologic features rules out the above benign lesions. Appropriate sampling of the lesion is, therefore, very important, because it may be difficult to make a proper diagnosis with limited specimens. Tumors with a pure glandular component with no UC component, either invasive or in situ, are diagnosed as adenocarcinoma. In difficult cases, the expression of MUC5AC apomucin may be useful as an immunohistochemical marker of glandular differentiation in urothelial tumors [15]. TERT mutations can also be used in the differential diagnosis of glandular lesions of the bladder which may be seen in approximately 70% of UC with glandular differentiation but are consistently negative in primary adenocarcinoma of the bladder [16]. Microcystic urothelial carcinoma does not show true glandular differentiation. Metastatic adenocarcinoma should be considered when the patient has a history of an adenocarcinoma elsewhere. Recognition of glandular differentiation is evident with H&E sections, and IHC is generally not necessary in this setting. If a diagnosis of adenocarcinoma is made, it is very important to distinguish a primary urinary adenocarcinoma from metastatic adenocarcinoma (particularly of colorectal origin), which is far more common than primary urinary adenocarcinoma and may require different surgical management.

Urothelial Carcinoma with Trophoblastic Differentiation

Since 1904, more than 30 cases of tumors with trophoblastic differentiation, including cases of the so-called pure choriocarcinoma, have been reported in the literature. In contrast to conventional high-grade UC which usually affects individuals in the fifth and older decades of life, this entity has been reported to affect individuals as young as 23 years old. The true incidence of HCG positivity within tumors is likely much greater than commonly understood and has been reported in up to 35% of high-grade UC [17, 18]. Therefore, HCG positivity alone does not indicate UC with trophoblastic differentiation.

This entity shows a wide morphological spectrum. Besides the component of conventional invasive UC, it also may demonstrate formation of syncytiotrophoblast, areas of hemorrhage and necrosis, and formation of areas resembling choriocarcinoma (Fig. 6.3), pure choriocarcinoma, and UC without morphological evidence of choriocarcinoma that express human chorionic gonadotropin (HCG). The latter group of tumors is morphologically UC, and the only evidence of trophoblastic differentiation is the production of HCG within tumor cells detected by IHC. These areas may be immediately juxtaposed with tumor cells that are morphologically identical but are negative for HCG expression. This group of tumors should not be classified as UC with trophoblastic differentiation. The remainder of tumors displays a variety of trophoblastic tissue patterns, ranging from scattered multinucleate giant cells to well-defined syncytiotrophoblastic cells that wrap around mononuclear cells. The latter pattern, indistinguishable from true choriocarcinoma, has been very rarely reported. To make the diagnosis of UC with trophoblastic differentiation, a UC component must be identified. Some tumors with advanced choriocarcinomatous growth may show minimal residual urothelial malignancy, and the only evidence of the origin of the tumor may be adjacent UC in situ.

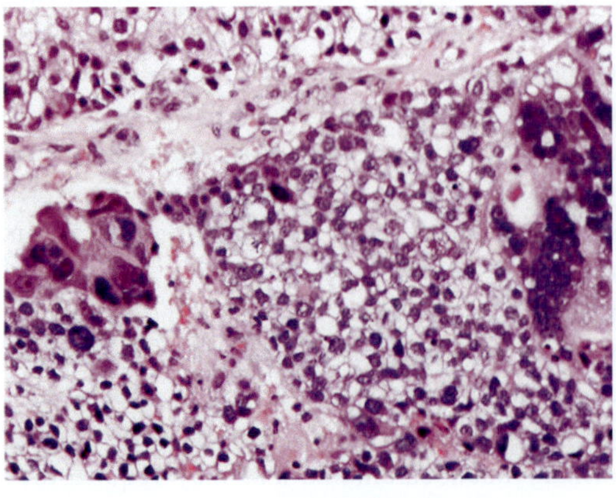

Fig. 6.3 Urothelial carcinoma with trophoblastic differentiation resembling choriocarcinoma

The frequent expression of HCG within urothelial carcinoma and the occasional presence of trophoblastic differentiation have prompted discussion as to the origin of tumors with trophoblastic characteristics. While some have proposed that this differentiation arises from primitive rests left behind during embryologic development, others believe that normal urothelium retains some ability for pluripotential development and that upon malignant transformation, this differentiation (or dedifferentiation) may become evident. Some authors propose that trophoblastic differentiation is a metaplastic phenomenon, supported by the occurrence of HCG positivity in all morphological varieties of trophoblastic differentiation and the frequency of metaplasia within urothelium along other cell lines, including squamous and glandular, as previously discussed [18].

The differential diagnosis for this UC variant includes the giant cell variant of UC (will be discussed below), UC with stromal osteoclast-like giant cell formation, and undifferentiated carcinomas. While all of these lesions may be characterized by the presence of large, pleomorphic cells, the true syncytiotrophoblast is distinguished by the cytoplasmic immunoreaction for HCG. Staining is intense within giant cells and may also be seen in surrounding urothelial cells. In addition to HCG production (and many subtypes of HCG), IHC may show positivity within tumor cells for other placental antigens including human placental lactogen (HPL) and pregnancy-specific beta-1 glycoprotein (SP-1). Additionally, cases of pure germ cell neoplasms may also occur in the bladder, without a UC precursor. The diagnosis of which may require a high copy number of the isochromosome 12p, as seen by fluorescence in situ hybridization (FISH), thus supporting germ cell differentiation [19]. However, primary pure germ cell neoplasms in the bladder are extremely rare, and early reported "primary choriocarcinoma of the bladder" probably represent UC with syncytiotrophoblasts.

The presence of syncytiotrophoblasts within UC portends a poor prognosis, but the significance of trophoblastic differentiation marked only by the presence of HCG production is unclear, and many feel it has no prognostic significance [17, 18, 20]. It has been associated more commonly with high-grade lesions and may be associated with a poorer response to chemotherapy and radiation therapy than tumors without trophoblastic differentiation. Because of these findings, the presence of trophoblastic differentiation and the estimated percentage within the tumor should be documented in the report. Clinically, patients with trophoblastic differentiation have the same presentation and symptoms as patients without it. The tumoral production of HCG has been related to gynecomastia in some patients, while others have shown no endocrinologic manifestations. Elevated serum and urine HCG may be seen in some patients and can be used as a helpful serum tumor marker of response to treatment in these patients.

Other Rare Types of Urothelial Carcinoma with Divergent Differentiation

Rarely, UC demonstrates small cell differentiation (minor component small cell carcinoma coexists with conventional UC). Any amount of small cell carcinoma should be reported, as this is relevant in guiding therapy. If the small cell carcinoma component constitutes the majority of the tumor, the diagnosis of small cell carcinoma should be made (see other section). More rarely, Müllerian differentiation and different lines of germ cell differentiation can be seen in an otherwise conventional UC [1].

Nested Urothelial Carcinoma

This variant is characterized by the banal appearance of the tumor cells with a nested growth pattern, which may be confused with von Brunn nests, cystitis cystica, and nephrogenic adenoma. The definition of nested UC has been expanded to include other tumors showing deceptively benign histology, such as the large nested carcinoma and the UC with small tubules, earlier considered separate entities [1, 21].

UC nested variant is very rare with an estimated incidence of 0.3%. The most frequent clinical manifestation is of hematuria, urgency, or signs of urinary obstruction. Almost all the patients within this group are males in their later adulthood (53–97 years old).

Histologically, although the overlying urothelium is not ordinarily involved by the neoplastic cells, tumor cells are arranged in nests and abortive tubules that infiltrate the lamina propria and muscularis propria. The tumor cells are deceptively benign in appearance. Therefore, some pathologists use "carcinoma with deceptively bland features" to describe this variant (Fig. 6.4).

However, scattered, more atypical tumor cells are found in every reported case. Also helpful in recognizing this variant of UC is the fact that the degree of nuclear atypia increases along with the depth of invasion. To appreciate the invasive pattern is a key to accurately diagnose this entity.

The aggressive clinical behavior of this variant of UC is discordant with its deceptively

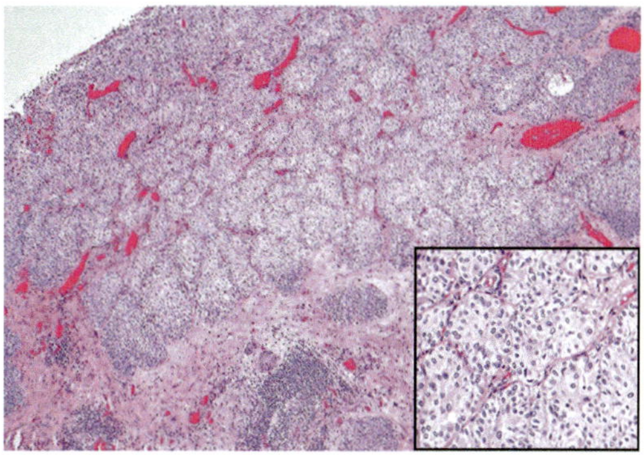

Fig. 6.4 Nest variant urothelial carcinoma. Insert showing bland nuclear features

bland cytological appearance. Several series have shown that these tumors commonly present at high stage including nodal invasion. While it is documented that nested variant tumors are associated with progressive or recurrent disease, its clinical outcome is similar to conventional UC, with no difference in recurrence rate or survival when treated surgically [22–25]. Nonetheless, nested variant is an aggressive tumor and should, therefore, be treated accordingly.

The major differential diagnoses for the nested variant of UC are the benign lesions including von Brunn nests, cystitis glandularis, cystitis cystica, inverted papilloma, inverted low-grade UC, nephrogenic adenoma, paraganglionic tissue, and paraganglioma. If the tumor cells are found to be invading into muscularis propria, the distinction from a benign lesion should be easier to make. Most invasive UCs exhibit irregular infiltration by atypical cells, often accompanied by invasion-induced stromal response. The invasive cell nests are confluent, lack a central lumen, and are usually closely opposed to the overlying urothelial surface. Von Brunn nests, cystitis cystica, and cystitis glandularis are typically well circumscribed, lack nuclear atypia, and are not associated with a desmoplastic response or invading into muscularis propria. Nephrogenic adenoma is characterized by the presence of a single layer of cells lining the tubules with a collagen cuffing, in contrast to the nested variant of urothelial carcinoma, which consists of multiple layers. PAX2/PAX 8 is positive in nephrogenic adenoma and negative in UC, which can be useful to separate these two entities.

Prostatic adenocarcinoma and urinary bladder adenocarcinoma occasionally may be included in the differential diagnosis. Prostatic adenocarcinoma can be excluded by its location, nuclear features, and positive reactions for prostate-specific antigen and prostatic acid phosphatase. Adenocarcinoma of the urinary bladder frequently exhibits colonic differentiation with distinct gland formation lined by columnar cells, which is morphologically distinct from the nested variant of UC.

FISH studies using UroVysion probes are found to be very useful in separating UC with nested variant from von Brunn nests on paraffin-embedded bladder specimens, documented by a group of pathologists from Mayo Clinic [26]. TERT promoter mutation assay may be used to distinguish nest variant UC from benign mimickers by the presence of TERT promoter mutation associated with this tumor [27].

Microcystic Urothelial Carcinoma

Microcystic variant is another deceptively benign-looking UC which often presents at late stage. This variant, also known as urothelial carcinoma with gland-like lumens, is defined by formation of round to oval microcysts, macrocysts (1–2 mm in diameter), and tubular structures containing granular eosinophilic material and necrotic cellular debris (Fig. 6.5). Luminal secretions may have a targetoid appearance. This material displays mucinous qualities that can be highlighted by periodic acid-Schiff (PAS) and Alcian blue staining. Intracytoplasmic mucin deposits are also seen with PAS stain. Calcifications may also be present within cyst walls. A cyst lining is variably present and consists of flattened to plump urothelial cells, which have the same cytologic features of typical urothelial cells. The cystic lining cells are cytologically bland but can exhibit variation in size, resembling the solid nests of UC, which is a key feature in differentiating this neoplasm from benign lesions. The stromal response to surrounding tumor nests is variable,

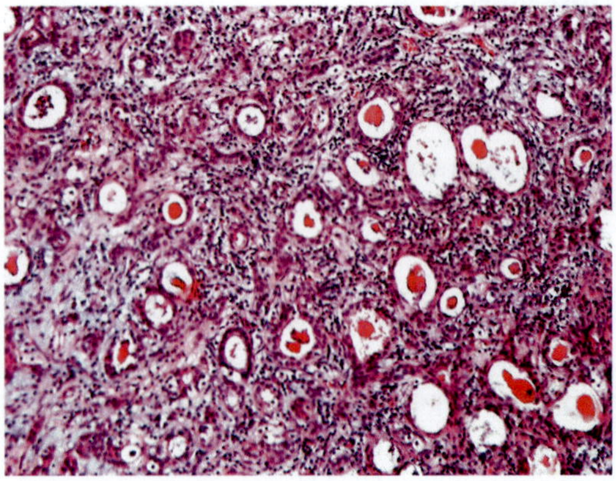

Fig. 6.5 Microcystic urothelial carcinoma

ranging from conspicuous, extremely cellular to scant stroma. Reported cases typically demonstrate a high-grade tumor (grades 2 or 3), and the microcystic component may compose a majority or a minority of the invasive lesion, though the designation of the term "microcystic variant" is reserved for cases with prominent microcystic architecture. The exact percentage required to make this diagnosis has not been determined.

The differential diagnosis of this lesion is important, as it may resemble many benign histological patterns, and thus could easily be misdiagnosed. Cystitis cystica and cystitis glandularis in particular may be difficult to differentiate from the microcystic variant of UC, especially in small biopsy specimens. The dramatic variation in nuclear size, in addition to other atypical characteristics, is helpful in distinguishing feature of the microcystic variant of UC. Also, the invasive nature of the lesion helps to rule out benign processes. Microcystic UC shows a haphazard, deeply infiltrating growth pattern, unlike cystitis cystica or cystitis glandularis, which remain superficial. Nephrogenic adenoma (nephrogenic metaplasia) may also resemble this variant, but the invasive growth pattern and cytologic characteristics of the microcystic carcinoma should make the distinction. While nephrogenic adenoma has the same tubular architecture as microcystic UC, the former tends to form a well-circumscribed lesion with confinement to the lamina propria. In general, invasion of the muscularis propria is the best means of differentiating microcystic UC from any of the abovementioned benign disease processes. In cases of doubt, IHC may be needed as nephrogenic adenoma stains with PAX2/PAX8 while UC stains with GATA3 and P63.

Another diagnostic consideration is primary or metastatic adenocarcinoma. Although the cysts of the microcystic variant may resemble small infiltrating glands and may produce mucin, the architecture and cytology of the lining epithelium are distinctly urothelial in nature. The nested variant of UC with tubular differentiation may also resemble the microcystic variant, but the nested areas will not be present in the latter. Immunohistochemical findings have been studied in the few reported cases and are identical to those seen in other UCs. The cases reported show little difference in presentation and prognosis from conventional invasive UC [28, 29].

Micropapillary Urothelial Carcinoma

This variant is characterized by a conventional infiltrating UC with an admixed micropapillary growth pattern. Since the MD Anderson group first reported micropapillary UC, this tumor is well known as an aggressive morphological variant of UC [30]. There is a clear male predominance (M: F = 3:1), and the peak incidence is in the sixth decade of life. This variant UC accounts for 0.6–2.2% of all UC, but it has been suggested that the incidence may be higher than currently reported.

There are two distinct and characteristic histological features: small nests or slender fusiform papillary processes that do not contain central true fibrovascular cores, contained within empty lacunar spaces (Fig. 6.6a). These spaces are most likely tissue fixation artifacts, as they lack a lining epithelium or endothelial cells, speculated to be secondary to tissue retraction. The lack of true fibrovascular cores is unique and different from traditional papillary carcinoma (Fig. 6.6b). Another very characteristic appearance of micropapillary pattern is inverted polarization of nuclei. The characteristic triad for micropapillary carcinoma is [1] multiple tight cell clusters in single lacunar spaces, [2] small cell nests (four or less than four cells thick) in lacunar spaces, and [3] inverted nuclear polarization (inside out).

The invasive component is strikingly similar to papillary serous carcinoma of the ovary. Cytologically, the tumor cells show variable pleomorphism but typically show prominent nucleoli with uneven distribution of chromatin. Cytoplasm is usually abundant, ranging from clear to eosinophilic. Mitoses may be few to numerous. The nuclear grade is high in most tumors.

IHC supports the contention that micropapillary UC is a variant of UC of the bladder. The tumor cells are positive for cytokeratin 7 (100%),

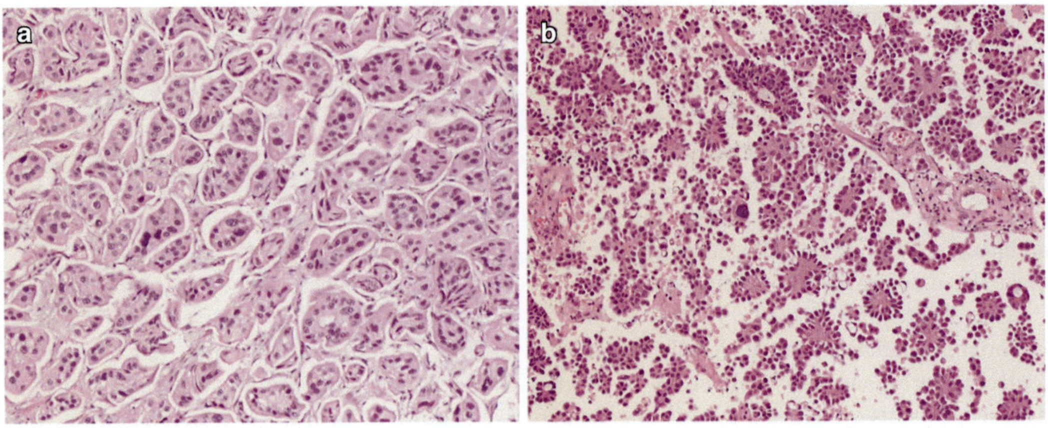

Fig. 6.6 (**a, b**) Micropapillary urothelial carcinoma

S100P (96%), uroplakin ii (90%), GATA3 (88%), P63 (70%), CK7 (95%), and CK20 (60%) [1, 28]. While conventional UCs demonstrate a very similar staining pattern, overexpression of CA-125 (positive in one-third of cases of micropapillary UC and barely in conventional UC) and MUC1 expression with reverse polarity is reported [31].

Micropapillary UC commonly presents at a high pathological stage and is associated with high frequency of LVI, frequent lymph node metastases, poor prognosis, and low survival rates. However, a stage-matched trial showed no significant difference comparing micropapillary variant and conventional UC in a 10-year survival after cystectomy [32, 33]. Some studies have observed that intravesical therapy is not effective for micropapillary UC and suggested a lower threshold for cystectomy, even in T1 patients with bacillus Calmette-Guérin-responsive disease. However, other data suggest that a more standard bladder-sparing approach is reasonable in selecting non-muscle invasive UC (NMIUC) patients [34, 35].

One important caveat for this variant of UC is that the use of "micropapillary" terminology to describe noninvasive UC. Micropapillary-like architecture may be seen in NMIUC and even rarely in UC in situ; however, it is not necessarily associated with worse outcomes compared with conventional noninvasive UC. Therefore, if the micropapillary component is limited to the noninvasive component, the tumor should not be classified as micropapillary carcinoma [1, 35, 36]. Additional discussion between the pathologist and the treating physician should be considered to avoid mismanagement in such instances.

HER2 alterations, including ERBB2 gene amplification or other mutations, occur at a much higher frequency in micropapillary UC than in conventional UC [37]. These patients have worse cancer-specific survival following radical cystectomy [38]. It also provides a potential role for HER2-targeted therapy in this variant, while definitive studies are lacking.

Micropapillary UC usually expresses markers of luminal phenotype (including FoxA1) which may have wild-type p53 and can be resistant to chemotherapy [39].

Micropapillary UC is not limited to the bladder, and it is considered as a morphological marker for aggressiveness. These features can be seen in the breast, colon, small bowel, pancreas, ovary, lung, and salivary glands. The differential diagnosis of micropapillary UC includes metastatic micropapillary adenocarcinoma of the lung, breast, and ovary. These tumors are morphologically identical to UC micropapillary variant. In the majority of these cases, there is a clinical history of lung, breast, or ovarian carcinoma; otherwise, a careful search for a primary tumor must be completed. IHC stains such as TTF-1 may be positive in lung tumors, ER and PR positive in breast carcinomas, or WT-1 maybe positive in ovarian tumors. Other metastatic adenocarcinomas; including colon and pancreas, may rarely display a micropapillary pattern and should be considered in the differential diagnosis. Malignant papillary mesothelioma is another possibility, but it is positive for WT-1 and negative for GATA3.

Lymphoepithelioma-like Urothelial Carcinoma

Lymphoepithelioma-like carcinoma (LELC) variant is defined as UC that histologically resemble lymphoepithelioma of the nasopharynx. The histology is characterized by proliferation of undifferentiated cells with a prominent, lymphocytic background (Fig. 6.7a). The major differential diagnoses are malignant lymphoma or chronic cystitis. Carcinomas with a similar morphology have also been described in other organs, including the salivary glands, thymus, cervix, skin, lung, and stomach. These carcinomas show a male predominance and mainly occur in late adulthood. The most frequent clinical presentation is hematuria. The tumor is solitary with an invasive growth pattern and is most often located in the bladder dome, posterior wall, or trigone.

The tumorigenesis of LELC variant is unclear. Unlike lymphoepithelioma of the nasopharynx, EBV virus is not found using either IHC or in situ hybridization technology. It has frequent P53 accumulations and most likely with similar pathogenesis to conventional UC, which are possibly derived from basal (stem) cells [40, 41].

Histologically, the tumor cells grow in a syncytial pattern. The individual cells display undifferentiated, large pleomorphic nuclei with prominent nucleoli and indistinct cytoplasmic

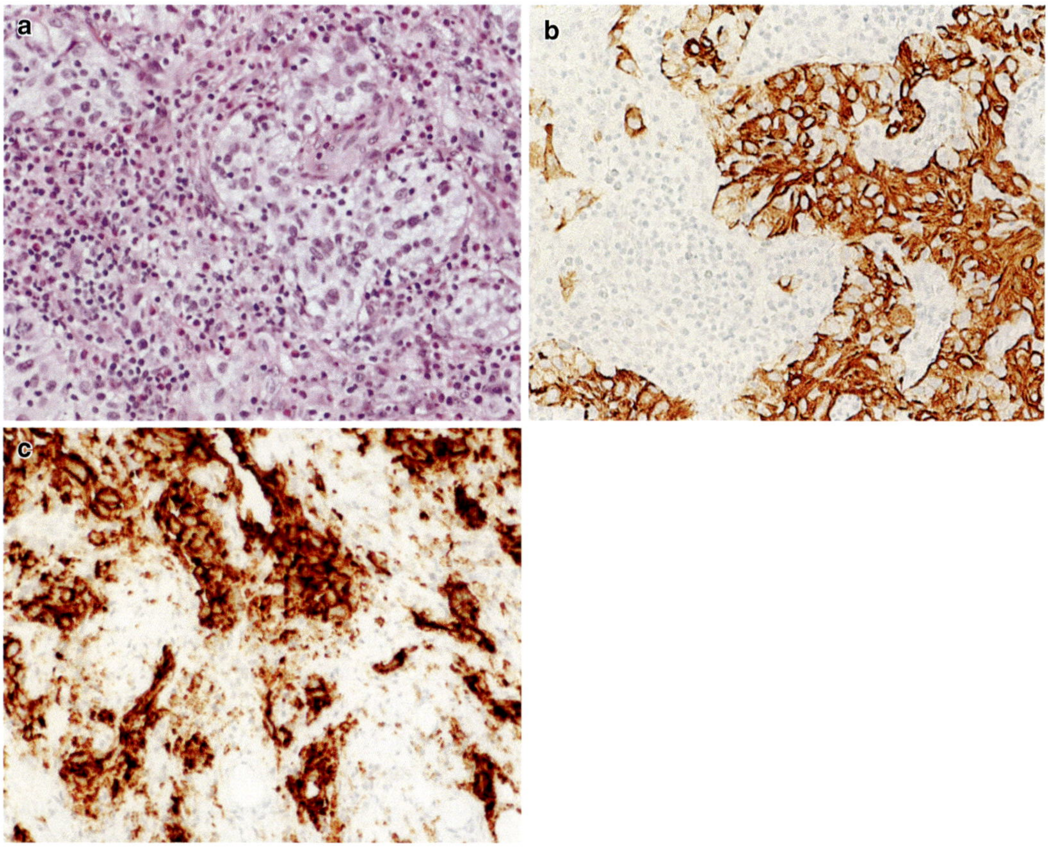

Fig. 6.7 (**a**) Lymphoepithelioma-like urothelial carcinoma. (**b**) Cytokeratin (AE1/3) highlights the tumor cells. (**c**) Tumor shows high PD-L1 expression

borders with syncytial growth. Mitoses are readily seen. The background is composed of a mixed population of inflammatory cells, predominantly lymphocytes, but plasma cells, histiocytes, and occasional neutrophils or eosinophils are also identified. Lymphocytes are seen not only at the periphery of tumor cell nests but also within tumoral nests and between tumor cells. A desmoplastic reaction is not seen. LELC can be pure, predominant, or focally admixed with conventional UC.

The major differential diagnosis includes large cell lymphoma, which is rare in the urinary bladder. Distinction from a lymphoma is extremely important, because the clinical management for lymphoma is dramatically different from UC. The presence of a syncytial pattern of large malignant cells is a clue to making the diagnosis. If necessary, immunohistochemistry can be very useful in this setting. The tumor cells are positive for epithelial markers, AE1/AE3 and CK7, but are rarely positive for CK20 (Fig. 6.7b). The lymphoid stroma is positive for CD45. CD3 and CD20 demonstrate a mixed population of B and T cells with T-cell predominance. Chronic cystitis may be confused with LELC when the tumor cells are scanty. It is particularly important to recognize this possibility in a small biopsy specimen containing prominent lymphoid stroma with a few neoplastic cells, which can be easily misdiagnosed as florid chronic cystitis. Therefore, a careful search for malignant cells using cytokeratin immunostaining is highly recommended for the differential diagnosis.

LELC, whether in pure or mixed form, has a similar prognosis to ordinary UC when treated by cystectomy [42].

Although no large-scale randomized clinical trials have been conducted to study the treatment of LELC, the available studies have shown that a combination of surgery and chemotherapy with radiation treatment has led to a very good clinical response. Because LELC of the urinary bladder is more sensitive to both chemotherapy and radiotherapy than conventional UC, radical cystectomy may not be necessary for all patients with muscle-invasive LELC of the urinary bladder, particularly its pure form [41, 43–45].

Recent study demonstrates that LELCs of the urinary bladder are enriched in a basal-like molecular subtype and share a high level of immune infiltration and PD-L1 expression, similar to basal tumors (Fig. 6.7c). The basal-like phenotype is consistent with the known sensitivity of LELC of the urinary bladder to chemotherapy and suggests that immune checkpoint therapy should be explored in this rare disease [46].

Plasmacytoid/Signet Ring Cell/ Diffuse Urothelial Carcinoma

Plasmacytoid variant of UC, also known as lymphoma-like, signet ring cell, and diffuse UC variant, exhibits the morphological features of lymphoma or plasmacytoma. Morphologically, the tumor is composed of single malignant cells without nesting. The tumor cells have eccentrically placed nuclei and abundant eosinophilic cytoplasm in variable amounts in the plasmacytoid variants. The cytologic atypia can be minimal (Fig. 6.8a and b). The plasmacytoid tumor component varies in published series, with most reported using a 30% or 50% cutoff [47–50].

Loss of E-cadherin represents a hallmark of plasmacytoid differentiation. The majority of plasmacytoid UCs demonstrate loss of membranous E, capital e-cadherin, which is consistent with the fact that they harbor IDH1 mutation or methylation. A univariate Cox regression analysis showed that nuclear E-cadherin accumulation in plasmacytoid UC was associated with a twofold increase in risk of death [51, 52].

Plasmacytoid features can also be seen in a variety of tumors affecting the bladder, which include large cell lymphoma, plasmacytoma, malignant melanoma, paraganglioma, neuroendocrine carcinoma, rhabdomyosarcoma, and metastatic carcinoma (such as adenocarcinoma of the breast or stomach). Those tumors with overlapping features are naturally the major differential diagnoses. Immunostains can be very useful in separating these entities. The tumor cells of the lymphoma-like and plasmacytoma-like UCs are positive for cytokeratin AE1/AE3 and CK7, with occasional positivity for CK20.

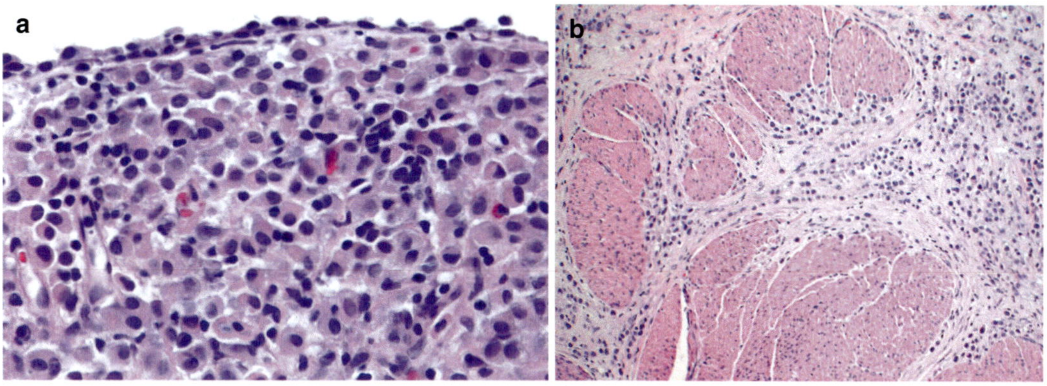

Fig. 6.8 Plasmacytoid urothelial carcinoma. (**a**) involves the lamina propria. (**b**) involves the muscularis propria

These cells are consistently negative for CD45 and other lymphoid markers (B and T cells). Likewise, melanocytic markers including S-100 protein, HMB-45, and Melan A are negative. In rhabdomyosarcoma, the tumor cells are positive for desmin, myogenin, and MyoD-1. Both plasmacytoid UC and metastatic breast lobular carcinoma are positive for GATA3. A panel of p63, HMWK, S100p, uroplakins, and ER, PR can be used to differentiate these two diseases [28, 53].

The patients with plasmacytoid UC typically present at an advanced stage with frequent positive surgical margin at cystectomy and peritoneal carcinomatosis [54]. The outcome is generally poor with high relapse and mortality comparing with conventional UC. Although plasmacytoid carcinoma appears to be chemotherapy-responsive, there are few long-term survivors [47–51, 55].

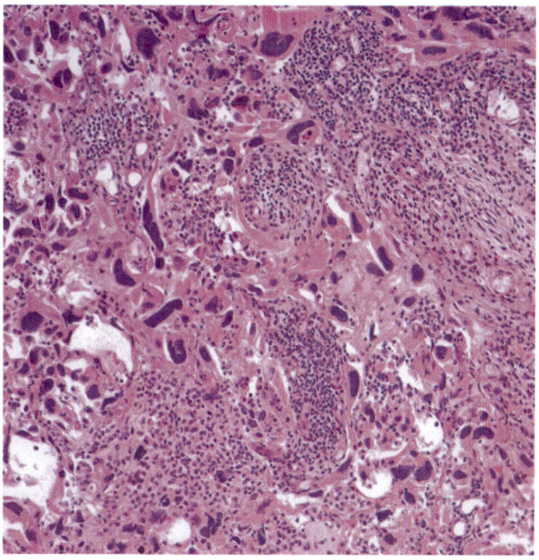

Fig. 6.9 Giant cell variant urothelial carcinoma

Giant Cell Variant of Urothelial Carcinoma

This variant of UC is characterized by the presence of epithelial tumor giant cells exhibiting marked nuclear atypia, along with a component of conventional UC, and was initially classified as an undifferentiated UC.

Microscopically, the giant cell variant of UC shows marked nuclear pleomorphism, typically with multiple nuclei, and consists of cohesive cells with abundant eosinophilic or amphophilic cytoplasm (Fig. 6.9). A component of conventional UC is present by definition. The tumor giant cells show positivity for epithelial/urothelial markers, including cytokeratin (CK7, CK8/CK18, CK20, Cam5.2), EMA, p63, GATA3, and negative for βHCG [56, 57].

These tumor giant cells are distinct from other giant cells described within other bladder tumors, including osteoclast-like giant cells occasionally seen in reactive lesions, syncytiotrophoblast, sarcomatoid variant of urothelial carcinoma, and giant cells of the so-called giant cell tumor of the bladder, which is indistinguishable from the giant cell tumor of bone and lacks urothelial differentiation.

Reactive and inflammatory stromal giant cells have little nuclear pleomorphism among their individual nuclei, with evenly distributed chromatin. These changes are seen in patients who have received intravesical bacillus Calmette-Guerin therapy (BCG), schistosomiasis, and, as a response to instrumentation, biopsy or resection. Langerhans-type giant cells are seen with BCG therapy, and the other conditions are usually associated with foreign body-type giant cells.

Osteoclast-like cells may also be seen within the stroma in urothelial carcinoma, and are not a component of the tumor itself. These cells have characteristic round nuclei without significant nuclear pleomorphism and overlapping and prominent nucleoli. The cytoplasm is amphophilic and may contain cellular debris, erythrocytes, or inflammatory cells. The osteoclast-like cells have also been described as an osteoclast-rich undifferentiated UC, which may also be considered in the differential diagnosis of the giant cell variant of UC, and are discussed below (undifferentiated carcinoma).

The true incidence of giant cell UC is not known, as it is a very rare entity. The significance of diagnosing the giant cell variant of UC is that it is associated with a poor prognosis and presents at an advanced stage.

Sarcomatoid Variant of Urothelial Carcinoma

This term describes UC with a component morphologically indistinguishable from sarcoma. The recent WHO classification has applied this term to all biphasic malignant tumors showing morphological and/or immunological evidence of urothelial and mesenchymal differentiation. It usually presents as advanced disease and has a poor prognosis and frequently expresses epithelial-to-mesenchymal transition markers, suggesting a possible mechanism associated with its aggressive behavior [1, 58, 59].

Clinical presentation is not different from other UCs, with hematuria as the usual presenting symptom. Previous radiation therapy and intravesical cyclophosphamide treatment was reported to be associated with tumor recurrence which shows sarcomatoid areas. Grossly, sarcomatoid carcinomas tend to be exophytic, polypoid lesions, filling the bladder lumen, with a dull gray, solid, fleshy appearance on cut section. There is no predilection for a specific site in the bladder walls, and these tumors have also been reported in the ureters and renal pelvis, as well. The morphology of the sarcomatoid components in sarcomatoid carcinoma may resemble a range of mesenchymal tumors, but the most common appearance is that it resembles a high-grade spindle cell sarcoma or malignant fibrous histiocytoma or undifferentiated sarcoma (Fig. 6.10). The background stroma may be myxoid, vascular, hemorrhagic, or desmoplastic. There may be heterologous differentiation, including in order of decreasing frequency: areas of osteosarcoma, chondrosarcoma, rhabdomyosarcoma, liposarcoma, angiosarcoma, or a mixture of these neoplasms. The respective volume and type of these areas should be included in the pathology report. The carcinoma component may be composed of urothelial, squamous, glandular, small cell types, or unclassified carcinoma. The mesenchymal and epithelial elements are intimately admixed, and gradual transition may be seen from one to the other. Ultrastructural studies show the presence of true desmosomes and cytoplasmic intermediate filaments suggestive of keratin within the sarcomatoid component, confirming its derivation from epithelial tissue.

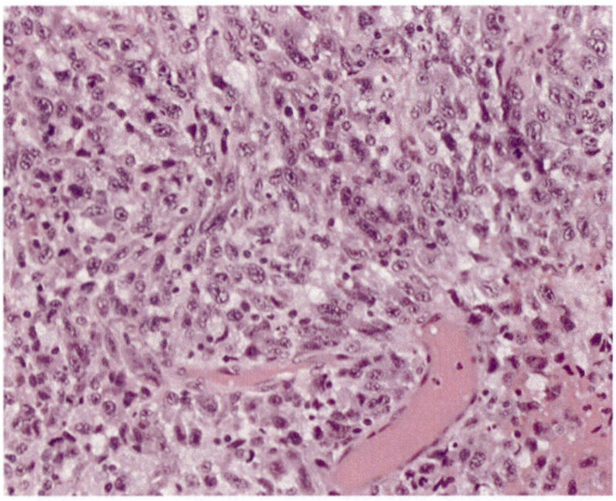

Fig. 6.10 Sarcomatoid urothelial carcinoma resembling a high-grade spindle cell sarcoma

The differential diagnosis includes many possibilities, such as pure sarcoma, giant cell variant of UC, trophoblastic variant of UC, osseous and chondroid stromal metaplasia in a UC, pseudosarcomatous stromal reaction, postoperative spindle cell nodule, inflammatory myofibroblastic tumors (pseudotumors), and spindle cell melanoma.

Diagnosis of a pure sarcoma can only be made in the absence of an epithelial malignancy, including UC in situ. A prior history of UC may provide sufficient evidence of this tumor being a sarcomatoid carcinoma, even though there is no apparent malignant epithelial component. Features that are helpful in making a decision include identification of nested or clustered tumor cells of the conventional UC component lying adjacent to sarcomatoid cells that also express cytokeratin. Positivity of diffuse epithelial markers (cytokeratin and EMA) is usually not seen in pure sarcoma, such as leiomyosarcoma or malignant fibrous histiocytoma, and may be helpful in distinguishing this entity from pure sarcomas. The markers that identify differentiation in the various forms of sarcoma will likewise be absent in sarcomatoid carcinoma. A common problem is a biopsy (transurethral resection of bladder tumor (TURBT)) of a bladder tumor exhibiting only sarcomatoid features without obvious epithelial elements. Although epithelial markers are commonly positive in the spindle cells, this reaction is not necessarily indicative of epithelial differentiation as intermediate filaments may be detected with these markers. It is well known that malignant fibrous histiocytoma of soft tissue and leiomyosarcoma can co-express epithelial markers. Positive expression of HMWK, p63, and GATA3 is more specific but with low sensitivity (GATA3-positive in 1/3 of sarcomatoid UC and negative in sarcoma) [60].

There are several entities generating a pseudosarcomatous pattern that may resemble the sarcomatoid variant of UC, some of which share overlapping features. High-grade invasive UC may incite formation of a brisk stromal reaction with atypical cells, termed pseudosarcomatous stromal reaction. These lesions are characterized by myxoid stroma containing slightly atypical cells and proliferating blood vessels adjacent to infiltrating carcinoma. It differs from the sarcomatoid variant of UC in that the spindle cell component expresses mesenchymal but not epithelial markers and also in that there is no transition from the spindle cell component to the UC. Inflammatory myofibroblastic tumors (also known as inflammatory pseudotumor, pseudosarcomatous fibromyxoid tumor, visceral form of nodular fasciitis, and pseudosarcomatous lesions) usually occur in younger patients and show a prominent chronic inflammatory infiltrate, stromal vascular proliferation, and extravasated red blood cells. In addition, the stroma may demonstrate marked myxoid change and/or edema. The spindle cell component may demonstrate mild cellular atypia as well as increased mitotic activity, but not atypical mitotic figures. Inflammatory myofibroblastic tumors are less likely to display necrosis and hemorrhage and do not have the potential to metastasize. They have minimal pleomorphism, hyperchromasia, mitotic activity, prominent nucleoli, and in general less cellular atypia than the sarcomatoid carcinoma [58, 61, 62].

It is important to note that myofibroblasts in inflammatory myofibroblastic tumor may show cytokeratin positivity, which should be considered when trying to differentiate these tumors from sarcomatoid carcinoma. Sarcomatoid carcinoma usually lacks the significant chronic inflammatory infiltrate seen in inflammatory myofibroblastic tumors and is more likely to have a neutrophilic component. Postoperative spindle nodules are very similar in histology and behavior to inflammatory myofibroblastic tumors, and some authors believe they are part of a spectrum of the same process. The diagnosis of postoperative spindle cell nodule requires appropriate history of surgery (usually 2–3 months, up to 6 years prior), and the lesion is frequently smaller than the abovementioned tumors and occurs in the same age group as UC. Melanoma is most easily distinguished through the use of IHC and demonstrates positivity for S-100 protein, HMB-45, and Melan A.

Undifferentiated Carcinoma

This category includes rare tumors that cannot be otherwise classified and usually exhibit high-grade malignant morphology. It spans a spectrum including tumors with mixed morphology such as small cell undifferentiated carcinoma, giant cell carcinoma, sarcomatoid carcinoma, undifferentiated carcinoma, not otherwise specified, and osteoclast-rich undifferentiated carcinoma [1].

Osteoclast-rich undifferentiated carcinoma is a group of tumors that have been recently described and may resemble extraosseous osteoclastic giant cell tumors, with biphasic composition of the osteoclastic giant cells and an associated mononuclear component, displaying marked atypia (Fig. 6.11) [63].

These tumors are still believed to be of urothelial origin, as the associated mononuclear component demonstrates epithelial/urothelial markers, association with a conventional UC component, and p53 positivity. It is recommended that these neoplasms be described as osteoclast-rich undifferentiated UC. The osteoclast-like giant cells were negative for epithelial/urothelial markers (GATA3, uroplakin II, thrombomodulin, and AE1/AE3) and indicate a reactive origin for these cells. This subtype of UC different from the giant cell variant of UC shows marked nuclear pleomorphism of the giant cells, whereas giant cell nuclei in the osteoclast-rich undifferentiated UC are cytologically bland [64].

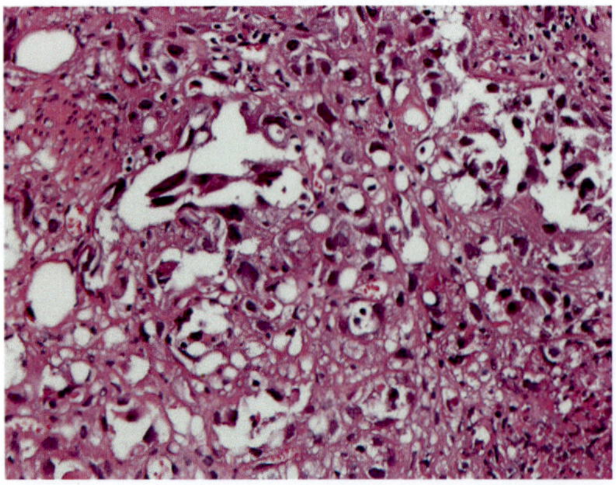

Fig. 6.11 Undifferentiated carcinoma

Clear Cell (Glycogen-Rich) Urothelial Carcinoma

It is not uncommon for UC with focal clear cell to change resulting from cytoplasmic glycogen accumulation. A diagnosis of clear cell (glycogen-rich) variant UC is made only when tumor shows predominant or exclusive clear cells, which is very rarely seen (Fig. 6.12). The clear cell pattern may involve in situ or invasive carcinomas. The underlying architecture is that of conventional UC, exhibiting variable morphology, from papillary to solid forms [1].

The clinical presentation and behavior do not differ from those of conventional UC. The distinction is still important, however, because of the resemblance to primary clear cell adenocarcinoma of the bladder as well as to adenocarcinoma from other sites, including renal, ovarian, and prostatic carcinomas. Clear cell adenocarcinoma of the bladder and female urethra is characterized by the formation of tubules, fine papillae, cysts, and hobnail cells, while clear cell urothelial carcinoma lacks these features. Additionally, the presence of urothelial dysplasia in sections of mucosa adjacent to the clear cell tumor suggests that the tumor is a UC and not adenocarcinoma. Immunohistochemistry can be helpful in differentiating clear cell UC from some forms of adenocarcinoma. The former typically shows immunophenotype similar to conventional UC (positive for CK7, CK20, S100P, p63, and GATA3) [28].

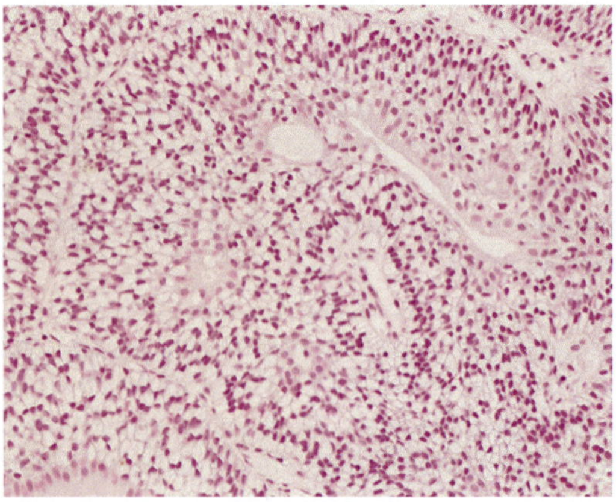

Fig. 6.12 Clear cell urothelial carcinoma

Lipid-Rich Urothelial Carcinoma

This is another very rare variant UC characterized by the presence of large cells containing large or multiple clear vacuoles exhibiting lipoblast-like cells and resembling liposarcoma (Fig. 6.13) [1]. It is usually associated with high-grade conventional UC, and the lipid-rich area comprises from less than 10% to up to 50%. Because of its rarity and the tumor cells' appearance, the lipoid cell variant may be misdiagnosed and must be distinguished from liposarcoma or signet ring cell carcinoma. Immunohistochemical staining showed that the lipid cell component was positive for CK7, CK20, CAM 5.2, HMWK, AE1/AE3, EMA, and thrombomodulin; vimentin and S100P were negative. A multi-institutional study of 27 patients showed that the lipoid cell variant of UC was associated with an aggressive behavior and a poor prognosis [65, 66].

New Variants of Urothelial Carcinoma

There are several recently proposed variants of UC not included in the current WHO classification. These include:

- *Pseudoangiosarcomatous variant of urothelial carcinoma* is characterized by tumor cell discohesion (acantholytic) that creates pseudolumina formations surrounded by attached residual tumor cells. The tumor is frequently associated with a dense variable collagen matrix. It is rare and usually accompanied by other UC variants. The neoplastic cells were found to be positive for GATA3 and cytokeratin 7, whereas CD34, CD31, and vimentin were negative [67, 68].
- *Urothelial carcinoma with chordoid or myxoid/mucinous stroma* is a unique subtype of UC showing extensive mucinous myxoid stroma and chordoid-like appearance with prominent cellular cording in a myxoid matrix, a pattern that may resemble extraskeletal myxoid chondrosarcoma, myoepithelioma, chordoma, or yolk sac tumor (Fig. 6.14). These carcinomas usually present with high-stage disease but maintain an immunophenotype of urothelial lineage. An unusual feature for this variant is the presence of invasive low-grade UC or associated low-grade papillary UC in approximately 50% of the cases [69, 70].
- ***Urothelial carcinoma with rhabdoid features*** is characterized by large and round or oval tumor cells with abundant cytoplasm, containing eosinophilic bodies that are composed of intermediate filaments. Most tumors have features of conventional UC at least focally and are characterized by an aggressive clinical course, with survival averaging around 5 months. Some authors classified it as undifferentiated carcinoma and found that loss of

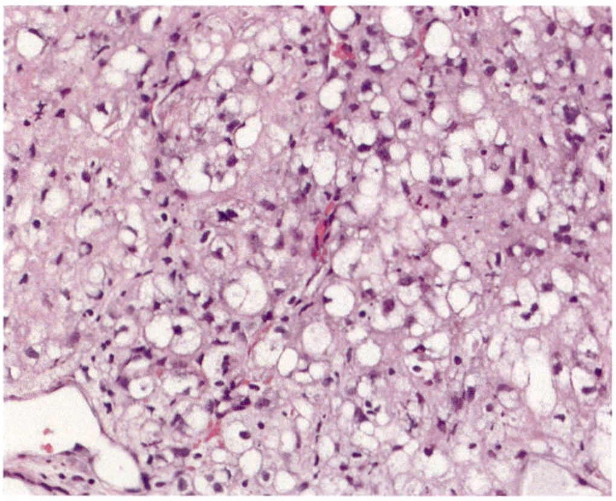

Fig. 6.13 Lipid-rich urothelial carcinoma exhibiting lipoblast-like cells and resembling liposarcoma

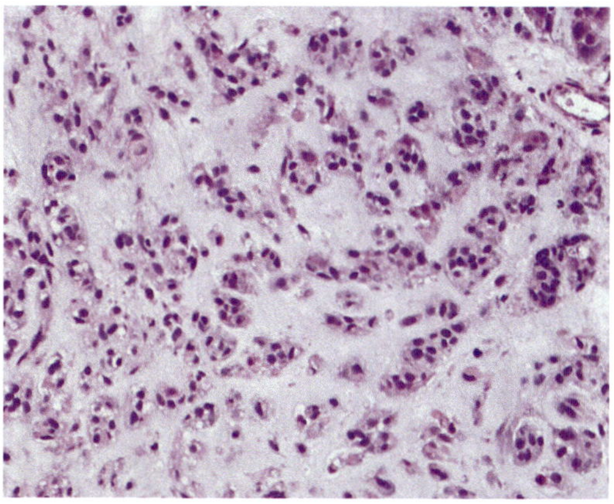

Fig. 6.14 Urothelial carcinoma with chordoid stroma mimicking chordoma

expression of the SWI/SNF complex is a frequent event in this type of tumors [71–73].

Neuroendocrine carcinoma includes small cell carcinoma and large cell neuroendocrine carcinoma, which are discussed in Chap. 9.

Summary

We have reviewed the morphological features of the variants of infiltrating UC and also highlighted major differential diagnoses for each variant, as well as the diagnostic pearls and pitfalls. It is important to recognize these variants in our daily practice that may impact clinical management and patient prognosis evaluation.

References

1. Moch H, Humphrey PA, Ulbright TM, Reuter V. WHO classification of tumors of the urinary system and male genital organs. Lyon: International Agency for Research on Cancer; 2016.
2. Krasnow RE, Drumm M, Roberts HJ, Niemierko A, Wu CL, Wu S, Zhang J, Heney NM, Wszolek MF, Blute ML, Feldman AS, Lee RJ, Zietman AL, Shipley WU, Efstathiou JA. Clinical outcomes of patients with histologic variants of urothelial Cancer treated with Trimodality bladder-sparing therapy. Eur Urol. 2017 Jul;72(1):54–60.
3. Zargar-Shoshtari K, Sverrisson EF, Sharma P, et al. Clinical outcomes after neoadjuvant chemotherapy and radical cystectomy in the presence of urothelial carcinoma of the bladder with squamous or glandular differentiation. Clin Genitourin Cancer. 2016;14:82–8.
4. Gofrit ON, Yutkin V, Shapiro A, et al. The response of variant histology bladder cancer to intravesical immunotherapy compared to conventional cancer. Front Oncol. 2016;15:43.
5. Wasco MJ, Daignault S, Zhang Y, Kunju LP, Kinnaman M, Braun T, Lee CT, Shah RB. Urothelial carcinoma with divergent histologic differentiation (mixed histologic features) predicts the presence of locally advanced bladder cancer when detected at transurethral resection. Urology. 2007 Jul;70(1):69–74.
6. Gulmann C, Paner GP, Parakh RS, et al. Immunohistochemical profile to distinguish urothelial from squamous differentiation in carcinomas of urothelial tract. Hum Pathol. 2013;44:164–72.
7. Alexander RE, Hu YC, Kum JB, et al. p16 expression is not associated with human papillomavirus in urinary bladder squamous cell carcinoma. Mod Pathol. 2012;25:1526–33.
8. Liu Y, Bui MM, Xu B. Urothelial carcinoma with squamous differentiation is associated with high tumor stage and pelvic lymph-node metastasis. Cancer Control. 2017;24:78–82.
9. Martin JE, Jenkins BJ, Zuk RJ, Blandy JP, Baithun SI. Clinical importance of squamous metaplasia in invasive transitional cell carcinoma of the bladder. J Clin Pathol. 1989;42:250–3.
10. Logothetis CJ, Dexeus FH, Chong C, Sella A, Ayala AG, Ro JY, Pilat S. Cisplatin, cyclophosphamide and doxorubicin chemotherapy for unresectable urothelial tumors: the M.D. Anderson experience. J Urol. 1989 Jan;141(1):33–7.
11. Choi W, Porten S, Kim S, Willis D, Plimack ER, Hoffman-Censits J, Roth B, Cheng T, Tran M, Lee IL, Melquist J, Bondaruk J, Majewski T, Zhang S, Pretzsch S, Baggerly K, Siefker-Radtke A, Czerniak B, Dinney CP, McConkey DJ. Identification of distinct basal and luminal subtypes of muscle-invasive bladder cancer with different sensitivities to frontline chemotherapy. Cancer Cell. 2014 Feb 10;25(2):152–65.
12. McConkey DJ, Choi W, Shen Y, Lee IL, Porten S, Matin SF, Kamat AM, Corn P, Millikan RE, Dinney C, Czerniak B, Siefker-Radtke AO. A prognostic gene expression signature in the molecular classification of chemotherapy-naïve urothelial Cancer is predictive of clinical outcomes from neoadjuvant chemotherapy: a phase 2 trial of dose-dense methotrexate, vinblastine, doxorubicin, and cisplatin with bevacizumab in urothelial Cancer. Eur Urol. 2016 May;69(5):855–62.
13. Wasco MJ, Daignault S, Zhang Y, et al. Urothelial carcinoma with divergent histologic differentiation (mixed histologic features) predicts the presence of locally advanced bladder cancer when detected at transurethral resection. Urology. 2007;70:69–74.
14. Kim SP, Frank I, Cheville JC, et al. The impact of squamous and glandular differentiation on survival after radical cystectomy for urothelial carcinoma. J Urol. 2012;188:405–9.
15. Kunze E, Francksen B, Schulz H. Expression of MUC5AC apomucin in transitional cell carcinomas of the urinary bladder and its possible role in the development of mucus-secreting adenocarcinomas. Virchows Arch. 2001;439:609–15.
16. Vail E, Zheng X, Zhou M, et al. Telomerase reverse transcriptase promoter mutations in glandular lesions of the urinary bladder. Ann Diagn Pathol. 2015;19:301–5.
17. Martin JE, Jenkins BJ, Zuk RJ, et al. Human chorionic gonadotrophin expression and histological findings as predictors of response to radiotherapy in carcinoma of the bladder. Virchows Arch A Pathol Anat Histopathol. 1989;414:273–7.
18. Grammatico D, Grignon DJ, Eberwein P, Shepherd RR, Hearn SA, Walton JC. Transitional cell carcinoma of the renal pelvis with choriocarcinomatous differentiation. Immunohistochemical and immunoelectron microscopic assessment of human chorionic gonado-

tropin production by transitional cell carcinoma of the urinary bladder. Cancer. 1993 Mar 1;71(5):1835–41.
19. Monn MF, Jaqua KR, Bihrle R, Cheng L. Primary choriocarcinoma of the bladder: a case report and review of literature. Clin Genitourin Cancer. 2017;15:188–91.
20. Young RH, Eble JN. Unusual forms of carcinoma of the urinary bladder. Hum Pathol. 1991;22:948–65.
21. Lopez-Beltran A, Henriques V, Montironi R, Cimadamore A, Raspollini MR, Cheng L. Variants and new entities of bladder cancer. Histopathology. 2019 Jan;74(1):77–96.
22. Drew PA, Furman J, Civantos F, Murphy WM. The nested variant of transitional cell carcinoma: an aggressive neoplasm with innocuous histology. Mod Pathol. 1996;9:989–94.
23. Lopez Beltran A, Cheng L, Montironi R, et al. Clinicopathological characteristics and outcome of nested carcinoma of the urinary bladder. Virchows Arch. 2014;465:199–205.
24. Linder BJ, Frank I, Cheville JC, Thompson RH, Thapa P, Tarrell RF, Boorjian SA. Outcomes following radical cystectomy for nested variant of urothelial carcinoma: a matched cohort analysis. J Urol. 2013 May;189(5):1670–5.
25. Mally AD, Tin AL, Lee JK, Satasivam P, Cha EK, Donat SM, Herr HW, Bochner BH, Sjoberg DD, Dalbagni G. Clinical outcomes of patients with T1 nested variant of urothelial carcinoma compared to pure urothelial carcinoma of the bladder. Clin Genitourin Cancer. 2017 Jul;14. S1558-7673(17)30199-4
26. Oberg TN, Kipp BR, Campion MB, Voss JS, Jimenez RE, Sebo TJ, Cheville JC, Halling KC, Zhou M, Zhang J. Utilization of FISH to distinguish urothelial carcinoma with nested variant growth pattern from von Brunn's nests. Mod Pathol. 2010;23(Suppl 1):934.
27. Zhong M, Tian W, Zhuge J, Zheng X, Huang T, Cai D, Zhang D, Yang XJ, Argani P, Fallon JT, Epstein JI. Distinguishing nested variants of urothelial carcinoma from benign mimickers by TERT promoter mutation. Am J Surg Pathol. 2015 Jan;39(1):127–31.
28. Paner GP, Annaiah C, Gulmann C, Rao P, Ro JY, Hansel DE, Shen SS, Lopez-Beltran A, Aron M, Luthringer DJ, De Peralta-Venturina M, Cho Y, Amin MB. Immunohistochemical evaluation of novel and traditional markers associated with urothelial differentiation in a spectrum of variants of urothelial carcinoma of the urinary bladder. Hum Pathol. 2014 Jul;45(7):1473–82.
29. Lopez Beltran A, Montironi R, Cheng L. Microcystic urothelial carcinoma: morphology, immunohistochemistry and clinical behaviour. Histopathology. 2014 May;64(6):872–9.
30. Amin MB, Ro JY, el-Sharkawy T, Lee KM, Troncoso P, Silva EG, Ordóñez NG, Ayala AG. Micropapillary variant of transitional cell carcinoma of the urinary bladder. Histologic pattern resembling ovarian papillary serous carcinoma. Am J Surg Pathol. 1994 Dec;18(12):1224–32.
31. Sangoi AR, Higgins JP, Rouse RV, Schneider AG, McKenney JK. Immunohistochemical comparison of MUC1, CA125, and Her2Neu in invasive micropapillary carcinoma of the urinary tract and typical invasive urothelial carcinoma with retraction artifact. Mod Pathol. 2009 May;22(5):660–7.
32. Lopez-Beltran A, Montironi R, Blanca A, Cheng L. Invasive micropapillary urothelial carcinoma of the bladder. Hum Pathol. 2010 Aug;41(8):1159–64.
33. Wang JK, Boorjian SA, Cheville JC, Kim SP, Tarrell RF, Thapa P, Frank I. Outcomes following radical cystectomy for micropapillary bladder cancer versus pure urothelial carcinoma: a matched cohort analysis. World J Urol. 2012 Dec;30(6):801–6.
34. Spaliviero M, Dalbagni G, Bochner BH, Poon BY, Huang H, Al-Ahmadie HA, Donahue TF, Taylor JM, Meeks JJ, Sjoberg DD, Donat SM, Reuter VE, Herr HW. Clinical outcome of patients with T1 micropapillary urothelial carcinoma of the bladder. J Urol. 2014 Sep;192(3):702–7.
35. Willis DL, Fernandez MI, Dickstein RJ, Parikh S, Shah JB, Pisters LL, Guo CC, Henderson S, Czerniak BA, Grossman HB, Dinney CP, Kamat AM. Clinical outcomes of cT1 micropapillary bladder cancer. J Urol. 2015 Apr;193(4):1129–34.
36. Amin A, Epstein JI. Noninvasive micropapillary urothelial carcinoma: a clinicopathologic study of 18 cases. Hum Pathol. 2012 Dec;43(12):2124–8.
37. Ching CB, Amin MB, Tubbs RR, Elson P, Platt E, Dreicer R, Fergany A, Hansel DE. HER2 gene amplification occurs frequently in the micropapillary variant of urothelial carcinoma: analysis by dual-color in situ hybridization. Mod Pathol. 2011 Aug;24(8):1111–9.
38. Schneider SA, Sukov WR, Frank I, Boorjian SA, Costello BA, Tarrell RF, Thapa P, Houston Thompson R, Tollefson MK, Jeffrey Karnes R, Cheville JC. Outcome of patients with micropapillary urothelial carcinoma following radical cystectomy: ERBB2 (HER2) amplification identifies patients with poor outcome. Mod Pathol. 2014 May;27(5):758–64.
39. Guo CC, Dadhania V, Zhang L, Majewski T, Bondaruk J, Sykulski M, Wronowska W, Gambin A, Wang Y, Zhang S, Fuentes-Mattei E, Kamat AM, Dinney C, Siefker-Radtke A, Choi W, Baggerly KA, McConkey D, Weinstein JN, Czerniak B. Gene expression profile of the clinically aggressive micropapillary variant of bladder cancer. Eur Urol. 2016 Oct;70(4):611–20.
40. Gulley ML, Amin MB, Nicholls JM, Banks PM, Ayala AG, Srigley JR, Eagan PA, Ro JY. Epstein-Barr virus is detected in undifferentiated nasopharyngeal carcinoma but not in lymphoepithelioma-like carcinoma of the urinary bladder. Hum Pathol. 1995 Nov;26(11):1207–14.
41. Lopez-Beltrán A, Luque RJ, Vicioso L, Anglada F, Requena MJ, Quintero A, Montironi R. Lymphoepithelioma-like carcinoma of the urinary bladder: a clinicopathologic study of 13 cases. Virchows Arch. 2001 Jun;438(6):552–7.
42. Tamas EF, Nielsen ME, Schoenberg MP, Epstein JI. Lymphoepithelioma-like carcinoma of the uri-

nary tract: a clinicopathological study of 30 pure and mixed cases. Mod Pathol. 2007 Aug;20(8):828–34.
43. Yoshino T, Ohara S, Moriyama H. Lymphoepithelioma-like carcinoma of the urinary bladder: a case report and review of the literature. BMC Res Notes. 2014 Nov 4;7:779. https://doi.org/10.1186/1756-0500-7-779.
44. Dinney CP, Ro JY, Babaian RJ, Johnson DE. Lymphoepithelioma of the bladder: a clinicopathological study of 3 cases. J Urol. 1993 Apr;149(4):840–1.
45. Amin MB, Ro JY, Lee KM, Ordóñez NG, Dinney CP, Gulley ML, Ayala AG. Lymphoepithelioma-like carcinoma of the urinary bladder. Am J Surg Pathol. 1994 May;18(5):466–73.
46. Manocha U, Kardos J, Selitsky S, Zhou M, Johnson SM, Breslauer C, Epstein JI, Kim WY, Wobker SE. RNA expression profiling of Lymphoepithelioma-like carcinoma of the bladder reveals a basal-like molecular subtype. Am J Pathol. 2020 Jan;190(1):134–44.
47. Ro JY, Shen SS, Lee HI, Hong EK, Lee YH, Cho NH, Jung SJ, Choi YJ, Ayala AG. Plasmacytoid transitional cell carcinoma of urinary bladder: a clinicopathologic study of 9 cases. Am J Surg Pathol. 2008 May;32(5):752–7.
48. Nigwekar P, Tamboli P, Amin MB, Osunkoya AO, Ben-Dor D, Amin MB. Plasmacytoid urothelial carcinoma: detailed analysis of morphology with clinicopathologic correlation in 17 cases. Am J Surg Pathol. 2009 Mar;33(3):417–24.
49. Keck B, Stoehr R, Wach S, Rogler A, Hofstaedter F, Lehmann J, Montironi R, Sibonye M, Fritsche HM, Lopez-Beltran A, Epstein JI, Wullich B, Hartmann A. The plasmacytoid carcinoma of the bladder – rare variant of aggressive urothelial carcinoma. Int J Cancer. 2011 Jul 15;129(2):346–54.
50. Fox MD, Xiao L, Zhang M, Kamat AM, Siefker-Radtke A, Zhang L, Dinney CP, Czerniak B, Guo CC. Plasmacytoid urothelial carcinoma of the urinary bladder: a clinicopathologic and immunohistochemical analysis of 49 cases. Am J Clin Pathol. 2017 May 1;147(5):500–6.
51. Keck B, Wach S, Kunath F, Bertz S, Taubert H, Lehmann J, Stöckle M, Wullich B, Hartmann A. Nuclear E-cadherin expression is associated with the loss of membranous E-cadherin, plasmacytoid differentiation and reduced overall survival in urothelial carcinoma of the bladder. Ann Surg Oncol. 2013 Jul;20(7):2440–5.
52. Al-Ahmadie HA, Iyer G, Lee BH, Scott SN, Mehra R, Bagrodia A, Jordan EJ, Gao SP, Ramirez R, Cha EK, Desai NB, Zabor EC, Ostrovnaya I, Gopalan A, Chen YB, Fine SW, Tickoo SK, Gandhi A, Hreiki J, Viale A, Arcila ME, Dalbagni G, Rosenberg JE, Bochner BH, Bajorin DF, Berger MF, Reuter VE, Taylor BS, Solit DB. Frequent somatic CDH1 loss-of-function mutations in plasmacytoid variant bladder cancer. Nat Genet. 2016 Apr;48(4):356–8.
53. Borhan WM, Cimino-Mathews AM, Montgomery EA, Epstein JI. Immunohistochemical differentiation of plasmacytoid urothelial carcinoma from secondary carcinoma involvement of the bladder. Am J Surg Pathol. 2017 Nov;41(11):1570–5.
54. Kim DK, Kim JW, Ro JY, Lee HS, Park JY, Ahn HK, Lee JY, Cho KS. Plasmacytoid variant urothelial carcinoma of the bladder: a systematic review and meta-analysis of clinicopathological features and survival outcomes. J Urol. 2020 Aug;204(2):215–23.
55. Dayyani F, Czerniak BA, Sircar K, Munsell MF, Millikan RE, Dinney CP, Siefker-Radtke AO. Plasmacytoid urothelial carcinoma, a chemosensitive cancer with poor prognosis, and peritoneal carcinomatosis. J Urol. 2013 May;189(5):1656–61.
56. Lopez-Beltran A, Blanca A, Montironi R, Cheng L, Regueiro JC. Pleomorphic giant cell carcinoma of the urinary bladder. Hum Pathol. 2009 Oct;40(10):1461–6.
57. Samaratunga H, Delahunt B, Egevad L, Adamson M, Hussey D, Malone G, Hoyle K, Nathan T, Kerle D, Ferguson P, Nacey JN. Pleomorphic giant cell carcinoma of the urinary bladder: an extreme form of tumour de-differentiation. Histopathology. 2016 Mar;68(4):533–40.
58. Cheng L, Zhang S, Alexander R, Maclennan GT, Hodges KB, Harrison BT, Lopez-Beltran A, Montironi R. Sarcomatoid carcinoma of the urinary bladder: the final common pathway of urothelial carcinoma dedifferentiation. Am J Surg Pathol. 2011 May;35(5):e34–46.
59. Sanfrancesco J, McKenney JK, Leivo MZ, Gupta S, Elson P, Hansel DE. Sarcomatoid urothelial carcinoma of the bladder: analysis of 28 cases with emphasis on clinicopathologic features and markers of epithelial-to-mesenchymal transition. Arch Pathol Lab Med. 2016 Jun;140(6):543–51.
60. Chang A, Brimo F, Montgomery EA, Epstein JI. Use of PAX8 and GATA3 in diagnosing sarcomatoid renal cell carcinoma and sarcomatoid urothelial carcinoma. Hum Pathol. 2013 Aug;44(8):1563–8.
61. Lopez-Beltran A, Luque RJ, Mazzucchelli R, Scarpelli M, Montironi R. Changes produced in the urothelium by traditional and newer therapeutic procedures for bladder cancer. J Clin Pathol. 2002;55:641–7.
62. Jones EC, Young RH. Myxoid and sclerosing sarcomatoid transitional cell carcinoma of the urinary bladder: a clinicopathologic and immunohistochemical study of 25 cases. Mod Pathol. 1997;10:908–16.
63. Baydar D, Amin MB, Epstein JI. Osteoclast-rich undifferentiated carcinomas of the urinary tract. Mod Pathol. 2006;19:161–71.
64. Priore SF, Schwartz LE, Epstein JI. An expanded immunohistochemical profile of osteoclast-rich undifferentiated carcinoma of the urinary tract. Mod Pathol. 2018 Jun;31(6):984–8.
65. Leroy X, Gonzalez S, Zini L, Aubert S. Lipoid-cell variant of urothelial carcinoma: a clinicopathologic and immunohistochemical study of five cases. Am J Surg Pathol. 2007 May;31(5):770–3.
66. Lopez-Beltran A, Amin MB, Oliveira PS, Montironi R, Algaba F, McKenney JK, de Torres I, Mazerolles C, Wang M, Cheng L. Urothelial carcinoma of the bladder,

lipid cell variant: clinicopathologic findings and LOH analysis. Am J Surg Pathol. 2010 Mar;34(3):371–6.
67. Paner GP, Cox RM, Richards K, Akki A, Gokden N, Lopez-Beltran A, Krausz T, McKenney JK, Steinberg GD. Pseudoangiosarcomatous urothelial carcinoma of the urinary bladder. Am J Surg Pathol. 2014 Sep;38(9):1251–9.
68. Yıldız P, Behzatoğlu K, Hacıhasanoğlu E, Okcu O, Durak H, Yücetaş U. Histological, immunohistochemical features and pathogenesis of pseudoangiosarcomatous urothelial carcinoma. Ann Diagn Pathol. 2017 Oct;30:17–20.
69. Cox RM, Schneider AG, Sangoi AR, Clingan WJ, Gokden N, McKenney JK. Invasive urothelial carcinoma with chordoid features: a report of 12 distinct cases characterized by prominent myxoid stroma and cordlike epithelial architecture. Am J Surg Pathol. 2009 Aug;33(8):1213–9.
70. Tavora F, Epstein JI. Urothelial carcinoma with abundant myxoid stroma. Hum Pathol. 2009 Oct;40(10):1391–8.
71. Kumar S, Kumar D, Cowan DF. Transitional cell carcinoma with rhabdoid features. Am J Surg Pathol. 1992;16:515–21.
72. Parwani AV, Herawi M, Volmar K, Tsay SH, Epstein JI. Urothelial carcinoma with rhabdoid features: report of 6 cases. Hum Pathol. 2006;37:168–72.
73. Agaimy A, Bertz S, Cheng L, Hes O, Junker K, Keck B, Lopez-Beltran A, Stöckle M, Wullich B, Hartmann A. Loss of expression of the SWI/SNF complex is a frequent event in undifferentiated/dedifferentiated urothelial carcinoma of the urinary tract. Virchows Arch. 2016 Sep;469(3):321–30.

Other Types of Carcinoma

7

Kosuke Miyai, Hussam Abu-Farsakh, and Jae Y. Ro

Squamous Cell Carcinoma

Introduction

The 2016 World Health Organization (WHO) classification defines urinary bladder squamous cell carcinoma (SCC) as a carcinoma derived from the urothelium with a histologically pure squamous cell phenotype [1]. Therefore, if elements of an invasive or noninvasive urothelial carcinoma (UC) are present, the tumor should be classified as urothelial carcinoma with squamous differentiation. Although there are several potential etiologic factors, such as prolonged catheterization and smoking, which lead to the development of urinary bladder SCC, the most significant factor is chronic bilharzial infection. In Western countries where bilharzial infection is not endemic, pure SCC is an uncommon variant of urinary bladder cancer. In contrast, urinary bladder SCC is the most prevalent histological type of bladder cancer in the Middle Eastern and African countries, where its pathogenesis is linked to an endemic, chronic bilharzial infection. A comparison between non-bilharzial and bilharzial SCC is summarized in Table 7.1.

Epidemiology

Primary SCC in non-bilharzial urinary bladder is uncommon. In Western countries, pure SCC of the bladder represents 2.1–6.7% of all bladder malignancies [2–5]. The tumors are most often diagnosed in the seventh decade [2, 3, 5]. The male-to-female ratio for non-bilharzial SCC is slightly lower than that reported for UC and varies from 1.3:1 to 1.8:1 [2–4].

The incidence of bilharzial bladder SCC is highest in Egypt, yet other countries, including Iraq, parts of Saudi Arabia, Yemen, and Sudan, also share a high incidence of this cancer type. In an earlier case series reported by Ghoneim et al., SCC accounts for 608 (59%) of 1026 cystectomy specimens collected in Egypt over a 21-year span [6]. However, a more recent report from Egypt has indicated that UC is currently more common than SCC, which corresponds to a decrease in bilharziasis incidence [7]. The male-to-female ratio is 5:1, and patients with bilharzial SCC are on an average 10–20 years younger than those diagnosed with non-bilharzial SCC, which is

K. Miyai (✉)
National Defense Medical College, Department of Basic Pathology, Saitama, Japan
e-mail: mykusu228@nifty.com

H. Abu-Farsakh
Department of Pathology, First Medical Lab, Amman, Jordan

J. Y. Ro
Department of Pathology and Genomic Medicine, Weill Medical College of Cornell University/Houston Methodist Hospital, Houston, TX, USA
e-mail: JaeRo@houstonmethodist.org

H. Zhou et al. (eds.), *Urinary Bladder Pathology*, https://doi.org/10.1007/978-3-030-71509-0_7

Table 7.1 Comparison between non-bilharzial and bilharzial SCC of the urinary bladder [4]

Features	Non-bilharzial SCC	Bilharzial SCC
Epidemiology, causes, and clinical findings		
Geographical distribution	Western countries	Middle East, Africa, Southeast Asia, South America
% in all bladder malignancies	2.1–6.7%	59%
Age	Seventh decade	Fifth decade
Male/female	1.3–1.8:1	5:1
Principal predisposing factor	Prolonged catheterization in patients with spinal cord injury	Bacterial infections associated with bilharziasis
Principal symptom	Hematuria	Irritative bladder
Pathological findings		
Commonest gross feature	Ulcerative	Nodular
Predominant site	Lower part of the bladder	Upper part of the bladder
Differentiation	Most are moderately to poorly differentiated	Most are well to moderately differentiated
Stage	Most are advanced	Most are advanced
Nodal involvement	8–10%	15–20%
Treatment and prognosis		
Standard treatment	Radical cystectomy	Radical cystectomy
5-year survival	50–55%	43–57%

SCC, squamous cell carcinoma

most likely related to an increased occupational bilharzial exposure in men who work in the fields infested with these parasites [8, 9].

Etiology

In the United States, SCC of the bladder often occurs in patients with a spinal cord injury who are subjected to prolonged placement of indwelling catheters [10]. In these patients, diagnosis of non-bilharzial SCC is linked to bladder inflammation caused by chronic urinary tract irritation from bacterial infections, foreign bodies, bladder calculi, or chronic bladder outlet obstructions. These recent studies reveal that the declining bladder cancer incidence may be associated with a change in catheterization procedures from chronic indwelling catheters to clean intermittent catheterization [11]. In addition to catheterization-associated bladder SCC, there are several other potential causes that give rise to this cancer. There has been one case report of an SCC of the bladder diagnosed consequently to intravesical immunotherapy with bacillus Calmette-Guérin (BCG) in a patient with preexisting squamous dysplasia [12].

Bilharzial SCC carcinogenesis is most likely related to the secondary bacterial infections that accompany bilharzial infestation, rather than the parasite itself. This chronic bacterial infection has two distinct sequelae: (1) nitrates and secondary amines in the urine are reduced to carcinogenic nitrosamines through bacterial catalysis, and (2) bacterial infection is implicated in the secretion of the β-glucuronidase enzyme, which may split conjugated carcinogens to yield free carcinogenic products [13, 14]. These carcinogens then act upon the mucosal epithelial cells of the bladder, resulting in irreversible and potentially carcinogenic changes in the DNA. Additionally, mechanical irritation and inflammation of the bladder caused by the parasite's eggs also appears to be an important tumor-promoting factor [7]. Finally, other contributing factors include liver dysfunction, vitamin A and B deficiency, smoking, chronic irritation due to urinary calculi, and exposure to pesticides [7, 14].

Clinical Features

Principal clinical features of non-bilharzial urinary bladder SCC are similar to those of UC. Hematuria is the most common symptom, seen in 63–100% of patients, and irritative bladder symptoms are seen in two-thirds of these patients. Weight loss, back or pelvic pain, and obstructive symptoms are often suggestive of advanced disease, seen in one-third of patients [2, 3]. At diagnosis, most patients have no previous history of urologic tumors. Finally, the tumor may occupy a diverticulum, and its relationship with bladder calculi has been well described [2, 3].

The clinical presentations of bilharzial SCC are similar to those of chronic cystitis: frequent and painful micturition, hematuria, suprapubic pain, and pyuria [8, 15]. Consequently, symptoms of regular bilharzial cystitis and early SCC significantly overlap, leading to a delay in cancer diagnosis. Therefore, almost all patients with SCC have at least some degree of muscle-invasive disease, and 25–30% of the patients are clinically inoperable at the time of diagnosis [8, 15].

Pathological Features

In terms of gross findings, non-bilharzial SCCs of the bladder are not much different from UC and tend to be ulcerated, infiltrating, and unifocal at the time of diagnosis (Fig. 7.1a), while 60–80% of the bilharzial SCC cases appear as nodular fungating tumors [8, 16]. In a study of 114 patients with non-bilharzial SCC, a predilection for the trigone and lateral wall has been recorded, occurring in 56 and 99 patients (including those with multiple tumors), respectively [3]. The tumor usually arises from the upper part of the urinary bladder at the posterior/lateral wall or vault. In contrast to the non-bilharzial SCC, trigonal tumors are rare. The cut surface usually demonstrates a firm, white tumor that spans the entire wall of the bladder, lamina propria, muscularis propria, and perivesical fat, and sometimes extends to adjacent organs (Fig. 7.1b).

Regardless of the existence of bilharzia, the histological hallmarks of bladder SCCs are polygonal tumors cells with individual keratinization or group keratinization (keratin-pearl formation), intercellular bridges, and keratotic cellular debris. Well-differentiated SCCs show tumor nests with marked squamous differentiation (Fig. 7.2a). In moderately differentiated SCCs, nests are more irregular in outline, and keratotic foci are smaller (Fig. 7.2b). Poorly differentiated SCCs consist of even smaller infiltrative nests, cords, trabeculae, or isolated anaplastic cells (Fig. 7.2c). Tumor necrosis is frequently seen and appears to inversely correlate with tumor differentiation. Keratinization of cells at the stromal interface is a sign of invasion. Most non-bilharzial SCCs are moderately to poorly differentiated, and well-differentiated SCCs comprise less than 10% of all cases [17]. In contrast to non-bilharzial SCC, almost half of the bilharzial SCCs are well-differentiated and show abundant keratinization with keratin pearl formation. Of the remaining tumors, 30–40% and 10–20% are moderately and poorly differentiated, respectively [8, 15, 16]. As shown in Fig. 7.2d, almost all of the bilharzial SCC specimens show histological evidence of bilharzial infection [8]. Active bilharzial granulomas are observed in 10% of the cases, although mature worms of *Schistosoma* species are rarely seen inside veins.

Both bilharzial and non-bilharzial SCCs are usually diagnosed at a muscle-invasive stage

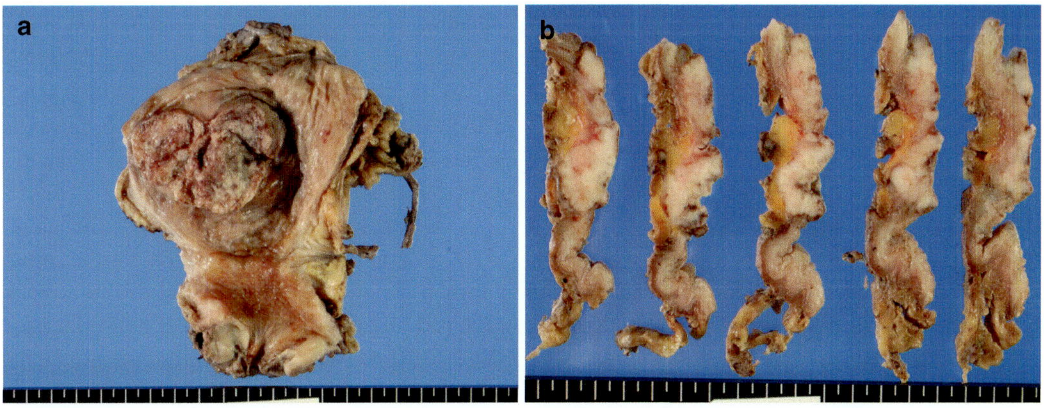

Fig. 7.1 Gross appearance (**a**) and cut surface (**b**) of squamous cell carcinoma of the urinary bladder

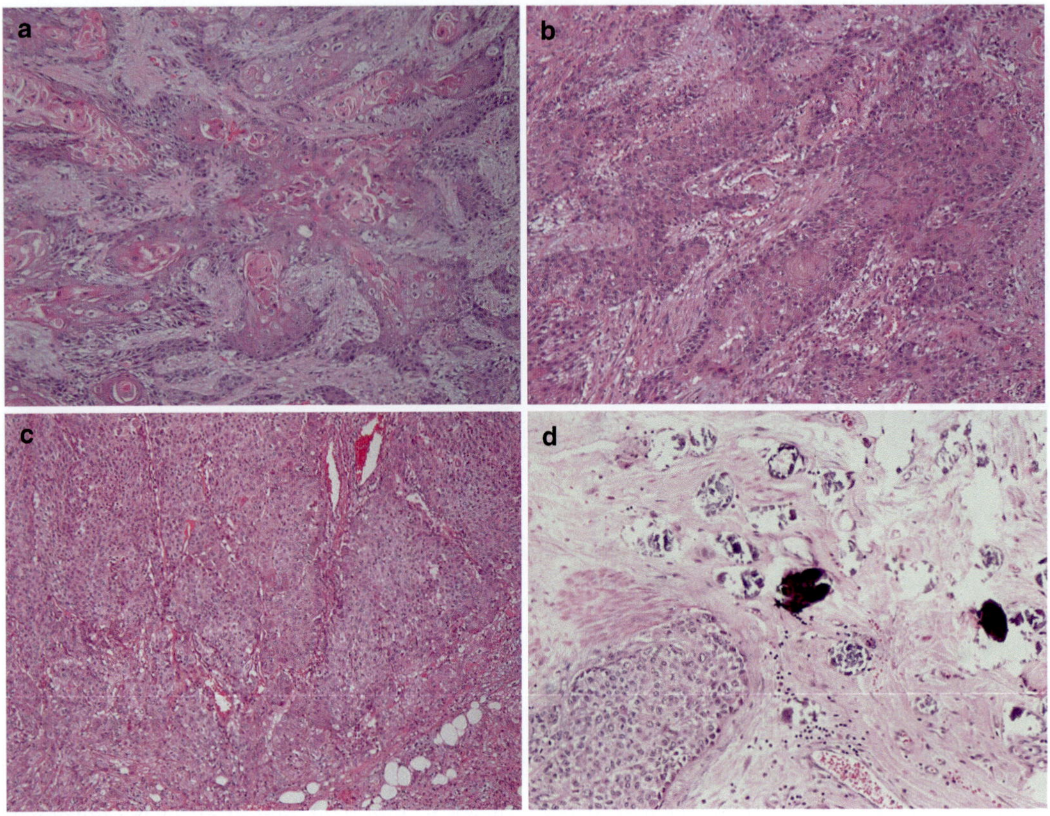

Fig. 7.2 Squamous cell carcinoma of the urinary bladder. Well-differentiated (**a**), moderately differentiated (**b**), and poorly differentiated (**c**) squamous cell carcinoma. (**d**) Bilharzial squamous cell carcinoma of the urinary bladder showing poorly differentiated features and ova of *Schistosoma* species. (Original magnification: **a**–**c**, x200; **d**, x100)

[18, 19]. Compared to pathological staging, clinical understaging has been reported in 30–60% of the cases [8, 19–21]. Importantly, in spite of the advanced T stages, the incidence of lymph node metastasis is relatively lower, in the order of 15–25% [8, 15–17, 19]. In addition, when compared to UC, SCC has a lower incidence of distant metastasis which is estimated to be present in 8–10% of all cases [1, 22].

Molecular and Genetic Aspects

The molecular data for SCC of the bladder has been compiled based mostly on the bilharziasis-associated cohort analysis. Several cytogenetic and classic molecular studies have showed gains of chromosomal material predominantly at 5p, 6p, 7p, 8q, 11q, 17q, and 20q, while losses are most frequent at 3p, 4q, 5q, 8p, 13q, 17p, and 18q [23–25]. Classic cytogenetics and comparative genomic hybridization (CGH) have been performed in only a few non-bilharzial SCC cases [26, 27]. Results of a single CGH study of 11 non-bilharzial SCCs show that the predominant chromosomal changes are gains at 1q, 8q, and 20q, as well as losses of 3p, 9p, and 13q [26]. With respect to the differences between SCC and UC, loss of 3p has been demonstrated as a relatively specific genetic aberration for SCC [26, 27].

In a recent mutational analysis for *TERT* gene, *TERT* promoter mutation, which is the most common genetic alteration in UC of the urinary tract, is detected in 12/15 (80%) of non-bilharzial SCCs [28]. As with UC, p53 immunopositivity and gene mutation have been observed in a wide range of bilharzial SCCs [29–31]. Specifically, *TP53* mutations in bilharzial SCC include more base transitions at CpG dinucleotides than those seen in UCs [30]. Other molecular aberrations known to occur in UCs, including *HRAS* mutations, EGFR overexpression, and HER2 expression, have also been detected in bilharzial SCC at comparable frequencies [31–33].

Treatment and Prognosis

Irrespective of the bilharzial status, there are few treatment options available for patients diagnosed with bladder SCC. In most cases, radical cystoprostatectomy or radical cystectomy is recommended as the only viable therapeutic approach, as radiation and chemotherapy offer limited therapeutic benefits [34, 35]. Consequently, the 5-year disease-free survival rate following a radical cystectomy is 43–57%, with poor prognosis attributed to an advanced tumor stage and lymph node involvement at diagnosis [18, 19, 35]. Most bladder SCC patients die due to failure of locoregional tumor control: about 90% of the bladder SCC deaths are caused by a locoregional recurrence within 3 years of diagnosis. As shown by a recent study, the pathologic stage is the most important prognostic parameter for patients diagnosed with the bilharzial SCC of the bladder: in a series of 154 bilharzial SCC cases, the overall 5-year survival rate for patients with pT1 and pT2 tumors was 66.9%, compared to only 19% in those diagnosed with pT3 and pT4 tumors [36].

Histological Variants of Bladder SCC

Verrucous Carcinoma

Verrucous carcinoma is a rare, clinically indolent variant of invasive SCC, more commonly seen in the oral cavity, larynx, anus, and genital areas. Grossly, verrucous carcinoma appears as an exophytic, fungating, or filiform tumor. Microscopically, this tumor is characterized by a broad-pushing tongue-like stromal invasion by large-sized proliferations of very well-differentiated squamous epithelium, frequently associated with a dense infiltration of inflammatory cells at the interface between the atypical squamous proliferation and the underlying stroma [1]. Additionally, verrucous carcinoma tumor cells show lack of anaplastic features and frequent mitoses.

Pathologically, care should be taken to distinguish verrucous carcinomas from verrucous/pseudoepitheliomatous hyperplasia. Verrucous carcinomas exhibit a downgrowth of the well-differentiated squamous epithelium, which extends to a much wider and deeper extent than that encountered in verrucous/pseudoepitheliomatous hyperplasia. Therefore, in a superficial biopsy, the differentiation of these two conditions is almost impossible, mandating sampling of deeper tissue for a definitive distinction.

Basaloid SCC

Basaloid SCC is an aggressive and often deeply invasive neoplasm found mainly in the upper aerodigestive tract, penis, vulva, and cervix. The typical microscopic picture comprises of centrally necrotic, solid nests of small, poorly differentiated cells with scant cytoplasm resembling basal cell carcinoma, except that peripheral palisading is not conspicuous and numerous mitoses are often present. Only two cases of basaloid SCC of the bladder have been described [37, 38]. Specifically, Vakar-López et al. described a case of a 60-year-old woman with a bladder tumor that was morphologically characterized by small nests of basaloid cells with numerous mitoses [37]. However, the reported case also had microscopic foci of UC with squamous differentiation and SCC in situ. Neves et al. presented a case of the bladder basaloid SCC with a small amount (5%) of small cell carcinoma component [38]. The authors did not mention whether a concomitant UC component was detected. As seen in penile basaloid SCC, there is one case report suggesting the relationship between bladder basaloid SCC and human papilloma virus infection of the urinary tract [39].

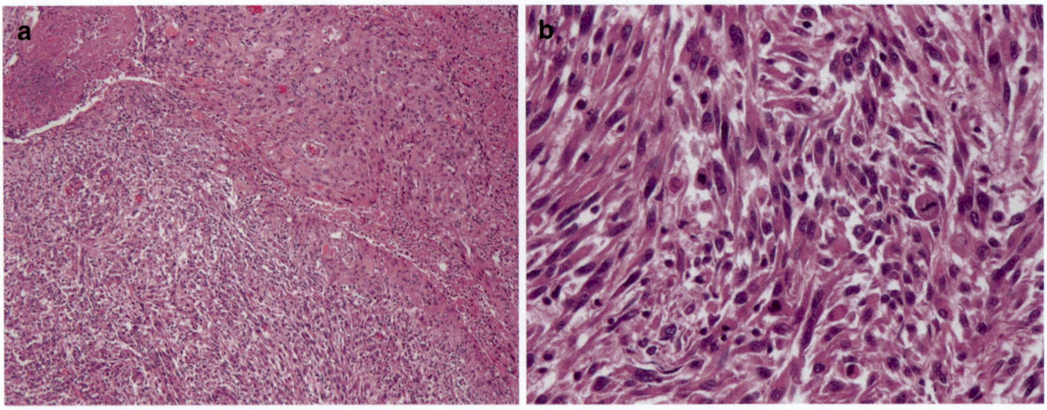

Fig. 7.3 (**a**) Sarcomatoid squamous cell carcinoma with a histological transition between typical squamous cell carcinoma (upper right) and sarcomatoid carcinoma (lower left). (**b**) Spindled tumor cells with marked cytological atypia and frequent mitoses. (Original magnification: **a**, x100; **b**, x400)

Sarcomatoid SCC

Sarcomatoid SCC is an aggressive variant of SCC predominantly composed of spindle and pleomorphic cells, with at least focal histological or immunohistochemical evidence of squamous differentiation (Fig. 7.3). In a case series of 45 bladder SCCs, 3 tumors showed a prominent focal spindled morphology [18]. However, the percentage of a sarcomatous component in comparison to the total tumor volume was not mentioned in the study. There has been a total of two reported cases of sarcomatoid carcinoma of the urinary bladder with SCC and small cell carcinoma components [40, 41].

Adenocarcinoma and Other Glandular Neoplasms

Introduction

Primary adenocarcinoma of the urinary bladder is derived from the urothelium but represents a pure glandular phenotype. Secondary adenocarcinomas involving the bladder either by direct invasion or by metastasis are more common than primary adenocarcinomas, and sometimes it may be challenging to distinguish each other, even with a comprehensive immunohistochemical study. Most urachal carcinomas are adenocarcinomas. Urachal adenocarcinoma is usually described together with bladder adenocarcinoma as they exhibit similar clinical and histological features. However, a classification system recently proposed delineates urachal glandular tumors into two broad categories: mucinous cystic tumors and non-cystic adenocarcinomas. The clinicopathological features and molecular aspects of these distinct glandular lesions are discussed in this chapter.

Primary Adenocarcinoma

Primary adenocarcinoma is an uncommon malignant neoplasm, accounting 0.5 to 2.0% of all bladder cancers. This neoplasm is usually seen in the patients' sixth decade of life with a male-to-female ratio of 2.7:1 [42]. Hematuria is the most common symptom, but some patients may present with irritative voiding symptoms and rarely mucusuria [43]. Although the pathogenesis is still unclear, several risk factors for primary bladder adenocarcinoma have been recognized, including bladder exstrophy, bilharziasis, cystocele, and bladder endometriosis [42].

There is no specific gross finding of primary bladder adenocarcinoma, except for a gelatinous appearance on cut surface in some cases. Primary adenocarcinoma can arise anywhere in the urinary bladder but most commonly involves the base (i.e., trigone and posterior wall). Histologically, bladder adenocarcinoma exhibits several different patterns, including enteric, mucinous, not otherwise specified (NOS), and mixed. The enteric type is similar to its gastrointestinal counterpart and is composed of pseudostratified nuclei and tall columnar cytoplasm (Fig. 7.4a). The mucinous type shows nests of infiltrating tumor cells floating in abundant extracellular mucin (Fig. 7.4b). In some cases of mucinous adenocarcinoma, signet ring cells with a large intracellular mucin vacuole that displace the nucleus to the periphery (Fig. 7.4c). Importantly, as carcinomas predominantly composed of signet ring cells without stromal mucin deposition have been reported to have a worse prognosis than do other histological types of adenocarcinoma [44], these are currently classified as plasmacytoid urothelial carcinoma [42]. Tumors with a mixture of the enteric and mucinous components are the most common histology of adenocarcinoma [42]. Other cases have nonspecific glandular growth; these are classified as the adenocarcinoma NOS type (Fig. 7.4d). There is no consensus on the grading system for bladder adenocarcinoma. Because immunohistochemistry is usually performed for the differential diagnosis between primary and secondary bladder adenocarcinoma, immunophenotype of the primary adenocarcinoma is integrally discussed in a section of secondary adenocarcinoma.

The molecular and genetic data on primary bladder adenocarcinoma are still limited. In a recent study using targeted next-generation sequencing for 15 primary adenocarcinomas, 11 exhibit at least one genomic alteration in *TP53*, *KRAS*, *PIK3CA*, *CTNNB1*, *APC*, *TERT*, *FBXW7*, *IDH2*, and *RB1*; however, all 3 adenocarcinomas with mucinous features show the distinct lack of genomic alterations across 51 cancer-related

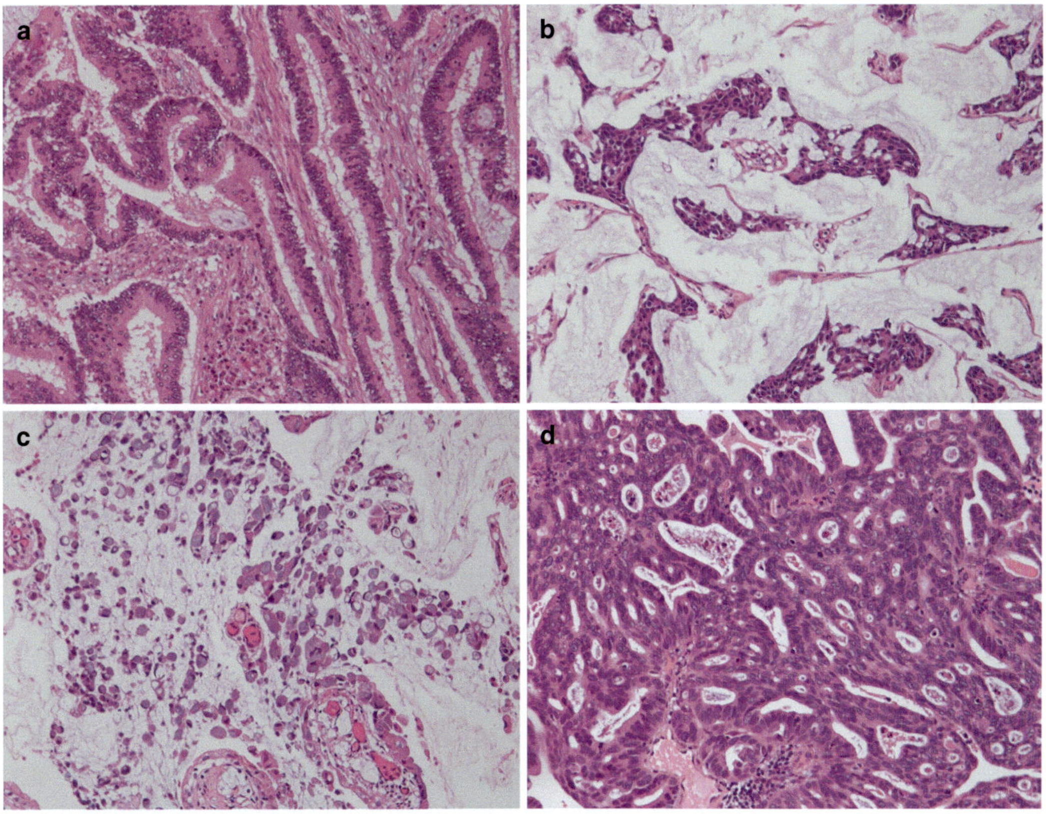

Fig. 7.4 Primary adenocarcinoma of the urinary bladder. Enteric type (**a**), mucinous type (**b**) with signet ring cells (**c**), and NOS type (**d**). (Original magnification, x200)

genes examined [45]. *TERT* mutation has also been reported in up to one-third of primary bladder adenocarcinoma [46].

Patients with bladder-invasive adenocarcinoma usually require radical cystectomy with pelvic lymph node dissection and urinary diversion. In some cases, partial cystectomy can be a treatment option, but a relatively high recurrence rate of the tumor after partial resection has been indicated [47]. Transurethral resection and intravesical BCG/mitomycin C therapy is generally ineffective for bladder adenocarcinoma. If the patient is not a candidate for surgery, radiation and chemotherapy may be considered. The prognosis for primary adenocarcinoma is generally poor, as most patients have advanced disease at diagnosis. The 5-year survival rate has been reported in the range of 40–50% [47, 48].

Secondary Adenocarcinoma

Secondary bladder involvement by adenocarcinoma of adjacent organs through direct extension or metastasis via a lymphovascular route is more common than primary bladder adenocarcinoma. The common primary organs to be considered include the colon, prostate, female genital tract, and breast.

Colorectal adenocarcinoma is the most frequent secondary tumor involving the bladder wall. It is generally difficult to differentiate primary bladder adenocarcinoma from secondary colorectal adenocarcinoma based on morphological features, especially on small biopsy specimens, as they share similar histological features. Immunohistochemistry has limited utility but is often used to help the differential diagnosis. Colorectal adenocarcinomas usually show nuclear and cytoplasmic/membranous staining for β-catenin, while primary bladder adenocarcinomas are negative or show only cytoplasmic/membranous staining [49]. Most bladder adenocarcinomas are immunoreactive for thrombomodulin and cytokeratin (CK) 7, whereas colorectal carcinomas are negative for thrombomodulin and CK7 [50]. CK20, CDX2, villin, and cadherin-17 are not useful, as they are commonly expressed in both colorectal and bladder adenocarcinomas [49]. Importantly, clinical history and colonoscopic findings are essential to identify the correct origin in most cases.

Prostatic adenocarcinoma also commonly invades the bladder, particularly the bladder neck and trigone regions. Because most prostatic adenocarcinomas are acinar type and demonstrate small atypical glands composed of relatively uniform malignant cuboidal cells, it is not difficult to distinguish them from bladder adenocarcinoma. However, a small subset of prostatic adenocarcinomas is ductal type with large tubulopapillary or cribriform gland with focal necrosis, resembling the enteric-type bladder adenocarcinoma. Although immunohistochemical study is extremely valuable in the differential diagnosis, a part of poorly differentiated or previously treated prostatic adenocarcinoma may not be immunoreactive for PSA and PSAP [51]. In this situation, the use of a panel together with additional prostate-specific markers including prostein and NKX3.1 is recommended [51].

Endometrial adenocarcinoma, especially endometrioid carcinoma, shows atypical glandular structures with occasional mucinous and squamous differentiations and may spread to the urinary bladder at advanced stages. Lobular-type breast carcinoma which seems to be more common involves the bladder than ductal type, although both types can involve the bladder. It may be challenging to distinguish these adenocarcinomas with bladder adenocarcinoma on a morphological analysis alone; however, immunohistochemical staining coupled with clinical history generally leads to the correct diagnosis [52]. Endometrioid carcinoma and breast adenocarcinoma are positive for estrogen receptor and progesterone receptor, whereas bladder adenocarcinomas are negative for these markers.

Urachal Adenocarcinoma

The urachus is a vestigial fibrous structure that connects the urinary bladder to the allantois during early embryogenesis. While the lumen of the urachus begins to be gradually obliterated during fetal development, incomplete obliteration can cause a tubular or cystic structure in the dome and elsewhere along the midline of the bladder in approximately one-third of adults at autopsy [53]. The urachal remnant is usually lined by urothelium; however, a vast majority of the urachal tumors are adenocarcinomas (occasionally UC or SCC). Urachal adenocarcinoma is less common than primary bladder adenocarcinoma, accounting less than 1% of all bladder carcinomas but approximately 10% of primary adenocarcinomas involving the bladder [43]. Most cases occur in the fifth or sixth decade of life, with the mean patient age of 51 years, about 10 years younger than that for bladder adenocarcinoma [43]. A male-to-female ratio of patients is 2:1 to 3:1. Patients may present with hematuria, pain, irritative symptoms, mucusuria, and umbilical discharge.

The clinicopathological criteria for diagnosis of urachal adenocarcinoma includes (1) location of the tumor in the bladder dome and/or anterior wall, (2) epicenter of carcinoma in the bladder wall, (3) absence of mucosal surface changes such as cystitis cystica and/or cystitis glandularis beyond the dome or anterior wall, and (4) absence of a known primary elsewhere [54]. The presence of a related urachal remnant supports the diagnosis, but its absence does not exclude this possibility. The cut surfaces of tumors are typically firm, whitish gray masses but occasionally are discrete, cystic, or cavitary tumors (Fig. 7.5).

A classification system, proposed by Amin et al. [55] and adopted by the 2016 WHO classification, delineates urachal glandular tumors into two broad categories, mucinous cystic tumors and non-cystic adenocarcinomas (Table 7.2).

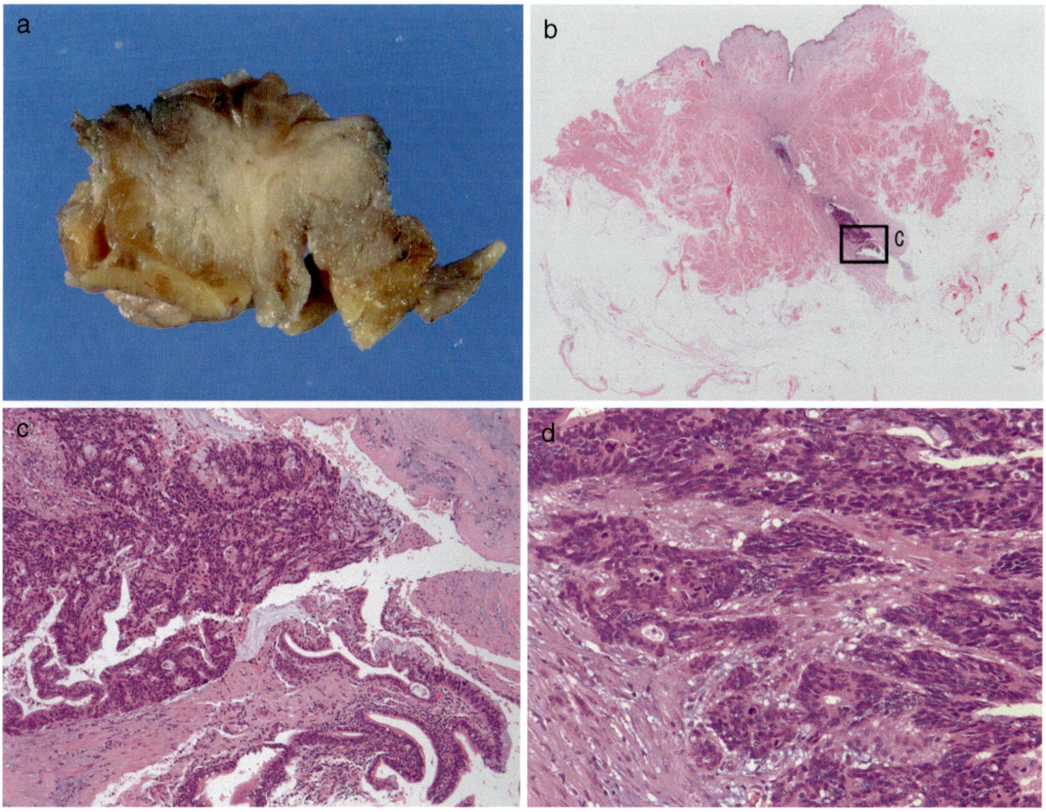

Fig. 7.5 Gross appearance (**a**) and a low-power view (**b**) of urachal non-cystic adenocarcinoma. Microscopically, enteric adenocarcinoma with focal urachal remnant (**c**) and stromal invasion (**d**) is noted. (Original magnification: **c**, x100; **d**, x200)

Non-cystic adenocarcinomas (accounting for 83% of cases) are more common than cystic tumors (17% of cases) [54, 55]. Non-cystic urachal adenocarcinomas exhibit a similar histology to primary bladder adenocarcinomas: enteric (Fig. 7.5), mucinous (with or without signet ring cells), and NOS types. On the other hand, mucinous cystic tumors demonstrate a morphological homology with mucinous tumors of the ovary: mucinous cystadenoma, mucinous cystadenoma of low malignant potential (MCTLMP) (with or without intraepithelial carcinoma), and mucinous cystadenocarcinoma with either microscopic or frank invasion [55]. Mucinous cystadenoma is a cystic tumor lined by a single layer of mucinous columnar cells with minimal cytological atypia and structural complexity. MCTLMP constitutes more than 50% of the mucinous cystic tumors and shows areas of epithelial proliferation, including formation of papillae and low-grade cytological atypia, resembling those of mucinous borderline tumor of the ovary (Fig. 7.6a, b and c). In a small subset of tumors, foci of intraepithelial

Table 7.2 Glandular tumors of the urachus [54]

Mucinous cystic tumors
Mucinous cystadenoma
Mucinous cystic tumor of low malignant potential with or without intraepithelial carcinoma
Mucinous cystadenocarcinoma with microscopic or frank invasion
Non-cystic adenocarcinoma
Enteric adenocarcinoma
Mucinous adenocarcinoma with or without signet ring cells
Adenocarcinoma, NOS
Mixed adenocarcinoma

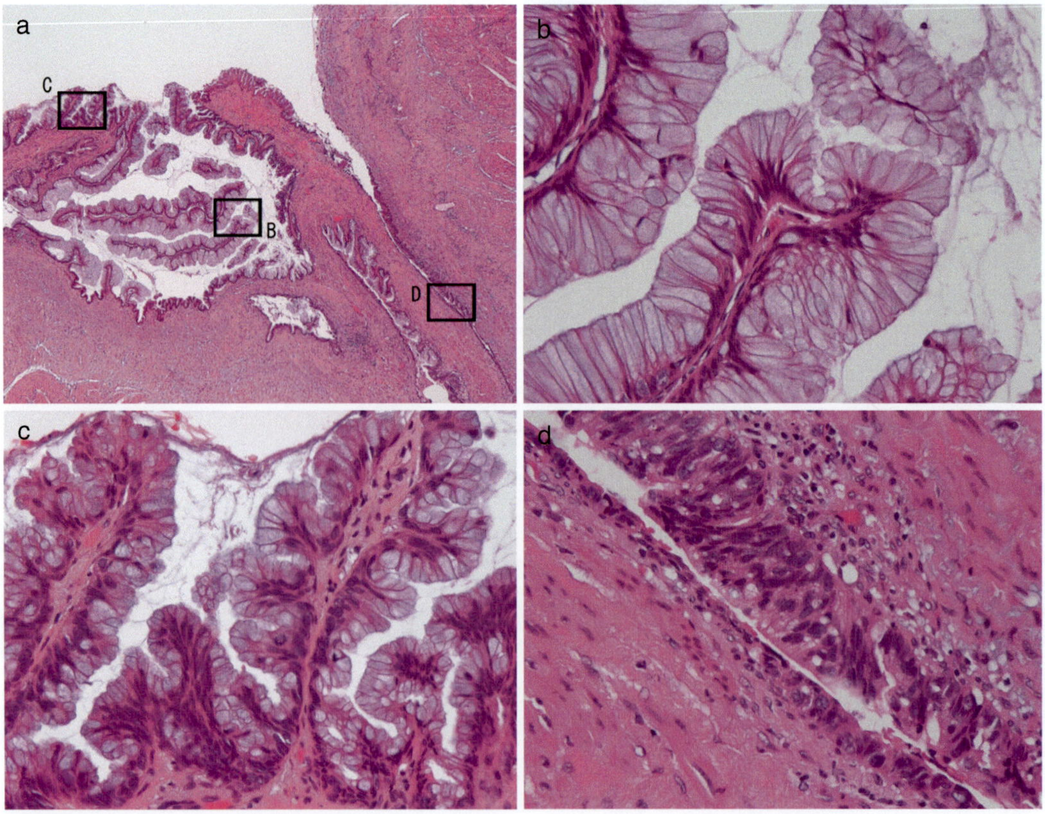

Fig. 7.6 Morphological spectrum of a single mucinous cystic tumor (**a**). Mucinous cystadenoma-like area (**b**), mucinous cystic tumor of low malignant potential (**c**), and a focal intraepithelial carcinoma component (**d**) are observed (original magnification: **a**, x40; **b**–**d**, x200)

carcinoma characterized by severe atypia, abundant mitoses, and complex architecture may be observed (Fig. 7.6d). For mucinous cystadenocarcinoma, Amin et al. defines lesions showing stromal invasion <2 mm and comprising <5% of the tumor as mucinous cystadenocarcinomas with microinvasion and lesions with more extensive invasion as those with frank invasion [55], although the interobserver reproducibility and clinical significance of this distinction have not been evaluated. Importantly, as the spectrum of atypia or only a small focus of invasive carcinoma may be present in individual cystic lesions (Fig. 7.6), rigorous sampling is necessary particularly when any degree of atypia is detected [56]. Immunohistochemical finding of non-cystic adenocarcinomas is essentially identical to that of mucinous cystic tumors; both types of tumors demonstrate variable (about 50%) CK7 and diffuse CK20 and CDX2 immunoreactivity [54, 55, 57]. There has been no helpful marker to distinguish between primary bladder adenocarcinoma and urachal adenocarcinoma. As with primary bladder adenocarcinoma, the lack of only focal positivity of nuclear β-catenin is potentially valuable in differentiating urachal adenocarcinoma from secondary bladder involvement of colorectal adenocarcinoma [57].

Recent studies using next-generation sequencing for urachal glandular tumors have revealed the molecular characteristics and genetic underpinnings of these rare neoplasms. Primary urachal adenocarcinomas harbor the spectrum of molecular alterations which are similar to those of primary bladder adenocarcinoma and colorectal adenocarcinoma, including *KRAS*, *NRAS*, *BRAF*, *APC*, *TP53*, *NF1*, and/or *SMAD4* mutations [58–60]. However, they generally lack *TERT* promoter and *PIK3CA* mutations, which are common in urothelial carcinoma [59, 61]. Of note, these sequencing studies to date have not subclassified urachal tumors according to the 2016 WHO classification; the molecular differences between urachal mucinous cystic tumors and non-cystic adenocarcinomas remain unclear.

The 5- and 10-year cancer-specific survival rates for patients with urachal adenocarcinoma are 40–64% and 31–49%, respectively [43, 62]. Importantly, progression-free survival of noninvasive mucinous cystic tumors is significantly better than that of non-cystic adenocarcinoma [55]. The Sheldon system is the most widely used staging system for urachal neoplasms and divides tumors as follows: confined to the urachal mucosa (pT1); extending into the urachal muscular layer (pT2); locally extending into the urinary bladder, abdominal wall, or other adjacent organs (pT3); and metastatic tumors (pT4) [63]. A variety of other similar staging systems, including Mayo and Ontario systems, have also suggested that clinically localized tumors have a good overall prognosis, whereas locally advanced and/or metastatic tumors have a poor overall prognosis [64, 65]. The current interest in staging for urachal carcinoma is a simplified dichotomous approach to divide tumors: (1) tumors confined to the urachus, bladder, and perivesical tissue and (2) tumors which spread to the peritoneum and other organs [66].

Clear Cell Carcinoma (Tumor of the Müllerian Type)

Clear cell carcinoma is a rare bladder carcinoma arising from preexisting Müllerian-type epithelium, typically endometriosis. Unlike other bladder glandular tumors, clear cell carcinoma occurs more frequently in females, and the mean age of patients is 57 years (ranging from 22 to 83 years) [67]. Patients usually present with hematuria, urinary frequency, or dysuria. Grossly, the tumor typically forms an exophytic and papillary mass. Histology of bladder clear cell carcinoma is similar to that of female genital tract, which is characterized by tubulocystic, papillary, and diffuse solid patterns of cuboidal or columnar tumor cells with clear and eosinophilic cytoplasm (Fig. 7.7). Hobnail cells are frequently observed. The nuclei are large with finely granular chromatin and prominent nucleoli (Fig. 7.7). Immunohistochemically, the tumor cells are usually positive for CK7, PAX8, AMACR, and CA-125, napsin A, and variably CK20, S100 protein, and PAX2 [67–70]. Nephrogenic adenoma,

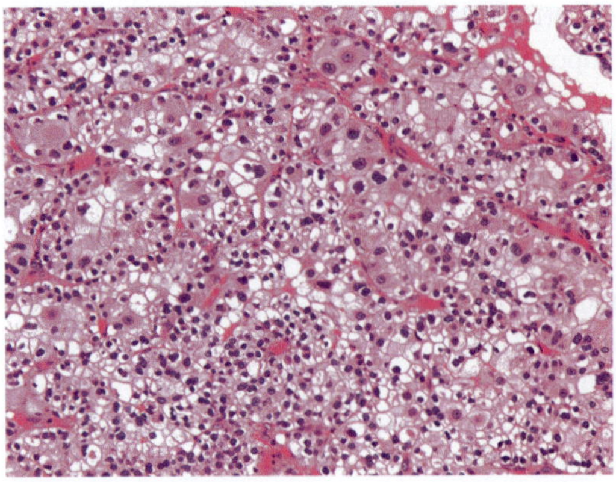

Fig. 7.7 Clear cell carcinoma of the urinary bladder. Densely packed tubulopapillary growth of tumor cells with clear and eosinophilic cytoplasm. (Original magnification, x200)

which also exhibits the proliferation of cuboidal or hobnail clear cells, should be differentiated from clear cell carcinoma [71]. Nephrogenic adenoma lacks prominent cytoarchitectural atypia and solid growth areas and more frequently affects males [71, 72]. Other differential diagnoses include metastatic clear cell carcinoma from the female genital tract and metastatic clear cell renal cell carcinoma. Overall, clinicoradiological correlations with careful immunohistochemical study are helpful for the correct diagnosis.

References

1. Shen SS, Al-Ahmadie H, Mahfouz SM. Squamous cell neoplasms. Tumours of the urinary system. In: Moch H, Humphrey PA, Ulbright TM, Reuter VE, editors. World Health Organization classification of tumours of the urinary system and male genital organs. Lyon: IARC Press; 2016. p. 108–10.
2. Johnson DE, Schoenwald MB, Ayala AG, Miller LS. Squamous cell carcinoma of the bladder. J Urol. 1976;115:542–4.
3. Rundle JS, Hart AJ, McGeorge A, Smith JS, Malcolm AJ, Smith PM. Squamous cell carcinoma of bladder. A review of 114 patients. Br J Urol. 1982;54:522–6.
4. Shokeir AA. Squamous cell carcinoma of the bladder: pathology, diagnosis and treatment. BJU Int. 2004;93:216–20.
5. Gschwend JE, Dahm P, Fair WR. Disease specific survival as endpoint of outcome for bladder cancer patients following radical cystectomy. Eur Urol. 2002;41:440–8.
6. Ghoneim MA, el-Mekresh MM, el-Baz MA, el-Attar IA, Ashamallah A. Radical cystectomy for carcinoma of the bladder: critical evaluation of the results in 1,026 cases. J Urol. 1997;158:393–9.
7. Salem HK, Mahfouz S. Changing patterns (age, incidence, and pathologic types) of schistosoma-associated bladder cancer in Egypt in the past decade. Urology. 2012;79:379–83.
8. El-Bolkainy MN, Ghoneim MA, Mansour MA. Carcinoma of the bilharzial bladder in Egypt: clinical and pathological features. Br J Urol. 1972;44:561–9.
9. El-Sebai I, Sherif M, El-Bolkainy MN, Mansour MA, Ghoneim MA. Verrucous squamous carcinoma of bladder. Urology. 1974;4:407–10.
10. Bejany DE, Lockhart JL, Rhamy RK. Malignant vesical tumors following spinal cord injury. J Urol. 1987;138:1390–2.
11. Pannek J. Transitional cell carcinoma in patients with spinal cord injury: a high-risk malignancy? Urology. 2002;59:240–4.
12. Brenner DW, Yore LM, Schellhammer PF. Squamous cell carcinoma of bladder after successful intravesical therapy with Bacillus Calmette-Guérin. Urology. 1989;34:93–5.
13. El-Aaser AA, El-Merzabani MM, Higgy NA, Kader MM. A study on the aetiological factors of bilharzial bladder cancer in Egypt. 3. Urinary beta-glucuronidase. Eur J Cancer. 1979;15:573–83.
14. Khales HM. Bladder cancer and bilharziasis today. Cancer J. 1993;6:65–71.
15. El-Said A, Omar S, Ibrahim S, Tawfik H, Eissa S, Ali S, et al. Bilharzial bladder cancer in Egypt, a review of 420 cases of radical cystectomy. Jpn J Clin Oncol. 1979;9:117–22.
16. Khafagy MM, El-Bolkainy MN, Mansour MA. Carcinoma of the bilharzial urinary bladder. A study of the associated mucosal lesions in 86 cases. Cancer. 1972;30:150–9.
17. Serretta V, Pomara G, Piazza F, Gange E. Pure squamous cell carcinoma of the bladder in western countries. Report on 19 consecutive cases. Eur Urol. 2000;37:85–9.
18. Lagwinski N, Thomas A, Stephenson AJ, Campbell S, Hoschar AP, El-Gabry E, et al. Squamous cell carcinoma of the bladder: a clinicopathologic analysis of 45 cases. Am J Surg Pathol. 2007;31:1777–87.
19. Khalaf I, Shokeir A, Shalaby M. Urologic complications of genitourinary schistosomiasis. World J Urol. 2012;30:31–8.
20. Richie JP, Waisman J, Skinner DG, Dretler SP. Squamous carcinoma of the bladder: treatment by radical cystectomy. J Urol. 1976;115:670–2.
21. Ghomneim MA, Mansour MA, El-Bolkainy MN. Staging of carcinoma of bilharzial bladder. Urology. 1974;3:40–2.
22. Wishnow KI, Dmochowski R. Pelvic recurrence after radical cystectomy without preoperative radiation. J Urol. 1988;140:42–3.

23. Aly MS, Khaled HM. Chromosomal aberrations in early stage bilharzial bladder cancer. Cancer Genet Cytogenet. 2002;132:41–5.
24. Fadl-Elmula I, Kytola S, Leithy ME, Abdel-Hameed M, Mandahl N, Elagib A, et al. Chromosomal aberrations in benign and malignant bilharzia-associated bladder lesions analyzed by comparative genomic hybridization. BMC Cancer. 2002;2:5.
25. Gonzalez-Zulueta M. Tumor suppressor gene alterations in squamous cell carcinoma of the bladder. J Natl Cancer Inst. 1995;87:1383–93.
26. El-Rifai W, Kamel D, Larramendy ML, Shoman S, Gad Y, Baithun S, et al. DNA copy number changes in Schistosoma-associated and non-Schistosoma-associated bladder cancer. Am J Pathol. 2000;156:871–8.
27. Molitor M, Junker K, Eltze E, Toma M, Denzinger S, Siegert S, et al. Comparison of structural genetics of non-Schistosoma-associated squamous cell carcinoma of the urinary bladder. Int J Clin Exp Pathol. 2015;8:8143–58.
28. Cowan M, Springer S, Nguyen D, Taheri D, Guner G, Rodriguez MA, et al. High prevalence of TERT promoter mutations in primary squamous cell carcinoma of the urinary bladder. Mod Pathol. 2016;29:511–5.
29. Ramchurren N, Cooper K, Summerhayes IC. Molecular events underlying schistosomiasis-related bladder cancer. Int J Cancer. 1995;62:237–44.
30. Warren W, Biggs PJ, el-Baz M, Ghoneim MA, Stratton MR, Venitt S. Mutations in the p53 gene in schistosomal bladder cancer: a study of 92 tumours from Egyptian patients and a comparison between mutational spectra from schistosomal and non-schistosomal urothelial tumours. Carcinogenesis. 1995;16:1181–9.
31. Abdulamir AS, Hafidh RR, Kadhim HS, Abubakar F. Tumor markers of bladder cancer: the schistosomal bladder tumors versus non-schistosomal bladder tumors. J Exp Clin Cancer Res. 2009;28:27.
32. Bue P, Wester K, Sjöström A, Holmberg A, Nilsson S, Carlsson J, et al. Expression of epidermal growth factor receptor in urinary bladder cancer metastases. Int J Cancer. 1998;76:189–93.
33. Berner A, Jacobsen AB, Fosså SD, Nesland JM. Expression of c-erbB-2 protein, neuron-specific enolase and DNA flow cytometry in locally advanced transitional cell carcinoma of the urinary bladder. Histopathology. 1993;22:327–33.
34. Swanson DA, Liles A, Zagars GK. Preoperative irradiation and radical cystectomy for stages T2 and T3 squamous cell carcinoma of the bladder. J Urol. 1990;143:37–40.
35. Ghoneim MA, Ashamallah AK, Awaad HK, Whitmore WF Jr. Randomized trial of cystectomy with or without preoperative radiotherapy for carcinoma of the bilharzial bladder. J Urol. 1985;134:266–8.
36. Elsobky E, El-Baz M, Gomha M, Abol-Enein H, Shaaban AA. Prognostic value of angiogenesis in schistosoma-associated squamous cell carcinoma of the urinary bladder. Urology. 2002;60:69–77.
37. Vakar-López F, Abrams J. Basaloid squamous cell carcinoma occurring in the urinary bladder. Arch Pathol Lab Med. 2000;124:455–9.
38. Neves TR, Soares MJ, Monteiro PG, Lima MS, Monteiro HG. Basaloid squamous cell carcinoma in the urinary bladder with small-cell carcinoma. J Clin Oncol. 2011;29:440–2.
39. Ginori A, Barone A, Santopietro R, Barbanti G, Cecconi F, Tripodi SA. Human papillomavirus-related basaloid squamous cell carcinoma of the bladder associated with genital tract human papillomavirus infection. Int J Urol. 2015;22:222–5.
40. Ishida M, Iwai M, Yoshida K, Kagotani A, Okabe H. Sarcomatoid carcinoma with small cell carcinoma component of the urinary bladder: a case report with review of the literature. Int J Clin Exp Pathol. 2013;6:1671–6.
41. Abrahams NA, Moran C, Reyes AO, Siefker-Radtke A, Ayala AG. Small cell carcinoma of the bladder: a contemporary clinicopathological study of 51 cases. Histopathology. 2005;46:57–63.
42. Grignon DJ, Cheville J, Ro JY, Tamboli P. Glandular neoplasms. Tumours of the urinary system. In: Moch H, Humphrey PA, Ulbright TM, Reuter VE, editors. World Health Organization classification of tumours of the urinary system and male genital organs. Lyon: IARC Press; 2016. p. 111–2.
43. Grignon DJ, Ro JY, Ayala AG, Johnson DE, Ordóñez NG. Primary adenocarcinoma of the urinary bladder. A clinicopathologic analysis of 72 cases. Cancer. 1991;67:2165–72.
44. Grignon DJ, Ro JY, Ayala AG, Johnson DE. Primary signet-ring cell carcinoma of the urinary bladder. Am J Clin Pathol. 1991;95:13–20.
45. Roy S, Pradhan D, Ernst WL, Mercurio S, Najjar Y, Parikh R, et al. Next-generation sequencing-based molecular characterization of primary urinary bladder adenocarcinoma. Mod Pathol. 2017;30:1133–43.
46. Cowan ML, Springer S, Nguyen D, Taheri D, Guner G, Mendoza Rodriguez MA, et al. Detection of TERT promoter mutations in primary adenocarcinoma of the urinary bladder. Hum Pathol. 2016;53:8–13.
47. Zaghloul MS, Nouh A, Nazmy M, Ramzy S, Zaghloul AS, Sedira MA, et al. Long-term results of primary adenocarcinoma of the urinary bladder: a report on 192 patients. Urol Oncol. 2006;24:13–20.
48. el-Mekresh MM, el-Baz MA, Abol-Enein H, Ghoneim MA. Primary adenocarcinoma of the urinary bladder: a report of 185 cases. Br J Urol. 1998;82:206–12.
49. Rao Q, Williamson SR, Lopez-Beltran A, Montironi R, Huang W, Eble JN, et al. Distinguishing primary adenocarcinoma of the urinary bladder from secondary involvement by colorectal adenocarcinoma: extended immunohistochemical profiles emphasizing novel markers. Mod Pathol. 2013;26:725–32.
50. Dadhania V, Czerniak B, Guo CC. Adenocarcinoma of the urinary bladder. Am J Clin Exp Urol. 2015;3:51–63.
51. Epstein JI, Egevad L, Humphrey PA, Montironi R, Members of the ISUP Immunohistochemistry in

Diagnostic Urologic Pathology Group. Best practices recommendations in the application of immunohistochemistry in the prostate: report from the International Society of Urologic Pathology consensus conference. Am J Surg Pathol. 2014;38:e6–e19.
52. Morichetti D, Mazzucchelli R, Lopez-Beltran A, Cheng L, Scarpelli M, Kirkali Z, et al. Secondary neoplasms of the urinary system and male genital organs. BJU Int. 2009;104:770–6.
53. Schubert GE, Pavkovic MB, Bethke-Bedürftig BA. Tubular urachal remnants in adult bladders. J Urol. 1982;127:40–2.
54. Gopalan A, Sharp DS, Fine SW, Tickoo SK, Herr HW, Reuter VE, et al. Urachal carcinoma: a clinicopathologic analysis of 24 cases with outcome correlation. Am J Surg Pathol. 2009;33:659–68.
55. Amin MB, Smith SC, Eble JN, Rao P, Choi WW, Tamboli P, et al. Glandular neoplasms of the urachus: a report of 55 cases emphasizing mucinous cystic tumors with proposed classification. Am J Surg Pathol. 2014;38:1033–45.
56. Paner GP, Lopez-Beltran A, Sirohi D, Amin MB. Updates in the pathologic diagnosis and classification of epithelial neoplasms of urachal origin. Adv Anat Pathol. 2016;23:71–83.
57. Paner GP, McKenney JK, Barkan GA, Yao JL, Frankel WL, Sebo TJ, et al. Immunohistochemical analysis in a morphologic spectrum of urachal epithelial neoplasms: diagnostic implications and pitfalls. Am J Surg Pathol. 2011;35:787–98.
58. Módos O, Reis H, Niedworok C, Rübben H, Szendröi A, Szász MA, et al. Mutations of KRAS, NRAS, BRAF, EGFR, and PIK3CA genes in urachal carcinoma: occurrence and prognostic significance. Oncotarget. 2016;7:39293–301.
59. Lee S, Lee J, Sim SH, Lee Y, Moon KC, Lee C, et al. Comprehensive somatic genome alterations of urachal carcinoma. J Med Genet. 2017;54:572–8.
60. Singh H, Liu Y, Xiao X, Lin L, Kim J, Van Hummelen P, et al. Whole exome sequencing of urachal adenocarcinoma reveals recurrent NF1 mutations. Oncotarget. 2016;7:29211–5.
61. Thiem S, Herold T, Krafft U, Bremmer F, Tolkach Y, Szász AM, et al. Telomerase reverse transcriptase (TERT) promoter mutations are rare in urachal cancer. Pathol Int. 2017;67:597–601.
62. Wright JL, Porter MP, Li CI, Lange PH, Lin DW. Differences in survival among patients with urachal and nonurachal adenocarcinomas of the bladder. Cancer. 2006;107:721–8.
63. Sheldon CA, Clayman RV, Gonzalez R, Williams RD, Fraley EE. Malignant urachal lesions. J Urol. 1984;131:1–8.
64. Molina JR, Quevedo JF, Furth AF, Richardson RL, Zincke H, Burch PA. Predictors of survival from urachal cancer: a Mayo Clinic study of 49 cases. Cancer. 2007;110:2434–40.
65. Pinthus JH, Haddad R, Trachtenberg J, Holowaty E, Bowler J, Herzenberg AM, et al. Population based survival data on urachal tumors. J Urol. 2006;175:2042–7.
66. Herr HW, Bochner BH, Sharp D, Dalbagni G, Reuter VE. Urachal carcinoma: contemporary surgical outcomes. J Urol. 2007;178:74–8.
67. Oliva E, Amin MB, Jimenez R, Young RH. Clear cell carcinoma of the urinary bladder: a report and comparison of four tumors of Mullerian origin and nine of probable urothelial origin with discussion of histogenesis and diagnostic problems. Am J Surg Pathol. 2002;26:190–7.
68. Gilcrease MZ, Delgado R, Vuitch F, Albores-Saavedra J. Clear cell adenocarcinoma and nephrogenic adenoma of the urethra and urinary bladder: a histopathologic and immunohistochemical comparison. Hum Pathol. 1998;29:1451–6.
69. Tong GX, Weeden EM, Hamele-Bena D, Huan Y, Unger P, Memeo L, et al. Expression of PAX8 in nephrogenic adenoma and clear cell adenocarcinoma of the lower urinary tract: evidence of related histogenesis? Am J Surg Pathol. 2008;32:1380–7.
70. Jassim SH, Khiyami A, Nguyen JK, Ganesan S, Tomashefski J Jr, Sawady J. Concordant clear cell "mesonephric" carcinoma of the bladder and lung adenocarcinoma with clear cell features – multiple primaries versus metastatic neoplasms: a case report. J Med Case Rep. 2017;11:133.
71. Oliva E, Young RH. Nephrogenic adenoma of the urinary tract: a review of the microscopic appearance of 80 cases with emphasis on unusual features. Mod Pathol. 1995;8:722–30.
72. Young RH. Tumor-like lesions of the urinary bladder. Mod Pathol. 2009;22:S37–52.

Mesenchymal Tumors

8

Michael J. Hwang and Pheroze Tamboli

Benign Mesenchymal Tumors

Benign mesenchymal tumors are similar to those observed in the soft tissue and other viscera. Most are straightforward to diagnose, as long as the pathologist includes these in their differential diagnosis, especially when faced with a tumor that appears to be "out of place" for the bladder and usual categories of bladder tumors.

Paragangliomas

Of all the benign tumors arising in the urinary bladder, paragangliomas are the ones most likely to be confused for urothelial carcinoma. As with other sites, chromaffin cells are considered the precursor cells of these tumors [1]. Paragangliomas have been reported in almost all age groups. In some series, they have been reported to be more common in women, with a male-to-female ratio of 1:3 [2]. Up to two-thirds of tumors are reported to express catecholamines, causing hypertension, headaches, tachycardia, and palpitations [1, 3].

Paragangliomas generally present as intramural masses, most often found in the bladder trigone and dome. Tumors have been reported to range from 1 cm to 9 cm, with an average of 4 cm [1]. Morphologic features of bladder paragangliomas are similar to those of pheochromocytoma of the adrenal gland and paragangliomas in other sites, including the typical *zellballen* appearance of tumor nests surrounded by a network of thin blood vessels (Fig. 8.1). Tumor cells tend to be uniform with moderate to abundant pale eosinophilic or clear cytoplasm and round or oval nuclei. Scattered cells with large bizarre nuclei may be present (Fig. 8.1). Mitoses are uncommon in most cases.

As expected, immunohistochemical stains of neuroendocrine differentiation including chromogranin, synaptophysin (Fig. 8.2), and CD56 are positive in the tumor cells. S-100 protein and SOX-10 highlight the sustentacular cells, although in some cases they may be hard to identify (Fig. 8.3). In recent years, paragangliomas have been reported to stain with the GATA-3 immunohistochemical stain (Fig. 8.4) in up to 90% of cases studied [4]. This fact needs to be kept in mind when GATA-3 is used in the differential diagnosis between urothelial carcinoma and paraganglioma. Epithelial markers, including cytokeratin, EMA, and carcinoembryonic antigen (CEA), are typically negative.

M. J. Hwang
Department of Pathology and Laboratory Medicine, Indiana University School of Medicine, Indianapolis, IN, USA

P. Tamboli (✉)
Department of Pathology, The University of Texas M. D. Anderson Cancer Center, Houston, TX, USA
e-mail: ptamboli@mdanderson.org

H. Zhou et al. (eds.), *Urinary Bladder Pathology*, https://doi.org/10.1007/978-3-030-71509-0_8

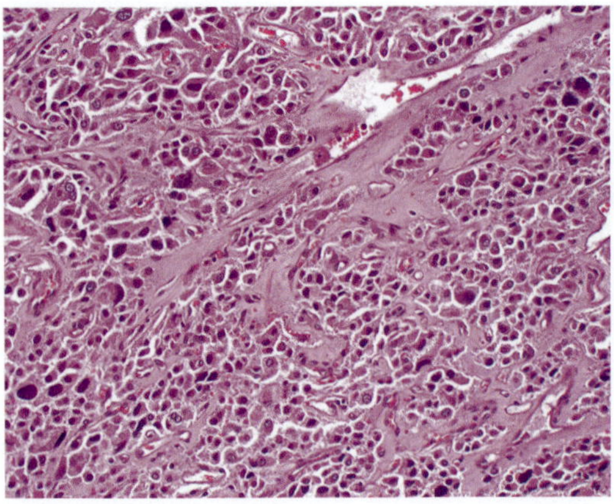

Fig. 8.1 Paraganglioma of the urinary bladder with tumor cells arranged in the *zenballen* configuration. Tumor cells have abundant eosinophilic cytoplasm. In contrast to the uniform round or oval nuclei of most tumor cells, some tumor cells have larger, variably sized, or pleomorphic nuclei

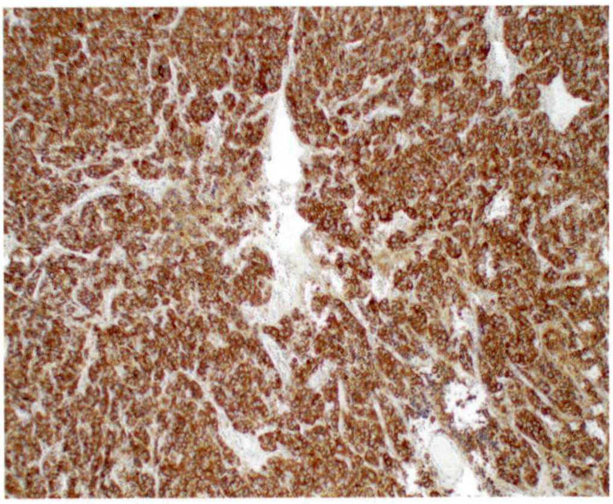

Fig. 8.2 Diffuse synaptophysin staining in paraganglioma

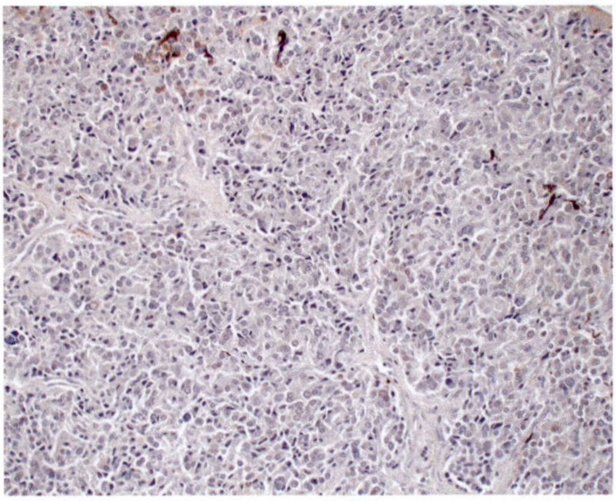

Fig. 8.3 S-100 stain in paraganglioma. Only scattered sustentacular cells are identified in the upper half of the image

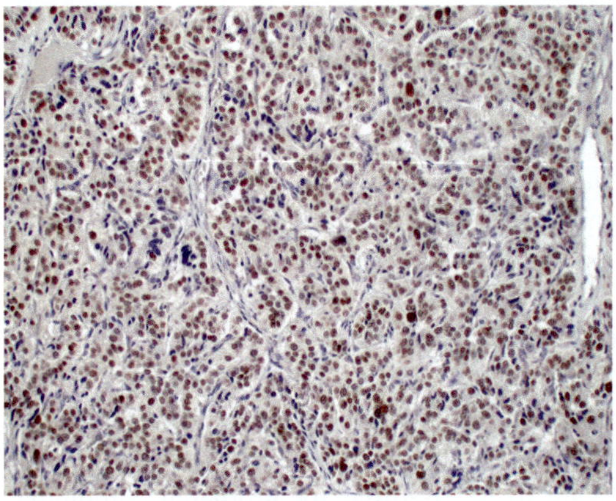

Fig. 8.4 GATA-3 stains the paraganglioma tumor cells

Paraganglioma may be misdiagnosed as urothelial carcinoma, especially the nested variant, which has an infiltrative growth pattern along with uniform tumor cells. Distorted paraganglioma cells deep in the bladder wall in small cauterized tissue fragments may also be confused for urothelial carcinoma (Fig. 8.5). Intact surface urothelium without dysplastic changes and appropriate use of immunohistochemical stains can help reach the correct diagnosis (Fig. 8.6).

Paragangliomas with necrosis, mitoses, and vascular invasion are reported to behave more aggressively [3]. However, as with pheochromocytomas, metastasis is the most reliable indicator of malignant behavior.

Similar to pheochromocytomas, mutations of succinate dehydrogenase (SDH) subunits B (SDHB) and D (SDHD) have been reported in a subset of patients with paragangliomas, resulting in severely reduced tumor SDH activity. Using the immunohistochemical stain for SDHB (Fig. 8.7), lack of expression in the tumor cells, as opposed to the nonneoplastic cells that serve as an internal positive control, can identify patients with germ line SDHB mutations [2]. SDH-deficient paragangliomas have similar morphologic features to those of SDH-intact tumors. However, the SDH-deficient tumors have been reported to be larger,

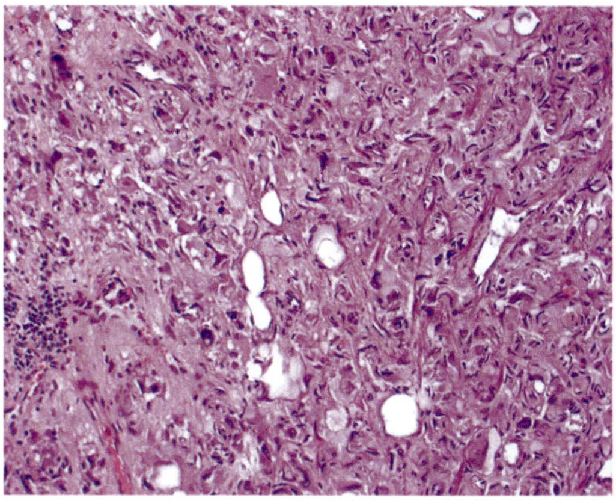

Fig. 8.5 Distorted and cauterized fragment of paraganglioma within the muscularis propria. There are distorted single tumor cells with large nuclei resembling high-grade urothelial carcinoma. When tumor cells are observed only within the lamina propria or muscularis propria with relatively intact urothelium, tumors other than urothelial carcinoma should be considered in the differential diagnosis

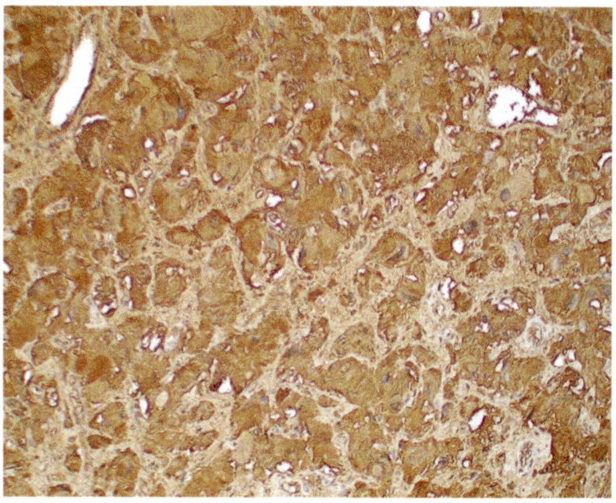

Fig. 8.6 Chromogranin stain highlights the paraganglioma cells, which are not clearly evident on the H&E in Fig. 8.5

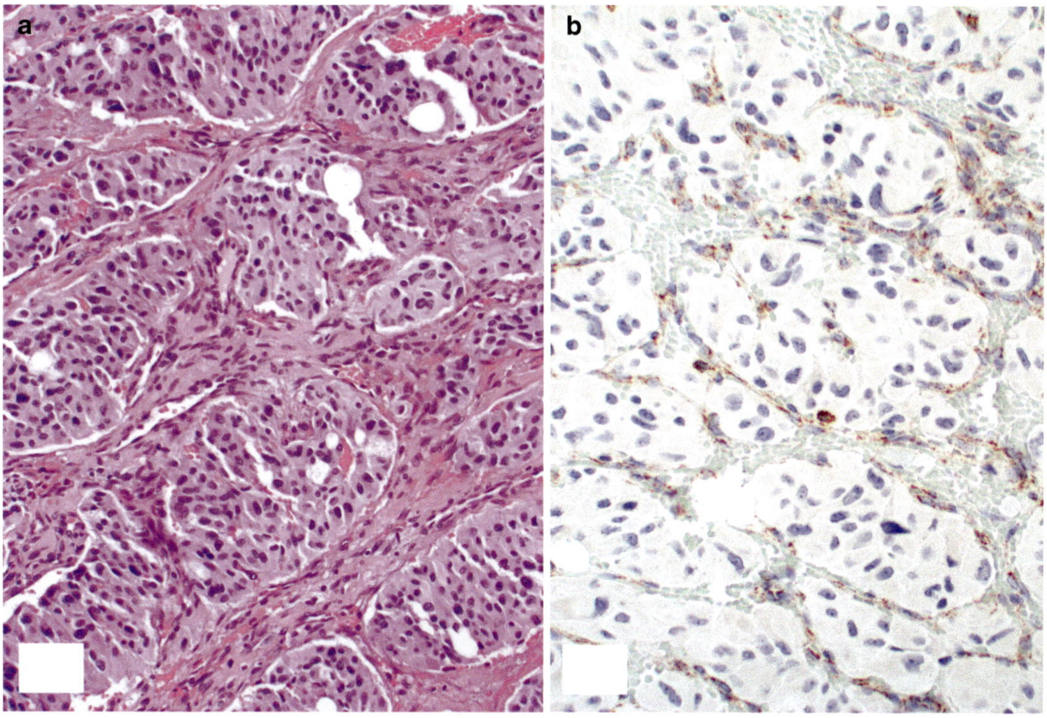

Fig. 8.7 Succinate dehydrogenase B (SDH-B)-negative paraganglioma. The H&E on the left (image A) shows typical morphologic features of a paraganglioma. The SDH-B immunohistochemical stain is negative in the tumor cells (right side, image B). Nonneoplastic cells, blood vessels in this image, serve as a internal positive control

with higher number of mitosis, frequent lymphovascular invasion, higher Ki67 labeling index, and are more likely to metastasize [5, 6].

Leiomyoma

This is the most common benign mesenchymal tumor of the urinary bladder. Most tumors occur in women and affect patients of all ages, including children [7]. These patients typically present with lower urinary tract symptoms (LUTS) such as hematuria, dysuria, and increased frequency of urination or urinary obstruction. At cystoscopy, they are observed as submucosal lesions, with normal-appearing surface mucosa in most cases. In rare cases, they may project into the bladder lumen as a pedunculated mass.

Grossly, they are similar to uterine leiomyomata with a firm, well-circumscribed, and whorled cut surface. Their morphologic features are typical of leiomyoma, the tumors are well-circumscribed (Fig. 8.8), with interlacing bundles of uniform smooth muscle cells with ovoid blunt-ended nuclei (Fig. 8.9). Some tumors may be more cellular with mild nuclear atypia. Rare mitoses may be present. Tumor necrosis is generally absent [8] but has been reported in rare tumors [7, 9]. In 2010, some tumors with degenerative nuclear atypia, but without mitotic activity, were referred to as symplastic leiomyomas. These cases were reported to have a benign clinical course [9].

As with all smooth muscle tumors, immunohistochemical stains for smooth muscle actin (SMA), calponin, caldesmon, desmin, CD34, and vimentin stains are positive. Estrogen and progesterone receptor staining has also been reported in few cases.

Low-grade leiomyosarcoma is the most important differential diagnosis for this tumor and is further discussed in the section on leiomyosarcoma below. Smooth muscle tumors lacking circumscription, those with one or more mitosis per 10 hpf, significant nuclear atypia, and necrosis should be considered as leiomyosarcomas [7]. The paucicellular foci of inflammatory myofibroblastic tumors (IMT) may be sometimes confused for smooth muscle cells in a small sample, especially since IMT also stain similar to smooth muscle cells. However, when viewed in the context of the entire tumor, the diagnosis is not difficult.

Most leiomyomas are treated by transurethral resection, less often by enucleation or partial cystectomy, and rarely by total cystectomy. As expected, these tumors have a benign clinical course [9].

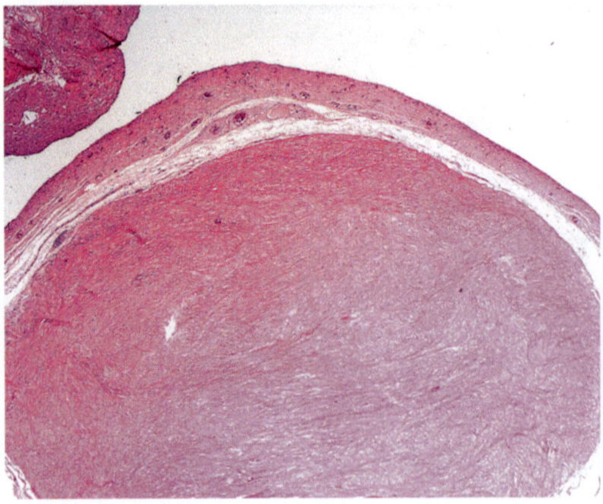

Fig. 8.8 Leiomyoma of the urinary bladder. There is a well-circumscribed uniform tumor nodule in the deep lamina propria, underneath the urothelial mucosa

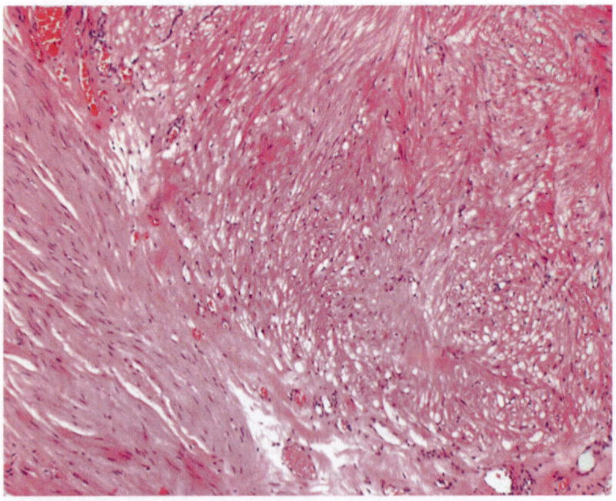

Fig. 8.9 Leiomyoma of the urinary bladder (upper right) contrasting with muscularis propria (lower left). The leiomyoma has interlacing bundles of uniform smooth muscle cells, and the tumor forms a distinct boundary with the muscularis propria

Neurofibroma

Although rare, neurofibroma is the third most common benign mesenchymal tumor of the urinary bladder. Approximately 60 cases have been reported in the literature [10, 11]. These tumors are most commonly seen in patients with type 1 neurofibromatosis (Fig. 8.10). They are present in the lamina propria and/or the muscularis propria, where they form plexiform mass(es). Tumors close to the urothelial mucosa may form a polypoid mass projecting into the bladder lumen. Large tumors extensively involving the urinary bladder have also been reported.

Their morphologic features are similar to other neurofibromas, with spindle cells that possess wavy eosinophilic cytoplasm and elongated cigar-shaped nuclei without nucleoli (Fig. 8.10). Morphologic features typically associated with cellular neurofibromas, such as pleomorphic nuclei with prominent nucleoli, may be present in some tumors. The differential diagnosis for the more cellular tumors includes malignant peripheral nerve sheath tumor (MPNST) [11] and rarely sarcomatoid urothelial carcinoma and inflammatory myofibroblastic tumor.

Other Benign Tumors

While leiomyoma and paraganglioma are the most common benign stromal tumors of the urinary bladder, there are other stromal tumors that rarely affect the urinary bladder. All of these also have similar morphologic features as their soft tissue counterparts.

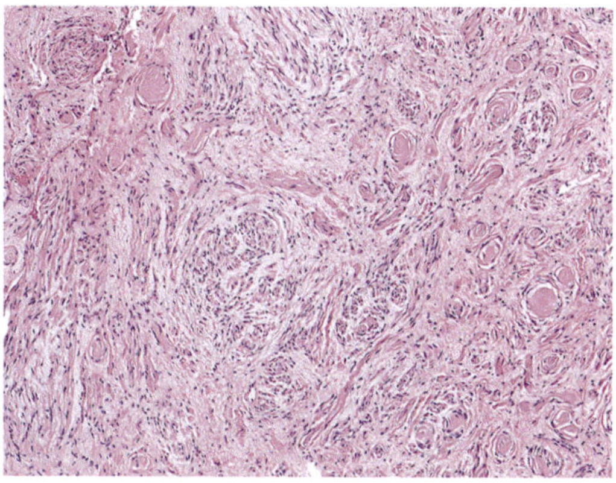

Fig. 8.10 Neurofibroma of the urinary bladder in a young child with history of neurofibromatosis. Tumor cells possess wavy eosinophilic cytoplasm and elongated cigar-shaped nuclei without prominent nucleoli

Schwannoma affecting the urinary bladder has been reported in a few patients who did not have neurofibromatosis [12]. As with other stromal tumors, they morphologically resemble schwannomas seen elsewhere in the body.

Granular cell tumor of the urinary bladder is rare, with fewer than 20 cases reported. Their morphology is similar to other granular cell tumors [13]. The granular eosinophilic cytoplasm may raise the differential diagnosis of urothelial carcinoma or squamous cell carcinoma. S-100 immunohistochemical stain is helpful, as it is typically positive in these tumors.

Lipomas of the urinary bladder are rare, with fewer than ten reported cases [14]. Morphologically, they resemble typical lipomas composed of mature adipose tissue.

Ganglioneuroma usually presents as a component of a composite paraganglioma-ganglioneuroma [15]. Nevertheless, they may occur as isolated tumors.

Gastrointestinal stromal tumor (GIST) has been reported in the urinary bladder and needs to be considered in the differential diagnosis of spindle cell tumors [16]. These extra-gastrointestinal GISTs are also consistently positive for CD117 (c-kit), with about 60–70% of tumors co-expressing CD34.

Other benign stromal tumors reported to involve the urinary bladder include *hemangioma, lymphangioma, solitary fibrous tumor*, and *rhabdomyoma*.

Malignant Mesenchymal Tumors

As with the benign stromal tumors, primary malignant mesenchymal tumors of the urinary bladder are rare. Most cases are reported either as isolated cases or as a small series of cases. Their morphologic features are no different than those of their counterparts in the soft tissue or other viscera.

Leiomyosarcoma

Leiomyosarcoma (LMS) is the most common sarcoma of the urinary bladder. These tend to occur later in life, usually in men between the ages of 60 and 70; however, there is a wide age range reported in the literature [7]. Some patients have a prior history of radiation therapy to the pelvic region, and few tumors have also been reported in patients treated with cyclophosphamide. As with other bladder tumors, patients present with lower urinary tract symptoms including gross hematuria, urinary frequency, and rarely pelvic pain.

Tumor size is variable, with 5 cm being the average reported in the literature [7, 17–19]. Tumors close to the urothelial mucosa may form a polypoid mass, sometimes with an ulcerated surface. These tumors tend to have an infiltrative growth pattern and are soft and fleshy. Necrosis, hemorrhage, and myxoid change may also be evident.

Morphologic features are similar to those of LMS in soft tissue or other viscera, including interlacing fascicles of malignant spindle cells and foci of necrosis. Cells have eosinophilic cytoplasm, hyperchromatic pleomorphic nuclei, and one or more nucleoli (Fig. 8.11). Myxoid stroma may be seen in a subset of tumors. Some tumors are predominantly composed of epithelioid cells [7, 17, 18]. Majority of cases are reported to have >5 mitoses per 10 high-power fields (HPF). Mitotic count and presence of necrosis provide important diagnostic clues to differentiate LMS from leiomyomas.

While most LMS are high-grade, a small number are considered low-grade. Unlike leiomyomas, low-grade LMS are not well-circumscribed, exhibit cytologic atypia and necrosis, and have mitoses, although with a lower mitotic count. In essence, tumors with an invasive growth pattern, significant nuclear atypia, necrosis, and mitoses should be diagnosed as LMS. The presence of mitoses is important; however, there are reports of low-grade LMS with only 1 mitosis per 10 hpf, affecting patients who died of metastatic disease [7]. It should be noted that there is no universally accepted grading or staging system for LMS of the urinary bladder. However, there are several proposed systems based on nuclear atypia, mitoses, tumor necrosis, tumor size, depth of invasion, and presence metastasis [20, 21].

In biopsies and TURBTs, it may be difficult to diagnose a low-grade LMS. These tumors are more cellular than a leiomyoma, have atypical nuclei and few or no visible mitoses, and lack necrosis. Fortunately, these tumors are rare and are best assigned a diagnosis of smooth muscle tumor of unknown malignant potential, with the caveat that the biologic behavior cannot be accurately predicted until the entire tumor can be evaluated (Figs. 8.12, 8.13 and 8.14).

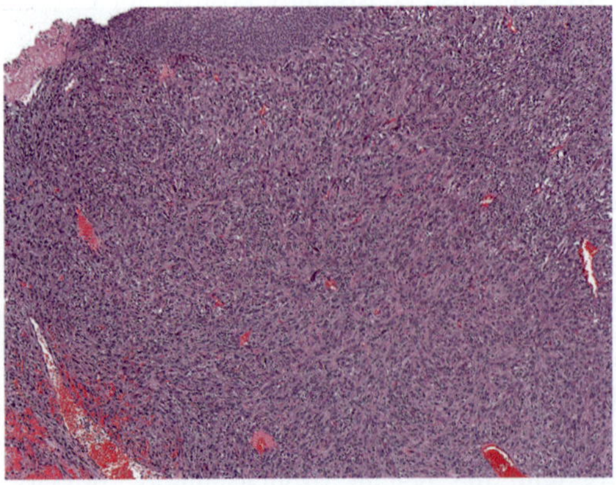

Fig. 8.11 Leiomyosarcoma of the urinary bladder. Morphologic features include fascicles of malignant spindle cells, with eosinophilic cytoplasm, hyperchromatic pleomorphic nuclei, and one or more prominent nucleoli. The overlying urothelial mucosal surface (upper left corner) is ulcerated

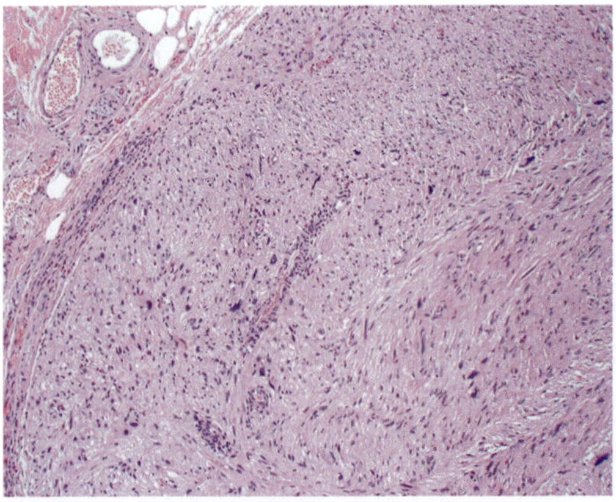

Fig. 8.12 Smooth muscle tumor of unknown malignant potential. In this limited TURBT sample, the tumor appears well circumscribed (upper left). Even at this low-power view, variably sized nuclei are visible

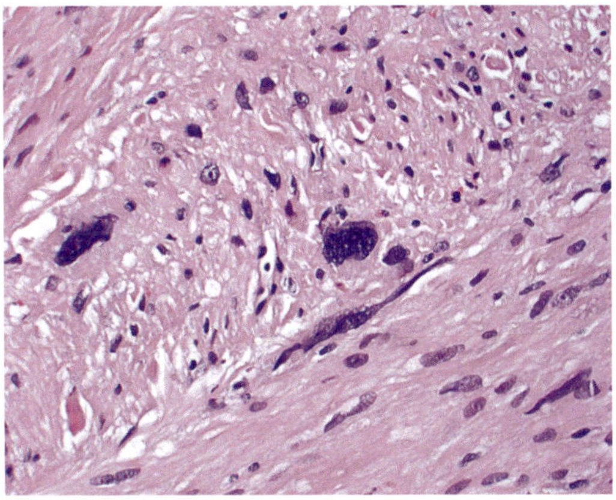

Fig. 8.13 Smooth muscle tumor of unknown malignant potential. Higher-power view (same tumor as in Fig. 8.12) shows variably sized nuclei, some of which are hyperchromatic and highly atypical

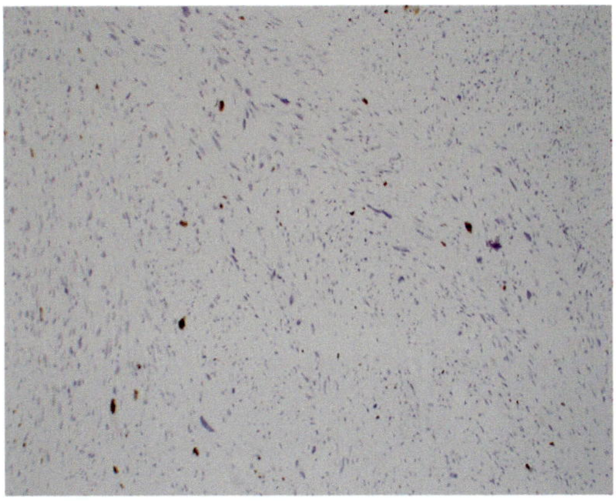

Fig. 8.14 Smooth muscle tumor of unknown malignant potential. Low Ki67 stain index

LMS stain positive with immunohistochemical stains for SMA, caldesmon, and calponin. Desmin is reported positive in less than half of these tumors. Epithelial markers such as cytokeratin and EMA may be focally positive in some tumors, especially the ones with epithelioid cells [22].

Inflammatory myofibroblastic tumor (described later in this chapter) and sarcomatoid urothelial carcinoma with smooth muscle differentiation are the two most common differential diagnostic considerations for high-grade LMS. Sarcomatoid urothelial carcinoma generally has a typical invasive carcinoma or carcinoma in situ component, in addition to the malignant spindle cell component. Immunohistochemical stains for cytokeratin cocktail, high molecular weight cytokeratin (HMWCK), p63, and GATA-3 may be useful to identify the urothelial carcinoma component. But prudence is required as some sarcomas may stain with cytokeratin, while sarcomatoid urothelial carcinoma may show only focal staining with epithelial markers of urothelial differentiation (Fig. 8.15).

Rhabdomyosarcoma

Rhabdomyosarcomas (RMS) are the most common malignant bladder tumors in children. However, few cases have also been reported in adults. They affect children of all ages and have a slight male preponderance [23, 24]. Most patients present with hematuria, accompanied by other urinary tract symptoms including frequency, dysuria, and sometimes urinary obstruction.

These tumors usually form a polypoid, soft, and fleshy mass, with necrosis and sometimes foci of hemorrhage. Morphologically, these are similar to RMS in other sites. Although all types of RMS have been reported to involve the bladder, embryonal RMS is by far the most common type. The botryoid subtype accounts for about a third of the embryonal RMS in the bladder. Spindle or stellate cells are present within myxoid stroma. Typical rhabdomyoblasts, with eosinophilic cytoplasm and cytoplasmic cross-striations, are present and are most readily visible in the botryoid subtype. Multiple mitoses are present, especially in the embryonal type. Alveolar RMS is less common, generally lacks the typical rhabdomyoblasts, and has fewer mitoses than the embryonal type [24]. Following chemotherapy, well-differentiated rhabdomyoblasts may be present. These cells have a large, smooth, single nucleus without significant pleomorphism or atypia and lack mitotic activity. These do not indicate the presence of persistent disease, and should not be confused for residual tumor, because the presence of residual tumor is an indication for continuation of chemotherapy [25].

Immunohistochemical stains used for diagnosis of RMS include myogenin, myo-D1, desmin,

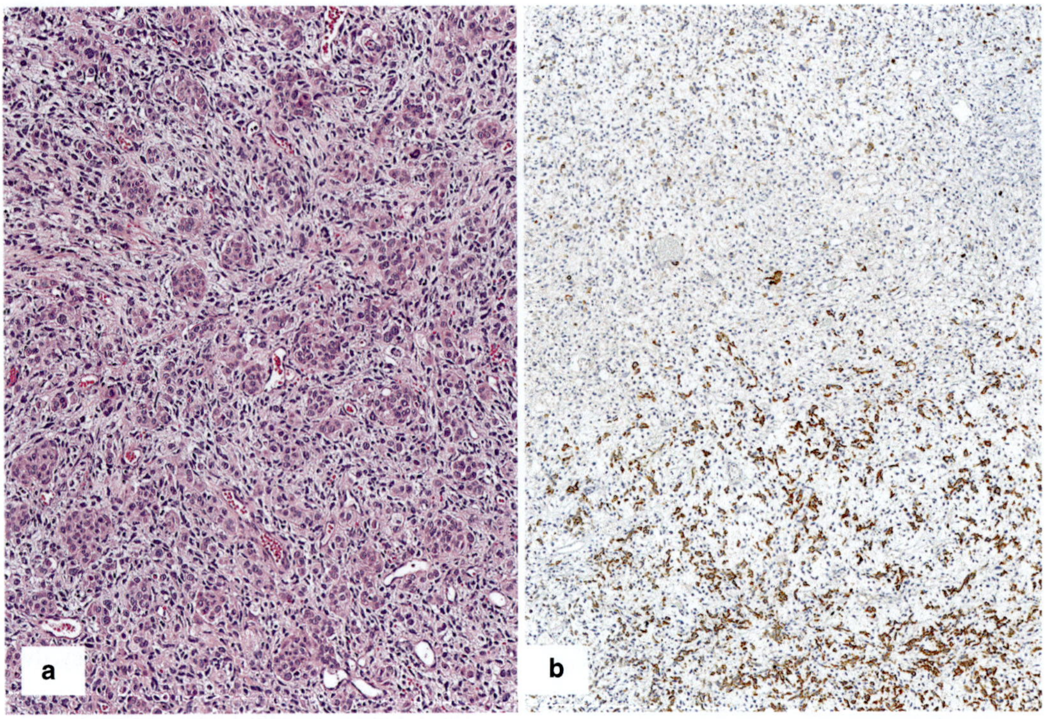

Fig. 8.15 Sarcomatoid urothelial carcinoma. The H&E on the left (image **a**) shows malignant spindle cells and nests of atypical epithelioid cells, resembling sarcoma. However, cytokeratin cocktail is only focally strongly positive in the spindle cells (right side, image **b**)

and myoglobin. Nuclear transcription factors myogenin and myo-D1 are the most sensitive and specific stains used for this diagnosis. Since these are nuclear stains, cytoplasmic staining is considered nonspecific and needs to be reported as negative. Embryonal RMS exhibits a heterogeneous pattern of staining, while alveolar RMS shows strong diffuse nuclear staining with myogenin and myo-D1.

Angiosarcoma

This sarcoma has been reported in fewer than 40 patients, a number of whom had a prior history of pelvic radiation therapy [26, 27]. These sarcomas are often deeply invasive into the muscularis propria. As with all primary bladder sarcomas, their morphologic features are similar to those of their visceral or soft tissue counterparts (Figs. 8.16 and 8.17).

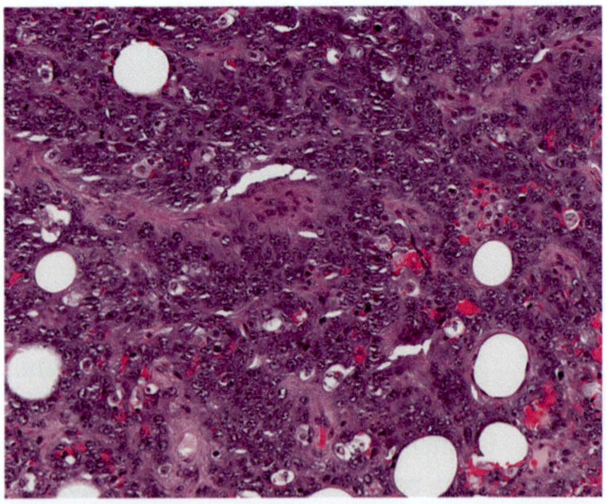

Fig. 8.16 Angiosarcoma of the urinary bladder in a patient with a prior history of pelvic radiation therapy. The tumor has more epithelioid features, resembling a high-grade urothelial carcinoma invading the adipose tissue. This case was diagnosed as high-grade urothelial carcinoma on the initial biopsy, due to the limited sample and the lack of clinical history

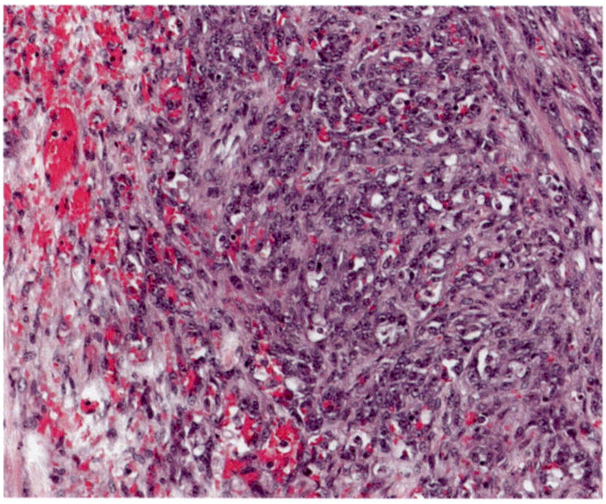

Fig. 8.17 Angiosarcoma of the urinary bladder in a patient with a prior history of pelvic radiation therapy. In this image, the tumor (same as in Fig. 8.16) has morphologic features more typical of angiosarcoma

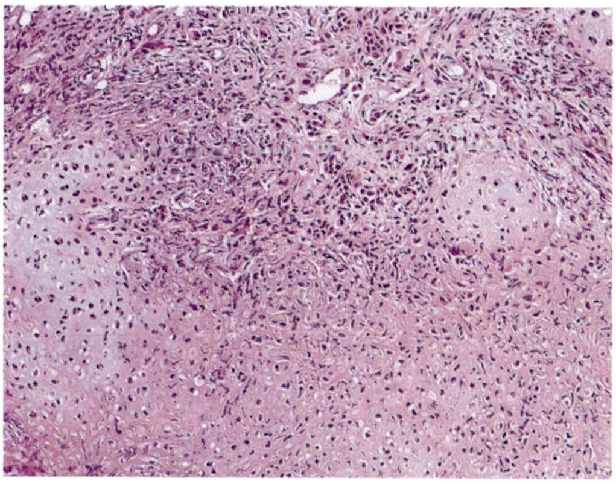

Fig. 8.18 Sarcomatoid urothelial carcinoma with divergent differentiation. The sarcomatoid component is almost entirely composed of cartilage

"Pseudoangiosarcomatous carcinoma" is an important differential diagnostic consideration in addition to sarcomatoid urothelial carcinoma, where urothelial carcinoma cells may form anastomosing channels and abortive pseudo-vascular spaces, due to acantholysis of tumor cells. CD31, ERG, and factor VIII immunohistochemical stains are positive in the angiosarcoma, while cytokeratin cocktail, GATA-3, cytokeratin 7, and p63 are positive in the urothelial carcinoma.

Miscellaneous Sarcomas of the Urinary Bladder

Other primary sarcomas arising in the urinary bladder are few and far between. These sarcomas have been reported as primary tumors; however, some of these, especially those reported in the early days of immunohistochemistry, may represent sarcomatoid urothelial carcinoma with divergent differentiation (Fig. 8.18). To reach the diagnosis of these primary sarcomas, sarcomatoid urothelial carcinoma and secondary involvement need to be ruled out. Extensive sampling may be required to rule out the presence of typical urothelial carcinoma and/or urothelial carcinoma in situ. For this reason, one should be cautious with making the diagnosis of primary sarcomas of the bladder in a limited sample.

Approximately 35 cases of primary *osteosarcoma* have been reported [28]. Their morphologic features are typical of other extra-skeletal osteosarcomas. Their differential diagnosis also includes urothelial carcinoma with osseous metaplasia.

Chondrosarcoma of the urinary bladder is rare and has the same morphologic features as those involving soft tissue [29]. However, as with osteosarcoma, heterologous cartilaginous component of sarcomatoid urothelial carcinoma is far more common (Fig. 8.18).

Only a few *malignant rhabdoid tumors* have been reported, all in children under 5 years of age [30]. Tumors have the typical morphologic features of extrarenal rhabdoid tumors and lack of expression of SMARCB1/INI1, which can be detected by immunohistochemical stain for BAF47 also known as INI-1.

Few cases of *malignant peripheral nerve sheath tumor (MPNST)* have been reported [31], mostly in adults with a history of neurofibromatosis.

Other rare sarcomas of the urinary bladder include malignant fibrous histiocytoma (MFH), fibrosarcoma, liposarcoma, hemangiopericytoma, Kaposi's sarcoma, and malignant paraganglioma (also see paraganglioma).

Myofibroblastic Lesions

Inflammatory myofibroblastic tumor (IMT) and postoperative spindle cell nodule (PSCN) are myofibroblastic lesions with overlapping morphologic features. The term PSCN, traditionally, has been reserved for lesions that occur in the bladder following a surgical procedure. IMT refers to myofibroblastic tumors that arise de novo without a history of prior instrumentation.

Postoperative Spindle Cell Nodule

Postoperative spindle cell nodule (PSCN) is a myofibroblastic proliferation at the site of prior instrumentation or trauma, which may include child birth and pelvic surgery on organs other than the bladder. These were first reported in 1990 [32] and since have been reported in a wide age range and are found to be more common in men [19, 33].

These proliferations form nodular masses at the site of a prior cystoscopic biopsy or transurethral resection. Most are less than 1.0 cm in greatest dimension although reported to range from 0.4 cm to 3.0 cm. Microscopically, there is a proliferation of spindle cells arranged in interlacing fascicles that may infiltrate between muscularis propria bundles (Fig. 8.19). The spindle cells are present within an edematous or myxoid stroma, with small delicate blood vessels and inflammatory cells. Due to its proliferative nature, numerous mitoses may be present; however, there is no or minimal nuclear pleomorphism and atypia. Dense acellular eosinophilic material may be present, sometimes surrounded by foreign body giant cells. The spindle cells stain for cytokeratin, SMA, and desmin, although staining may not be uniform [19].

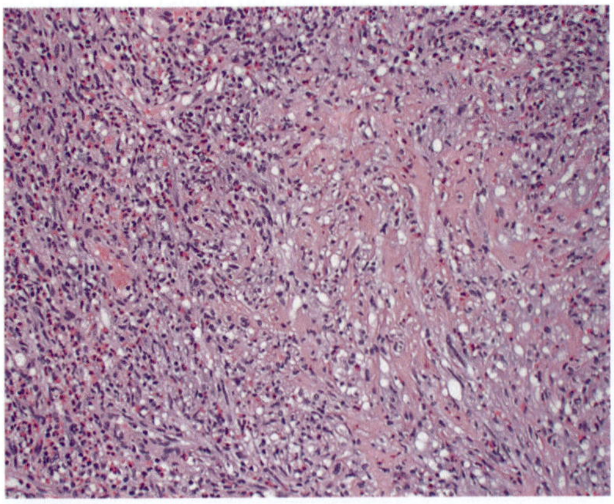

Fig. 8.19 Postoperative spindle cell nodule of the bladder. There is a proliferation of spindle cells, with small delicate blood vessels and inflammatory cells. Dense acellular eosinophilic material is present in the center

In some cases, PSCN may resemble low-grade leiomyosarcoma; however, PSCN has small blood vessels that are rare in LMS and lacks atypical mitotic figures. Both lesions may show overlapping immunohistochemical profiles, so reliance on stains may be misleading. Of course, knowledge of prior instrumentation is also helpful. Therefore, a clinicopathologic correlation is mandatory to render a proper diagnosis of PSCN. Since most PSCNs resolve spontaneously, conservative management is best.

Inflammatory Myofibroblastic Tumor

Inflammatory myofibroblastic tumor (IMT) is a neoplastic proliferation of myofibroblasts and fibroblasts mixed with inflammatory cells. The lung was involved in initial reports of this tumor; however, now we know that it affects numerous organs and even soft tissues. While IMT is the current name of this tumor, perusal of older literature will lead the reader to find a number of alternate names including inflammatory pseudotumor, pseudosarcomatous fibromyxoid tumor, pseudosarcomatous myofibroblastic tumor, pseudomalignant spindle cell proliferation, atypical myofibroblastic tumor, atypical fibromyxoid tumor, nodular fasciitis, and plasma cell granuloma [33, 34]. IMTs show a slight male preponderance and have been reported in almost all age groups, including children [33]. As with other bladder tumors, patients present with lower urinary tract symptoms, including hematuria.

IMTs usually form small nodules or ulcerated masses in the bladder mucosa. They may form a polypoid mass; tumors measuring up to 10 cm have been reported [33]. IMTs typically have haphazardly arranged spindle cells and are variably cellular (Fig. 8.20). The paucicellular foci may resemble granulation tissue, with the spindle cells within a myxoid stroma (Fig. 8.21). In the more cellular foci, spindle cells are arranged in fascicles (Fig. 8.22). The tumor may infiltrate in between muscularis propria bundles and sometimes may even extend into perivesical adipose tissue. The myxoid areas may have stellate and/or polygonal cells. Occasional strap-shaped cells or

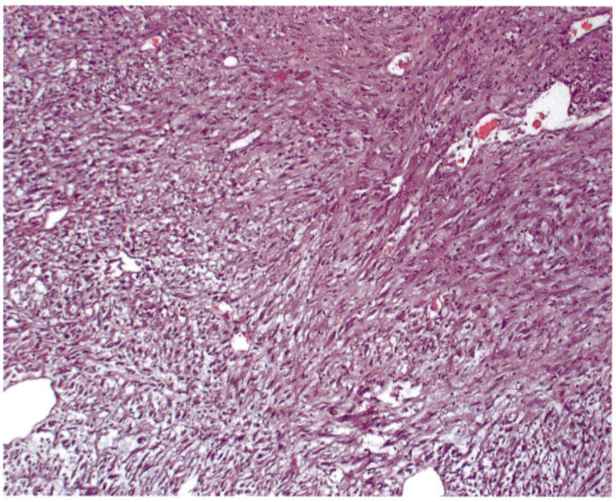

Fig. 8.20 Inflammatory myofibroblastic tumors typically have haphazardly arranged spindle cells and are variably cellular. This image shows the interface between the variably cellular foci. Top right has cellular foci of spindle cells arranged in fascicles, while bottom left has the paucicellular foci with spindle cells in a myxoid stroma

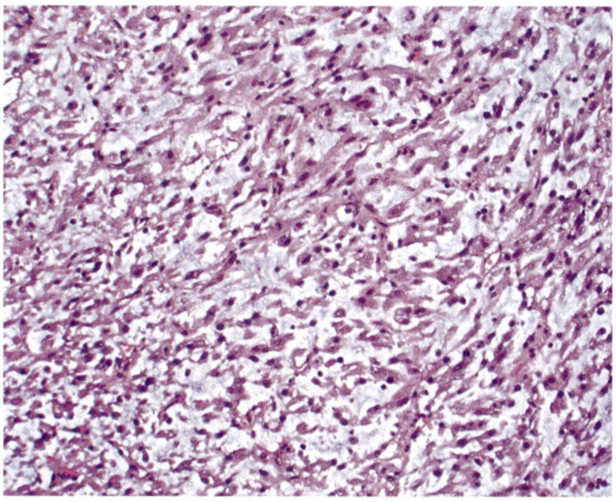

Fig. 8.21 Inflammatory myofibroblastic tumor, paucicellular focus with myxoid stroma. The spindle cells have eosinophilic cytoplasm. The nuclei are large and resemble those of tissue culture fibroblasts. Few strap-shaped cells with eosinophilic cytoplasm are also present

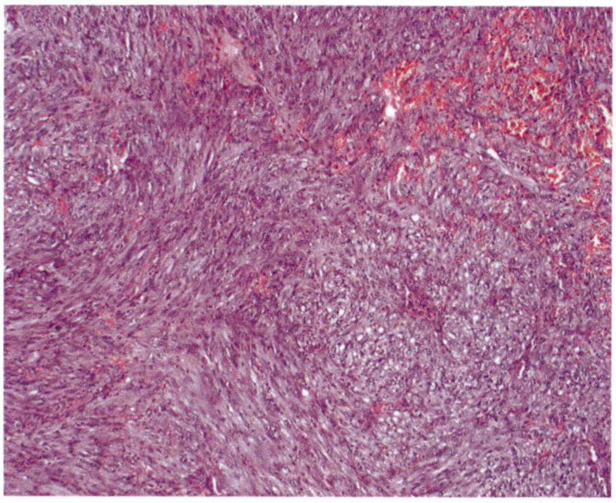

Fig. 8.22 Inflammatory myofibroblastic tumor. In the cellular foci, spindle cells are arranged in fascicles, almost resembling a leiomyosarcoma

"tadpole-like" cells with eosinophilic cytoplasm may be seen (Fig. 8.21). Tumor cells have eosinophilic or amphophilic cytoplasm. The nuclei are large and resemble those of tissue culture fibroblasts (Fig. 8.21). However, except for rare cases, they do not exhibit pleomorphism or hyperchromasia typically seen in sarcomas. Nucleoli are usually single, sometimes multiple, and small, while prominent nucleoli are the least common. Mitotic count is usually less than 5 mitoses per 10 hpf, but tumors with up to 20 mitoses per 10 hpf have been reported [33]. The lack of atypical mitoses is important to keep in mind, as their presence has not been reported in any of the published reports. The presence of atypical mitoses should lead to a critical evaluation of the tumor to rule out a sarcoma or sarcomatoid carcinoma [19, 33]. The inflammatory infiltrate is predominantly composed of lymphocytes, plasma cells, and eosinophils. The foci with myxoid stroma may show numerous red blood cells, which may form microscopic foci of hemorrhage.

Anaplastic lymphoma kinase 1 (ALK-1) is an important marker for IMT, as it is positive in approximately three-fourths of all cases using immunohistochemistry [33]. Antibody clone D5F3 has been reported to be superior in terms of intensity and extent of staining [35] (Fig. 8.23). There are three different types of staining patterns for ALK-1, which correspond to the ALK gene's distinct fusion partners.

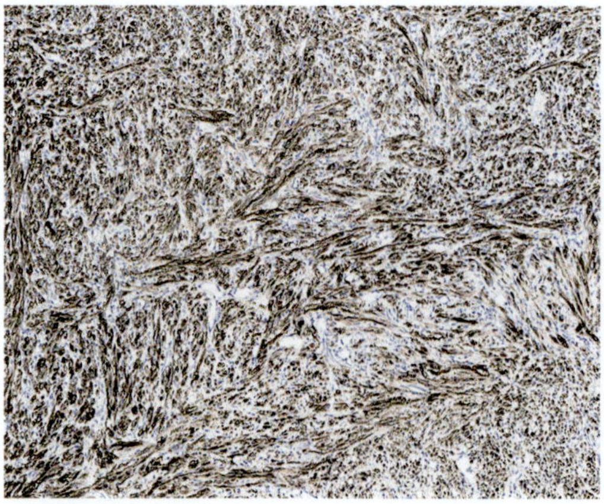

Fig. 8.23 Inflammatory myofibroblastic tumor. ALK-1 immunohistochemical stain (clone D5F3) shows strong and diffuse staining

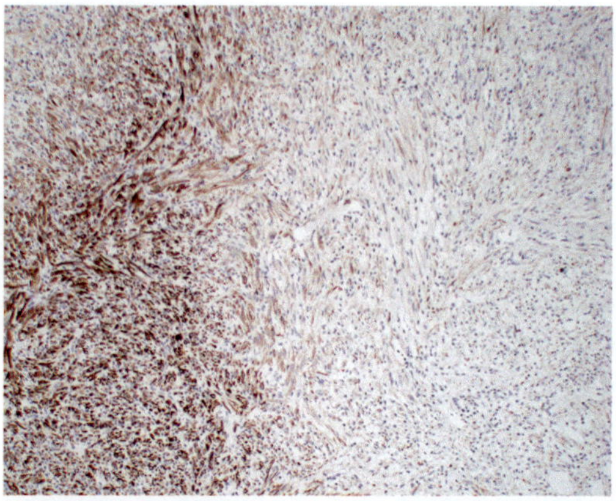

Fig. 8.24 Inflammatory myofibroblastic tumor. Cytokeratin cocktail stain is strongly positive in part of the tumor, while the rest is negative

TPM3-/TPM 4-ALK fusion is associated with diffuse smooth cytoplasmic staining, CLTC-ALK fusion is associated with granular cytoplasmic staining, and RANBP2-ALK fusion is associated with nuclear membrane staining [35]. In addition to ALK-1 immunohistochemical expression, ALK gene alterations have been reported in up to 70% of cases. Alterations of the ALK gene provide further evidence to suggest that these lesions are neoplastic in nature, rather than a reactive process [36, 37]. New molecular findings are reported for IMT of the lung, abdomen, esophagus, and pelvis. Recently, alterations of other kinase genes such as ROS1, RET, and NTRK3 gene fusions have been reported in IMT of the lung [38]. Rhabdomyosarcomas may also show ALK alterations, which needs to be kept in mind when RMS is in the differential diagnosis.

The myofibroblastic nature of the spindle cells is highlighted by staining for SMA and desmin; however, the staining may be variable within different foci of the same tumor. IMTs are usually negative for skeletal muscle-specific stains such as myogenin and myo-D1. Cytokeratin stain is positive, at least focally; but it may be strongly positive in some foci (Fig. 8.24), which can mislead one to assume the tumor is sarcomatoid carcinoma (Fig. 8.15).

Differential diagnosis of IMT includes sarcomatoid urothelial carcinoma, leiomyosarcoma, and rhabdomyosarcoma. Sarcomatoid urothelial carcinoma usually has a typical urothelial carcinoma component or in situ carcinoma. Cytokeratin stain may be misleading as it can be positive in both tumors. While IMTs stain with smooth muscle markers, sarcomatoid carcinomas are mostly negative. P63 and high molecular weight cytokeratin may be helpful since both are negative in IMT but may be positive in the epithelial component of sarcomatoid carcinoma. Leiomyosarcoma may also show focal staining for p63. Staining for p53 is often strong and diffuse in leiomyosarcoma and rhabdomyosarcoma, while it is usually weak or absent in IMT [35, 39]. The use of Ki67 staining for measuring proliferative activity to distinguish from sarcomas may be misleading, as IMT usually has a high proliferation index (Fig. 8.25).

Most IMTs are cured by transurethral resection. Local recurrence(s) may require partial or total cystectomy to achieve disease control in rare cases [19]. There are no credible reports of metastatic bladder IMTs. However, there are reports of malignant behavior of IMT arising in other organs. Therefore, the IMT lesions should be completely excised, and a close clinical follow-up is recommended.

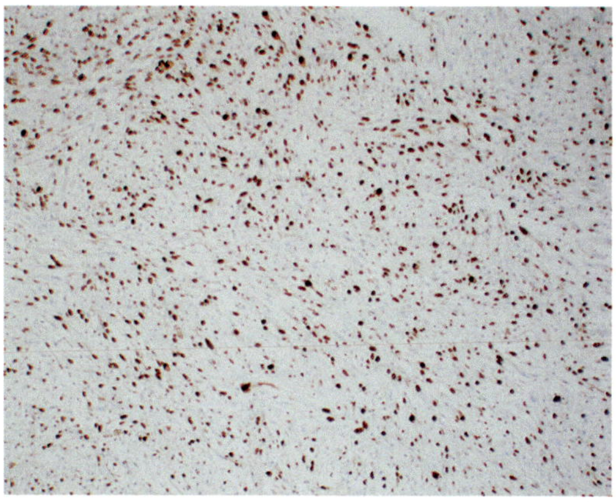

Fig. 8.25 Inflammatory myofibroblastic tumor. Ki67 stain shows the high proliferative activity of these tumors

Summary

The diagnosis of mesenchymal tumors in the urinary bladder is not difficult if the pathologist keeps these tumors in mind when looking at tumors that do not fit the morphologic features of typical urothelial carcinoma or its variants. Except for paraganglioma, which may be confused for high-grade urothelial carcinoma, the rest of the benign tumors are relatively straightforward to diagnose, as they resemble their counterparts in other organs. To avoid misdiagnosing paraganglioma as urothelial carcinoma, it is always a good practice to look for evidence of overlying urothelium with urothelial dysplasia or urothelial carcinoma in situ. Uniform nests of cells with pale or eosinophilic cytoplasm should raise the differential diagnosis of paraganglioma. Ultimately, immunohistochemical stains can easily help arrive at the correct diagnosis. As with benign tumors, sarcomas morphologically resemble those in other viscera and the soft tissue. Sarcomatoid urothelial carcinoma should be at the top of the differential diagnosis list for any malignant spindle cell tumor and should always be ruled out, before reaching the diagnosis of sarcoma or IMT.

References

1. Beilan JA, Lawton A, Hajdenberg J, Rosser CJ. Pheochromocytoma of the urinary bladder: a systematic review of the contemporary literature. BMC Urol. 2013;13:22.
2. Giubellino A, Lara K, Martucci V, Huynh T, Agarwal P, Pacak K, et al. Urinary bladder paragangliomas: how immunohistochemistry can assist to identify patients with SDHB germline and somatic mutations. Am J Surg Pathol. 2015;39(11):1488–92.
3. Cheng L, Leibovich BC, Cheville JC, Ramnani DM, Sebo TJ, Neumann RM, et al. Paraganglioma of the urinary bladder: can biologic potential be predicted? Cancer. 2000;88(4):844–52.
4. So JS, Epstein JI. GATA3 expression in paragangliomas: a pitfall potentially leading to misdiagnosis of urothelial carcinoma. Mod Pathol. 2013;26(10):1365–70.
5. Park S, Kang SY, Kwon GY, Kwon JE, Kim SK, Kim JY, et al. Clinicopathologic Characteristics and Mutational Status of Succinate Dehydrogenase Genes in Paraganglioma of the Urinary Bladder: A Multi-Institutional Korean Study. Arch Pathol Lab Med. 2017;141(5):671–7.
6. Mason EF, Sadow PM, Wagner AJ, Remillard SP, Flood TA, Belanger EC, et al. Identification of succinate dehydrogenase-deficient bladder paragangliomas. Am J Surg Pathol. 2013;37(10):1612–8.
7. Martin SA, Sears DL, Sebo TJ, Lohse CM, Cheville JC. Smooth muscle neoplasms of the urinary bladder: a clinicopathologic comparison of leiomyoma and leiomyosarcoma. Am J Surg Pathol. 2002;26(3):292–300.
8. Knoll LD, Segura JW, Scheithauer BW. Leiomyoma of the bladder. J Urol. 1986;136(4):906–8.
9. Lee TK, Miyamoto H, Osunkoya AO, Guo CC, Weiss SW, Epstein JI. Smooth muscle neoplasms of the urinary bladder: a clinicopathologic study of 51 cases. Am J Surg Pathol. 2010;34(4):502–9.
10. Kaefer M, Adams MC, Rink RC, Keating MA. Principles in management of complex pediatric genitourinary plexiform neurofibroma. Urology. 1997;49(6):936–40.
11. Cheng L, Scheithauer BW, Leibovich BC, Ramnani DM, Cheville JC, Bostwick DG. Neurofibroma of the urinary bladder. Cancer. 1999;86(3):505–13.
12. Cummings JM, Wehry MA, Parra RO, Levy BK. Schwannoma of the urinary bladder: a case report. Int J Urol. 1998;5(5):496–7.
13. Olaya M, Vicioso L, Hierro I, Quinonero A, Matilla A, Lopez-Beltran A. Granular cell tumor of the bladder: a case report. Anal Quant Cytopathol Histpathol. 2013;35(5):289–93.

14. Tsui JF, Weinberger JM, Kashan M, Weiss JP, Robinson BD, Blaivas JG. Bladder lipoma. J Urol. 2013;190(4):1387–8.
15. Chen CH, Boag AH, Beiko DT, Siemens DR, Froese A, Isotalo PA. Composite paraganglioma-ganglioneuroma of the urinary bladder: a rare neoplasm causing hemodynamic crisis at tumour resection. Can Urol Assoc J. 2009;3(5):E45–8.
16. Lasota J, Carlson JA, Miettinen M. Spindle cell tumor of urinary bladder serosa with phenotypic and genotypic features of gastrointestinal stromal tumor. Arch Pathol Lab Med. 2000;124(6):894–7.
17. Mills SE, Bova GS, Wick MR, Young RH. Leiomyosarcoma of the urinary bladder. A clinicopathologic and immunohistochemical study of 15 cases. Am J Surg Pathol. 1989;13(6):480–9.
18. Kunze E, Theuring F, Kruger G. Primary mesenchymal tumors of the urinary bladder. A histological and immunohistochemical study of 30 cases. Pathol Res Pract. 1994;190(4):311–32.
19. Iczkowski KA, Shanks JH, Gadaleanu V, Cheng L, Jones EC, Neumann R, et al. Inflammatory pseudotumor and sarcoma of urinary bladder: differential diagnosis and outcome in thirty-eight spindle cell neoplasms. Mod Pathol. 2001;14(10):1043–51.
20. Russo P, Brady MS, Conlon K, Hajdu SI, Fair WR, Herr HW, et al. Adult urological sarcoma. J Urol. 1992;147(4):1032–6.
21. Rosser CJ, Slaton JW, Izawa JI, Levy LB, Dinney CP. Clinical presentation and outcome of high-grade urinary bladder leiomyosarcoma in adults. Urology. 2003;61(6):1151–5.
22. Wick MR, Brown BA, Young RH, Mills SE. Spindle-cell proliferations of the urinary tract. An immunohistochemical study. Am J Surg Pathol. 1988;12(5):379–89.
23. Raney B Jr, Heyn R, Hays DM, Tefft M, Newton WA Jr, Wharam M, et al. Sequelae of treatment in 109 patients followed for 5 to 15 years after diagnosis of sarcoma of the bladder and prostate. A report from the Intergroup Rhabdomyosarcoma Study Committee. Cancer. 1993;71(7):2387–94.
24. Leuschner I, Harms D, Mattke A, Koscielniak E, Treuner J. Rhabdomyosarcoma of the urinary bladder and vagina: a clinicopathologic study with emphasis on recurrent disease: a report from the Kiel Pediatric Tumor Registry and the German CWS Study. Am J Surg Pathol. 2001;25(7):856–64.
25. Ortega JA, Rowland J, Monforte H, Malogolowkin M, Triche T. Presence of well-differentiated rhabdomyoblasts at the end of therapy for pelvic rhabdomyosarcoma: implications for the outcome. J Pediatr Hematol Oncol. 2000;22(2):106–11.
26. Tavora F, Montgomery E, Epstein JI. A series of vascular tumors and tumorlike lesions of the bladder. Am J Surg Pathol. 2008;32(8):1213–9.
27. Seethala RR, Gomez JA, Vakar-Lopez F. Primary angiosarcoma of the bladder. Arch Pathol Lab Med. 2006;130(10):1543–7.
28. Ghalayini IF, Bani-Hani IH, Almasri NM. Osteosarcoma of the urinary bladder occurring simultaneously with prostate and bowel carcinomas: report of a case and review of the literature. Arch Pathol Lab Med. 2001;125(6):793–5.
29. Torenbeek R, Blomjous CE, Meijer CJ. Chondrosarcoma of the urinary bladder: report of a case with immunohistochemical and ultrastructural findings and review of the literature. Eur Urol. 1993;23(4):502–5.
30. Savage N, Linn D, McDonough C, Donohoe JM, Franco A, Reuter V, et al. Molecularly confirmed primary malignant rhabdoid tumor of the urinary bladder: implications of accurate diagnosis. Ann Diagn Pathol. 2012;16(6):504–7.
31. Rober PE, Smith JB, Sakr W, Pierce JM Jr. Malignant peripheral nerve sheath tumor (malignant schwannoma) of urinary bladder in von Recklinghausen neurofibromatosis. Urology. 1991;38(5):473–6.
32. Huang WL, Ro JY, Grignon DJ, Swanson D, Ordonez NG, Ayala AG. Postoperative spindle cell nodule of the prostate and bladder. J Urol. 1990;143(4):824–6.
33. Harik LR, Merino C, Coindre JM, Amin MB, Pedeutour F, Weiss SW. Pseudosarcomatous myofibroblastic proliferations of the bladder: a clinicopathologic study of 42 cases. Am J Surg Pathol. 2006;30(7):787–94.
34. Ro JY, el-Naggar AK, Amin MB, Sahin AA, Ordonez NG, Ayala AG. Pseudosarcomatous fibromyxoid tumor of the urinary bladder and prostate: immunohistochemical, ultrastructural, and DNA flow cytometric analyses of nine cases. Hum Pathol. 1993;24(11):1203–10.
35. Choi E, Williamson SR, Montironi R, Zhang S, Wang M, Eble JN, et al. Inflammatory myofibroblastic tumour of the urinary bladder: the role of immunoglobulin G4 and the comparison of two immunohistochemical antibodies and fluorescence in-situ hybridization for the detection of anaplastic lymphoma kinase alterations. Histopathology. 2015;67(1):20–38.
36. Tsuzuki T, Magi-Galluzzi C, Epstein JI. ALK-1 expression in inflammatory myofibroblastic tumor of the urinary bladder. Am J Surg Pathol. 2004;28(12):1609–14.
37. Montgomery EA, Shuster DD, Burkart AL, Esteban JM, Sgrignoli A, Elwood L, et al. Inflammatory myofibroblastic tumors of the urinary tract: a clinicopathologic study of 46 cases, including a malignant example inflammatory fibrosarcoma and a subset associated with high-grade urothelial carcinoma. Am J Surg Pathol. 2006;30(12):1502–12.

38. Antonescu CR, Suurmeijer AJ, Zhang L, Sung YS, Jungbluth AA, Travis WD, et al. Molecular characterization of inflammatory myofibroblastic tumors with frequent ALK and ROS1 gene fusions and rare novel RET rearrangement. Am J Surg Pathol. 2015;39(7):957–67.

39. Westfall DE, Folpe AL, Paner GP, Oliva E, Goldstein L, Alsabeh R, et al. Utility of a comprehensive immunohistochemical panel in the differential diagnosis of spindle cell lesions of the urinary bladder. Am J Surg Pathol. 2009;33(1):99–105.

Neuroendocrine Tumors of the Urinary Bladder

9

Ahmed N. Shehabeldin and Jae Y. Ro

Neuroendocrine tumors (NETs) are commonly found in the lung, gastrointestinal tract, and pancreas. NETs of the lung are classified as small cell neuroendocrine carcinoma (SCNEC), large cell neuroendocrine carcinoma (LCNEC), and typical and atypical carcinoid tumors. NETs of the gastrointestinal tract and pancreas are subdivided based on their histological differentiation and Ki67 proliferation index into well-differentiated neuroendocrine tumors (WDNETs) grades 1, 2, and 3 or poorly differentiated neuroendocrine carcinomas (NEC) including SCNEC and LCNEC. In the urinary bladder, however, neuroendocrine neoplasms are classified into WDNETs, SCNEC, and LCNEC, in addition to paraganglioma [1]. The cell of origin of these tumors remains uncertain. Neuroendocrine cells found in the basement membrane of normal urothelium or reactive urothelial epithelium may give rise to WDNETs, while less differentiated NETs, including SCNEC and LCNEC, seem to arise from divergent differentiation of urothelial carcinoma [2]. Paragangliomas are thought to arise from chromaffin cells in the autonomic ganglia of the urinary bladder wall [3]. NETs of the urinary bladder are listed in Table 9.1 with clinical and pathologic features.

Well-Differentiated Neuroendocrine Tumors

Although the use of the term "carcinoid tumor" to describe WDNETs in the urinary bladder has been discouraged by the World Health Organization (WHO) [1], this term is still frequently used, especially when describing tumors with malignant features, such as "malignant carcinoid."

Epidemiology, Clinical Features, and Treatment

WDNETs of the urinary bladder are extremely rare, with fewer than 25 cases described in the literature [4]. Based on these few described cases, patient demographics are similar to those of urothelial carcinoma. WDNETs of the urinary bladder typically arise in middle-aged to elderly men who are, in most cases, asymptomatic; the tumors are found incidentally on cystoscopy or imaging studies performed for other reasons. In some cases, patients may present with nonspecific symptoms of hematuria and irritative urinary symptoms or with obstructive symptoms if the tumor is located

A. N. Shehabeldin
Department of Pathology and Genomic Medicine, Houston Methodist Hospital, Houston, TX, USA

J. Y. Ro (✉)
Department of Pathology and Genomic Medicine, Weill Medical College of Cornell University/Houston Methodist Hospital, Houston, TX, USA
e-mail: JaeRo@houstonmethodist.org

H. Zhou et al. (eds.), *Urinary Bladder Pathology*, https://doi.org/10.1007/978-3-030-71509-0_9

Table 9.1 A summary of the clinical and pathologic features of urinary bladder NETs

	WDNET	SCNEC	LCNEC	Paraganglioma
Clinical features				
Incidence	Extremely rare (~25 cases reported in the literature)	Rare (<1% of bladder tumors), 500 new cases per year	Extremely rare (~30 cases reported in the literature)	Rare (0.6% of bladder tumors)
Age range	Middle-aged to elderly	Elderly	Middle-aged to elderly	Young to middle-aged
Sex predilection	Male	Male	Male	Female
Syndrome association	None known	None known	None known	2/3 are sporadic; 1/3 are associated with inherited disorders (germline mutation in SDHB, VHL, NF-1, Carney triad, MEN 2A and MEN 2B, and familial paraganglioma syndrome)
Symptoms	Asymptomatic (discovered on cystoscopy or imaging performed for other purposes) or obstructive symptoms	Irritative and/or obstructive symptoms, symptoms of metastatic disease, and paraneoplastic syndromes	Irritative and/or obstructive symptoms and symptoms of metastatic disease	Hematuria, hypertension, and micturition syncope in approximately half of the cases, paroxysmal palpitation and diaphoresis less commonly seen
Prognosis	Cured by surgery in majority of cases; 1/4 of cases had aggressive local disease and LN or distant metastasis	Poor (5-year cancer-specific survival rate is 14–16%)	Poor	Cured by surgery in majority of cases; malignant features (extensive local disease and metastasis) in 20% of cases
Hypothesized cell of origin	NE cells found in the basement membrane of normal urothelium or reactive urothelial epithelium	Divergent differentiation of multipotent stem cells in the urothelial lining		Chromaffin cells in autonomic ganglia in the wall of the bladder
Pathologic features				
Gross appearance	Small (0.1–1.2 cm) smooth-surfaced nodules or polyps with hyperemic mucosa, located in the bladder neck or trigone area	Polypoid, nodular, or ulcerated appearance and variable degrees of muscular and perivesical fat invasion		Solitary, well-circumscribed, intravesical exophytic or intramural nodule, 2–5 cm at greatest dimension
Growth pattern	Nested, trabecular, glandular, or acinar architectures with frequent association with cystitis cystica and cystitis glandularis, Usually located in the lamina propria, Rarely involve the muscularis propria	Infiltrative sheets, cords, and occasional geographic necrosis		Characteristic discrete nests (Zellballen) with intervening vascular septa

Cytology	Abundant amphophilic granular cytoplasm (reminiscent of Paneth cells), bland nuclei with speckled chromatin, and absent to inconspicuous nucleoli Rarely, atypical cells with larger nuclei and conspicuous nucleoli can be seen, with rare to no mitoses, and no necrosis	Overlapping, small, round to oval, hyperchromatic nuclei with nuclear molding, speckled chromatin pattern, no or inconspicuous nucleoli, scant cytoplasm, high mitotic rate (>10 mitoses/10 high-power fields); Azzopardi phenomenon can be seen	Large, polygonal cells, low nuclear-cytoplasmic ratio, polymorphic nuclei, coarse chromatin, and prominent nucleoli; mitoses and necrosis are more pronounced than in SCNEC	Polygonal cells that have finely granular amphophilic cytoplasm and ovoid nuclei embedded in a richly vascularized fibrous stroma with sustentacular cells; nuclear pleomorphism and occasional mitotic figures can be seen, but do not reflect signs of malignancy
Immunohistochemistry	syn, chr, NSE, CD56+, c-Kit,CK7,uroplakin,TTF-1,PAP+/−,PSA-	syn, chr, NSE, CD56, INSM1+, CK7, EMA, CAM 5.2, CK, AE1/AE3 mostly + CK 34βE12, GATA3, TTF-1+/−, CK20, uroplakin, CD44v6, PSA, PAP-	syn, chr, NSE, CD56+, CK7, EMA, CAM 5.2, CK, AE1/AE3 mostly+ TTF-1-	Polygonal cells: syn,chr,NSE,CD56,GATA3+,CK,EMA- Sustentacular cells: S-100, SOX10
Ki-67 (Mib-1)	Low	High	High	Variable

NET neuroendocrine tumor, *WDNET* well-differentiated neuroendocrine tumor, *SCNEC* small cell neuroendocrine carcinoma, *LCNEC* large cell neuroendocrine carcinoma, *NE* neuroendocrine, *syn* synaptophysin, *chr* chromogranin, *NSE* neuron-specific enolase, *PAP* prostatic acid phosphatase, *PSA* prostate-specific antigen, *TTF*-1 thyroid transcription factor, *INSM1* insulinoma-associated protein 1, *EMA* epithelial membrane antigen, *CK* cytokeratin in the bladder outlet or the urethra. WDNETs of the urinary bladder are not hormonally active in most cases, and carcinoid syndrome has not been reported in association with these tumors [5]. However, paraneoplastic syndrome, in the form of calcitonin-producing WDNET, has been reported [6]. The majority of urinary bladder WDNETs behave in a benign fashion; however, cases with aggressive local disease, lymph node and/or distant metastasis, and death due to the disease have been described [1, 5].

Cystoscopic transurethral resection of low-grade WDNETs shows, in the few cases where long-term outcomes have been documented, no recurrence or disease progression [5]. For more aggressive disease, partial or radical cystectomy or cystoprostatectomy with systemic chemotherapy may be required [7, 8].

Pathologic and Immunohistochemical Features

On cystoscopic examination, most cases of WDNETs of the urinary bladder consist of small (0.1–1.2 cm) smooth-surfaced nodules or polyps with hyperemic mucosa located in the bladder neck or trigone area, although larger lesions (up to 5 cm) have been reported [7]. Histologically, WDNETs are usually located in the lamina propria. However, there are rare exceptions where the tumors involve the muscularis propria [9]. WDNETs demonstrate the typical pattern of carcinoid tumors found in other locations: trabecular, insular (Fig. 9.1a), pseudoglandular (Fig. 9.1b), or acinar architecture with frequent association with cystitis cystica and cystitis glandularis [9]. The neoplastic cells of WDNETs

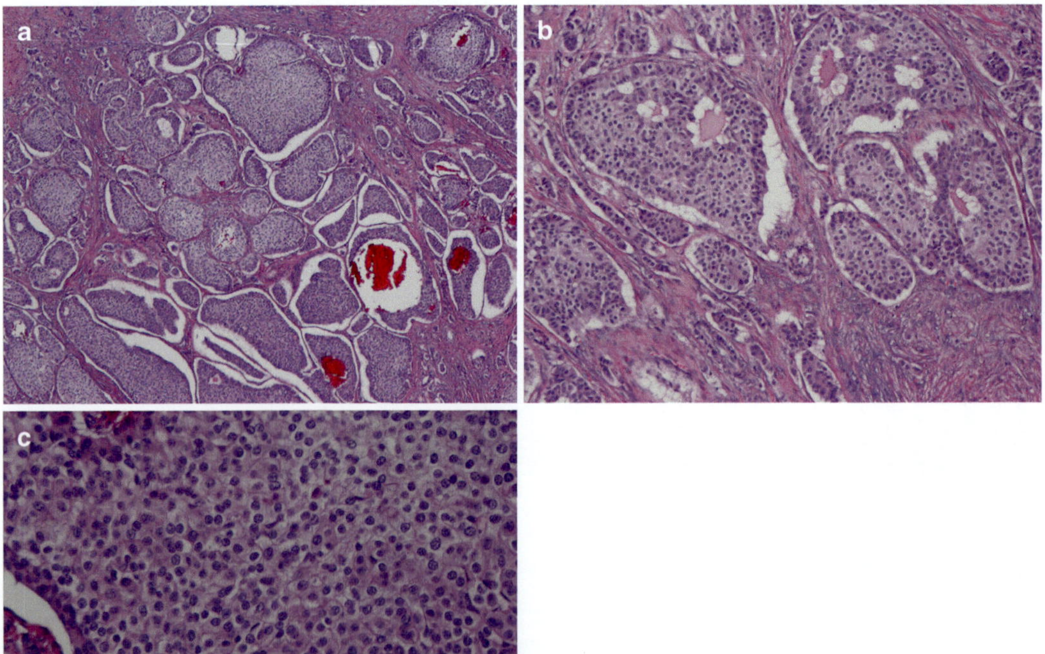

Fig. 9.1 (**a**) WDNET shows insular growth pattern with delicate fibrovascular stroma and artifactual stromal retraction (hematoxylin and eosin, 20x). (**b**) WDNET shows nested pattern with focal pseudoglandular architecture (hematoxylin and eosin, 100x). (**c**) WDNET cells have abundant amphophilic cytoplasm, bland nuclei with speckled chromatin, inconspicuous nucleoli, and no mitoses. Necrosis is not seen (hematoxylin and eosin, 200x)

have abundant amphophilic granular cytoplasm (reminiscent of Paneth cells), bland nuclei with speckled chromatin, and absent to inconspicuous nucleoli. Occasionally, atypical cells with large nuclei and conspicuous nucleoli can be seen. Mitoses are rare, and necrosis is generally absent (Fig. 9.1c). Although no defined criteria have been proposed for malignancy, malignant carcinoid tumors of the urinary bladder have been reported in the literature. In one case, transmural extension, serosal infiltration, and lymph node metastasis were seen [7]. In other cases, distant metastasis to the lungs and bones have been reported [8].

Urinary bladder WDNETs stain with commonly used neuroendocrine markers [synaptophysin, chromogranin, neuron-specific enolase (NSE), CD56, and CD57]. Additionally, some tumors show positive staining with c-Kit (CD117), cytokeratin-7, uroplakin, and thyroid transcription factor (TTF-1) [2, 5, 10]. Also, staining of the tumor cells with prostate acid phosphatase (PAP) presents a potential diagnostic pitfall where WDNETs can be confused with prostatic origin tumors. The lack of staining with other prostate-specific markers, including prostate-specific antigen (PSA) and NKX3.1, can be used to distinguish these entities [9].

In urinary bladder WDNETs, no further classification into grade 1, grade 2, and grade 3 based on a number of mitoses and Ki-67 proliferation index is officially recommended.

Small Cell Neuroendocrine Carcinoma

Epidemiology, Clinical Features, and Treatment

Previously known as oat cell carcinoma, SCNEC of the urinary bladder is more common than WDNET and LCNEC; however, it still only accounts for less than 1% of urinary bladder tumors [11], with approximately 500 new cases per year [2].

SCNECs of the urinary bladder, distinct from pulmonary SCNECs, are usually present as a combined form with urothelial carcinoma and SCNEC, and pure SCNECs are relatively rare. SCNECs typically affect older males with a history of smoking. Hematuria is the most commonly presenting symptom; irritative and obstructive symptoms are less commonly observed [11, 12]. Features of paraneoplastic syndrome, in the form of humoral hypercalcemia of malignancy secondary to the production of parathyroid hormone-related protein, have been observed [13]. Although urinary bladder SCNEC tends to have better prognosis than SCNEC of the lung or prostate [4], neuroendocrine differentiation of urothelial carcinoma confers a worse prognosis, with earlier distant metastases, than does conventional urothelial carcinoma [14, 15]. However, when SCNEC is compared to conventional urothelial carcinoma at similar stage, there is no difference in survival [16]. The 5-year cancer-specific survival rate for SCNEC is 14–16% [17, 18].

Surgical management with cystectomy has an important role in the management of patients with urinary bladder SCNEC, unlike SCNEC of the lung [11, 19–23]. SCNEC patients who receive chemotherapy, radiation therapy, and cystectomy achieve the best overall survival and cancer-specific survival outcomes compared to a single therapeutic modality [24]. Few cases of SCNEC arising in the ureter or the urethra have been reported in the literature, with similar histological features to SCNEC of the urinary bladder [25–27].

Molecular Genetics

These tumors are thought to arise from divergent differentiation of multipotent stem cells in the urothelial lining. This theory is supported by the exceedingly rare incidence of pure SCNEC of the urinary bladder and because these tumors are usually found in association with either urothelial carcinoma, squamous cell carcinoma, adenocarcinoma, or sarcomatoid carcinoma [11, 28–30]. In a series of 51 patients with SCNEC of the urinary bladder, the majority of cases had urothelial carcinoma; few patients had adenocarcinoma or squamous cell carcinoma components, and only 12% had pure SCNEC without other carcinoma components [31]. Additional studies demonstrated a common clonal origin of coexisting urothelial carcinoma and SCNEC, further substantiating the divergent differentiation model of SCNEC development. SCNEC of the urinary bladder shares common molecular aberrations with SCNEC of pulmonary origin. Deletions in 4q, 5q, 10q, and 13q; DNA gains in 5p, 6p, 8q, and 20q; and loss of heterozygosity in 3p25–26, 9p21, 9q32–33, and 17p13 have all been shown to lead to activation of oncogenes or suppression of tumor suppressor genes in SCNEC of the urinary bladder [32, 33]. Alteration in the tumor suppressor genes, RB1 and TP53, are found in 90% of SCNEC cases of the urinary bladder [16, 34]. However, alterations in these two genes are also prevalent in conventional high-grade urothelial carcinomas, which may lead to the conclusion that these mutations lead to the development of invasive tumors rather than drive neuroendocrine differentiation [35]. Activating mutations in TERT promoter gene are found in urinary bladder SCNEC and conventional urothelial carcinoma, but not lung or prostate SCNEC, further supporting the divergent differentiation model of SCNEC of the urinary bladder [36].

Pathologic Features

On cystoscopic examination, SCNEC can originate from anywhere in the urinary bladder, including urachal remnants. SCNEC has similar cystoscopic and gross pathologic features to urothelial carcinoma, with a polypoid, nodular, or ulcerated appearance; however, muscular and perivesical fat invasion is more commonly seen in SCNEC [4, 11, 37].

Histological examination shows the classical features of SCNEC in other organs, with morphologic triads: (1) small size of tumor cell nuclei (less than three resting lymphocytes (<20 microns); (2) scanty cytoplasm with overlapping, small, round to oval hyperchromatic nuclei and nuclear molding; and (3) speckled or "salt and pepper" chromatin pattern with no or inconspicuous nucleoli (Fig. 9.2a). In addition to these features, SCNECs always show a high mitotic rate (>10 mitoses/10 high-power fields) and single-cell necrosis or large areas of geographic necrosis (Fig. 9.2b and c). When small cell tumors do not show a high mitotic index and/or areas of necrosis, the diagnosis of SCNEC should be reserved for other ancillary diagnostic tests. Smudged, deeply basophilic material deposited in the blood vessels surrounding the tumor cells (Azzopardi phenomenon) can be observed. Most cases show lymphovascular and muscularis propria invasion [11, 14]. Coexisting non-small cell carcinoma components can be difficult to establish on biopsy specimens; however, resection specimens should be thoroughly sampled to look for more differentiated invasive urothelial carcinoma or urothelial carcinoma in situ (Fig. 9.3a and b).

In cases with crush artifacts or poorly prepared sections, non-small cell carcinoma may mimic SCNEC. In such cases, immunohistochemistry should be utilized to properly classify the tumor, as the classification has significant management implications.

Immunohistochemical Features

SCNEC of the urinary bladder typically expresses markers of epithelial and neuroendocrine differentiation. A panel of NSE, CD56, synaptophysin (Fig. 9.3c), and chromogranin (Fig. 9.3d) is typically used to demonstrate neuroendocrine differentiation. These neuroendocrine markers are not always expressed in SCNECs, and diagnosis can be based solely on examination of hematoxylin- and eosin-stained sections [1, 11, 14, 28]. Insulinoma-associated protein 1 (INSM1) is a recently described driver of neuroendocrine differentiation and a marker that has high sensitivity and specificity to neuroendocrine tumors and has been recently reported to be positive in 87% of SCNECs of the urinary bladder [38, 39]. Epithelial markers show variable positivity, with cytokeratin 7 (Fig. 9.3e), epithelial membrane antigen (EMA), cytokeratin AE1/AE3, and cytokeratin CAM 5.2 (perinuclear dot-like positivity) (Fig. 9.3f) seen in the majority of cases and cyto-

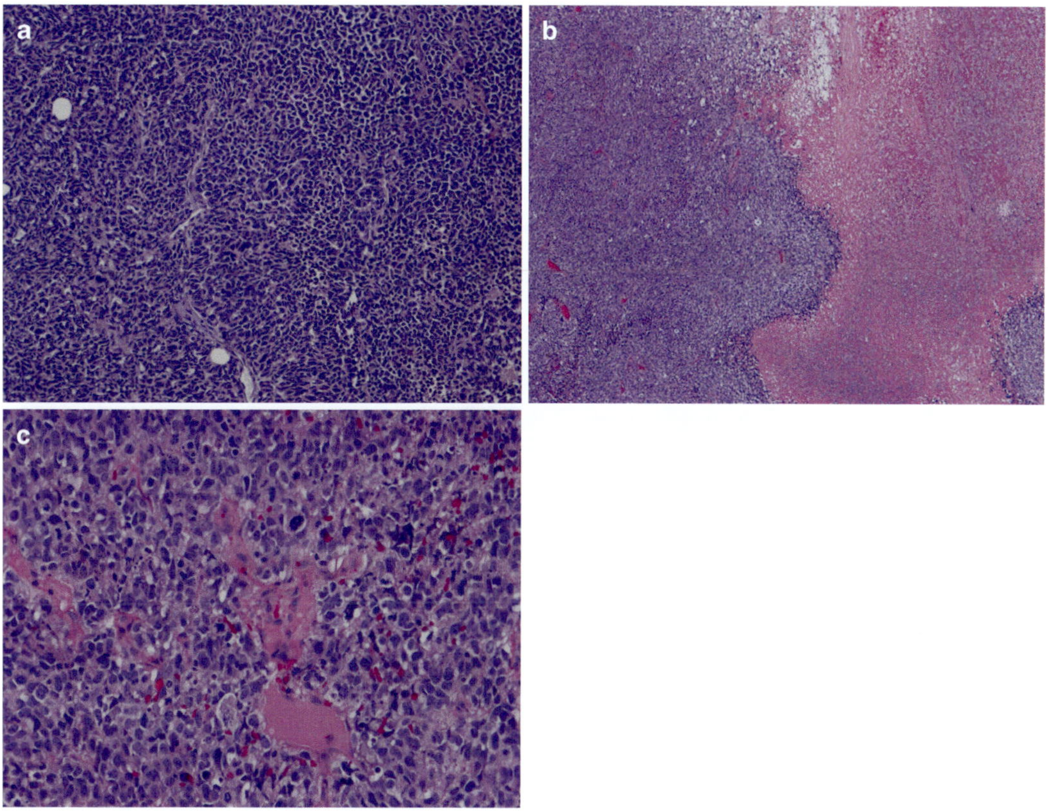

Fig. 9.2 (**a**) SCNEC cells have small nuclei, scanty cytoplasm, nuclear molding, and speckled chromatin pattern with no to inconspicuous nucleoli (hematoxylin and eosin, 100x). (**b**) SCNEC show large areas of geographic necrosis (hematoxylin and eosin, 40x). (**c**) SCNEC shows high mitotic activity (hematoxylin and eosin, 200x)

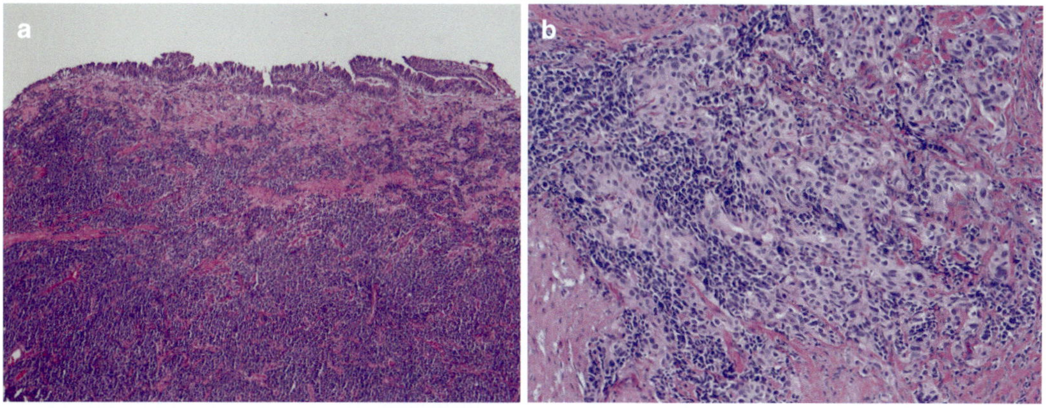

Fig. 9.3 (**a**) SCNEC (deeper in the urinary bladder wall) coexists with urothelial carcinoma in situ (on the surface) (hematoxylin and eosin, 40x). (**b**) SCNEC coexists with conventional invasive high-grade urothelial carcinoma (hematoxylin and eosin, 100x). (**c–g**) The conventional urothelial component from Fig. 9.3b shows positive membranous and cytoplasmic staining with CAM 5.2, CK7, and CK20 and no staining with NE markers. The SCNEC component shows cytoplasmic staining with synaptophysin but no staining with chromogranin. The cytokeratins show perinuclear dot-like positivity with CAM 5.2 and CK7 and no staining with CK20. ((**c**) synaptophysin, 100x; (**d**) chromogranin, 100x; (**e**) cytokeratin 7, 200x; (**f**) cytokeratin CAM 5.2, 200x; and (**g**) cytokeratin 20, 200x)

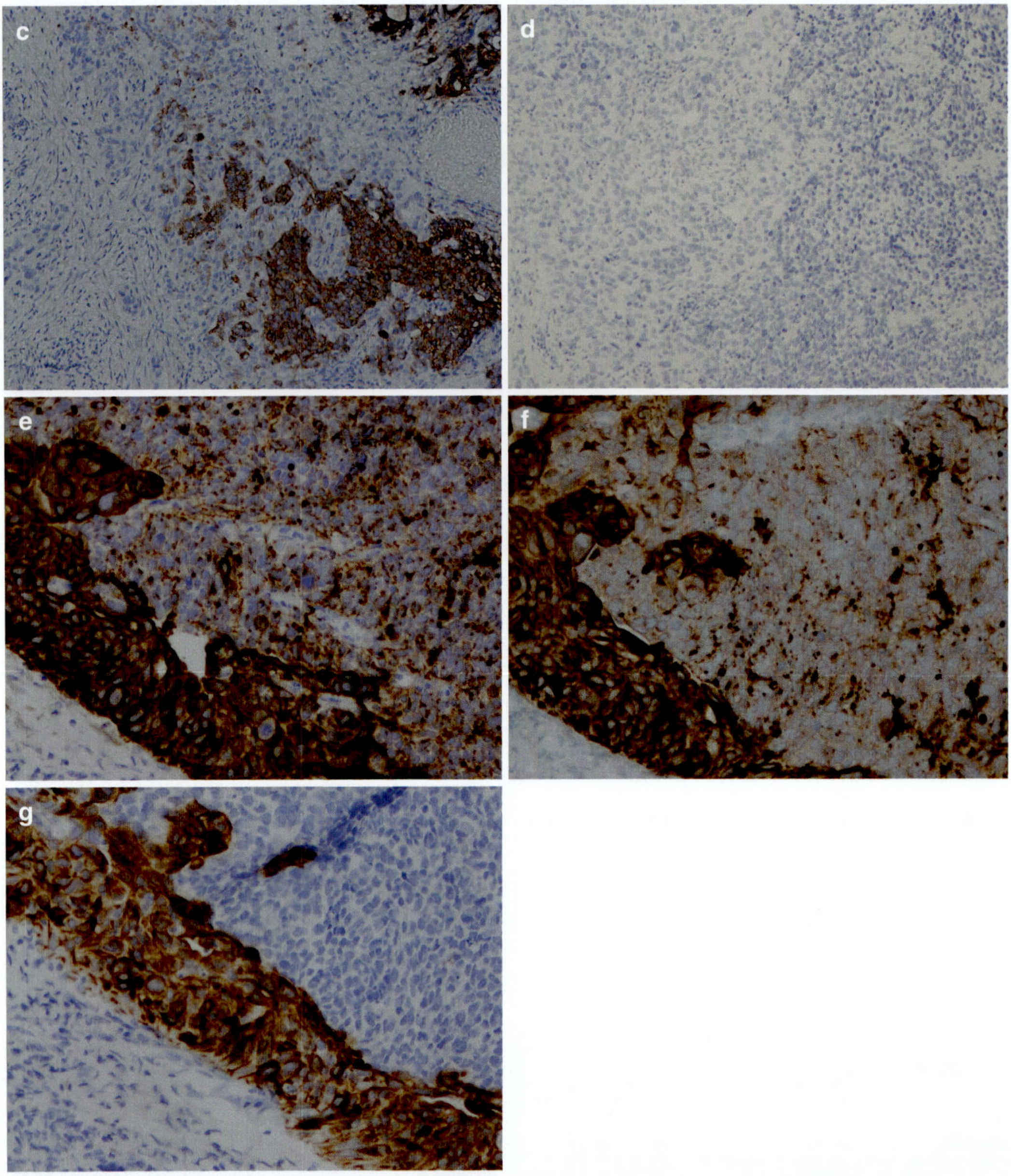

Fig. 9.3 (continued)

keratin 34βE12 in less than half of the cases [11, 14, 15, 28–31, 40–42]. Cytokeratin 20, which is commonly positive in urothelial carcinoma, is typically negative in SCNEC [2] (Fig. 9.3g). GATA3, a marker of conventional urothelial carcinoma, can be seen focally to diffusely positive in approximately one-third of SCNEC; however, this marker should be used with caution in cases of metastatic SCNEC, as lung origin tumors can show focal GATA3 expression in a minority of cases [43]. Uroplakin II and III, other known urothelial markers, mostly do not stain SCNEC [44]. TTF-1 is a marker classically thought to be lung- and thyroid-specific but is also expressed in up to

50% of SCNEC of the urinary bladder [1, 11, 45]. Detected expression of somatostatin receptors (SSTRs) type 2A and type 4 in SCNEC of the urinary bladder has been documented [46]. Varying rates of positivity for P53, P16, epidermal growth factor receptor (EGFR), and c-Kit (CD117) immunohistochemical staining have been documented [11]. Aberrant regulation of CD44 expression, a cell-cell and cell-matrix adhesion molecule, has been correlated with aggressive and metastatic variants of some tumors. The glycoprotein product of the v6 splice variant of CD44 (CD44v6) can be utilized to distinguish poorly differentiated urothelial carcinoma from SCNEC. Poorly differentiated urothelial carcinoma cases will show positive staining with CD44v6, while no staining is typically seen in SCNEC [47]. Differentiating between primary SCNEC of the urinary bladder and SCNEC arising in the prostate and involving the urinary bladder has important clinical implications. In most cases, the presence of a more differentiated, non-neuroendocrine carcinoma component helps in determining the origin of the SCNEC. However, in cases of pure SCNEC, distinguishing urothelial from prostatic origin can be challenging. In such cases, correlation with the clinical and imaging findings, in addition to immunohistochemistry, is required. PSA and PAP expression can be lost in prostatic SCNEC, but not in the more differentiated prostatic adenocarcinoma components. Thus, PSA,PAP, and NKX3.1 staining can be valuable differentiation tools [2, 48, 49]. Additionally, homeobox B13 (HOXB13) has been reported to be a specific and sensitive prostate marker that can be used, especially in poorly differentiated NETs [50].

Large-Cell Neuroendocrine Carcinoma (LCNEC)

Limited data is available regarding the cell of origin of this type of tumors; however, it is believed that LCNEC arises from similar pathways to SCNEC [2, 28].

Epidemiology, Clinical Features, and Treatment

LCNEC of the urinary bladder is rare, with fewer than 30 cases reported in the literature [51]. These tumors have a predilection to older males and generally have aggressive biological behavior and poor prognosis. Cases with pure LCNEC histology have a worse prognosis than cases where more conventional urothelial carcinoma is seen in combination with LCNEC [2, 51, 52]. Octreotide scanning commonly detects more differentiated NETs, but is not typically useful in detecting LCNEC. Thus, more conventional imaging modalities, like contrast-enhanced CT and PET/CT scans, are used in staging and in localizing distant metastasis [19]. Given the rarity of this tumor, treatment plans are based on extrapolation from the literature about pulmonary LCNEC [52].

A single case of primary LCNEC of the ureter has been reported. The tumor showed pure LCNEC morphology and stained with neuroendocrine markers and cytokeratin, but not with uroplakin or TTF-1 [53].

Pathologic and Immunohistochemical Features

Similar to LCNEC in the lung, microscopic examination of LCNEC of the urinary bladder shows neuroendocrine morphology, such as organoid nesting, trabecular growth, rosette-like structures, and peripheral palisading patterns with comedo-type central necrosis. The tumor cells are large and polygonal with low nuclear-cytoplasmic ratio, pleomorphic nuclei, coarse chromatin, and prominent nucleoli [54] (Fig. 9.4a). Mitoses and necrosis are more pronounced in LCNEC than in SCNEC [2]. Like SCNEC, mixed histology with LCNEC and urothelial, squamous, adenocarcinoma, or sarcomatoid carcinoma are commonly encountered [21]. Pure LCNEC is extremely rare. Like other tumors with neuroendocrine features, synaptophysin

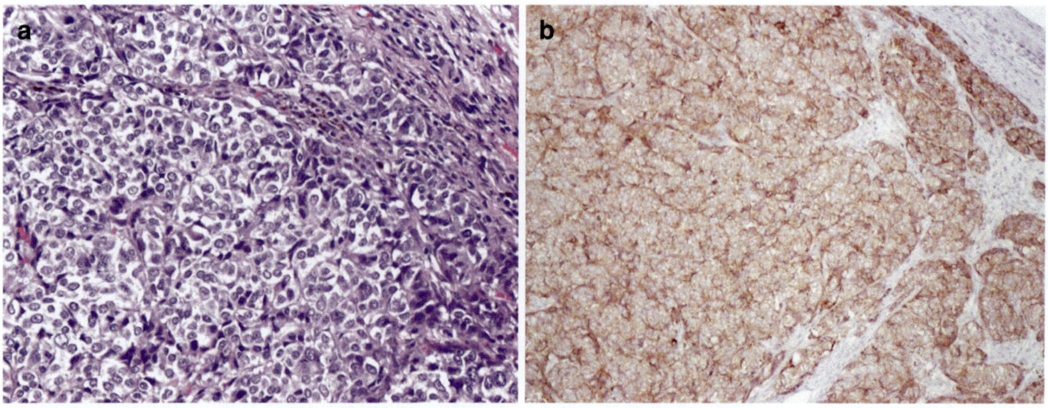

Fig. 9.4 (**a**) LCNEC shows large and polygonal tumor cells with low nuclear-cytoplasmic ratio, polymorphic nuclei, coarse chromatin, and focal prominent nucleoli (hematoxylin and eosin, 100x). (**b**) LCNEC shows cytoplasmic staining with synaptophysin (100x)

(Fig. 9.4b), chromogranin, CD56, and NSE are usually positive in these tumors, along with epithelial markers like cytokeratin AE1/AE3, cytokeratin CAM 5.2, and EMA. Unlike SCNEC, LCNEC of the urinary bladder are not TTF-1-positive [54]. Of note, chromogranin is less sensitive in LCNEC than in SCNEC in the urinary bladder [2]. The exceptionally high Ki-67 index in LCNEC (>95% in some cases), along with positive staining with neuroendocrine markers, serves to confidently distinguish this entity from urothelial carcinoma [54, 55].

The molecular alterations that occur in LCNEC of the urinary bladder have not been studied. Common molecular alterations seen in LCNEC of pulmonary origin, especially those with targetable mutations like EGFR, should be examined in these tumors [56].

Paraganglioma

Extra-adrenal paraganglioma, also known as extra-adrenal pheochromocytoma, is a relatively rare neuroendocrine tumor that arises from chromaffin cells in the autonomic ganglia. In the genitourinary tract, paraganglioma is most common in the bladder but has been reported in the kidney, renal pelvis, ureter, urethra, prostate, spermatic cord, and seminal vesicles [3, 57–64].

Epidemiology, Clinical Features, and Treatment

Despite being the most common site of paraganglioma in the genitourinary tract, urinary bladder paragangliomas represent less than 0.6% of urinary bladder tumors. Unlike other tumors with neuroendocrine differentiation in the urinary bladder, younger females are more likely to develop paragangliomas of the urinary bladder, with a 1:3 male-to-female ratio and a mean age of 45 years [65]. These tumors are either found incidentally on imaging or cystoscopy or present with the classic symptoms of hypertension, hematuria, and micturition syncope in only half of the cases, with paroxysmal palpitation and diaphoresis less commonly seen [19, 66–72].

About two-thirds of the paragangliomas arising in the genitourinary tract are sporadic, and one-third are seen in association with inherited disorders, including germline mutation in succinate dehydrogenase B (SDHB), von Hippel-Lindau disease (VHL), type 1 neurofibromatosis (NF-1), Carney triad, multiple endocrine neoplasia type 2A (MEN 2A) and 2B (MEN 2B), and familial paraganglioma syndrome [3, 73–76].

CT and MRI scans can be used to detect paragangliomas, but both have a lower sensitivity and specificity than radioisotope scanning with ^{131}Iodine metaiodinebenzylguinidine (MIBG)

[66, 67, 77, 78]. Complete surgical resection is the mainstay of treatment in genitourinary paragangliomas [66, 67, 73, 77, 79–81].

Although the majority of paragangliomas have good prognosis and are considered benign, malignant features, defined by metastasis or extensive local disease (i.e., deep local invasion or invasion of adjacent structures, lymph nodes, or distant metastases), are seen in 15–20% of cases. Tumors associated with mutations in SDHB are more likely to show malignant characteristics [2, 65, 73, 82–84].

Pathologic and Immunohistochemical Features

Urinary bladder paragangliomas grossly appear as solitary, well-circumscribed, intravesical exophytic, or intramural nodules that is 2–5 cm in greatest dimension (Fig. 9.5a). The ubiquitous nature of paraganglia in the bladder makes staging such tumors difficult, as paragangliomas arising in the paraganglia present in the muscular wall should not be interpreted as a muscle-invasive tumor (Fig. 9.5b).

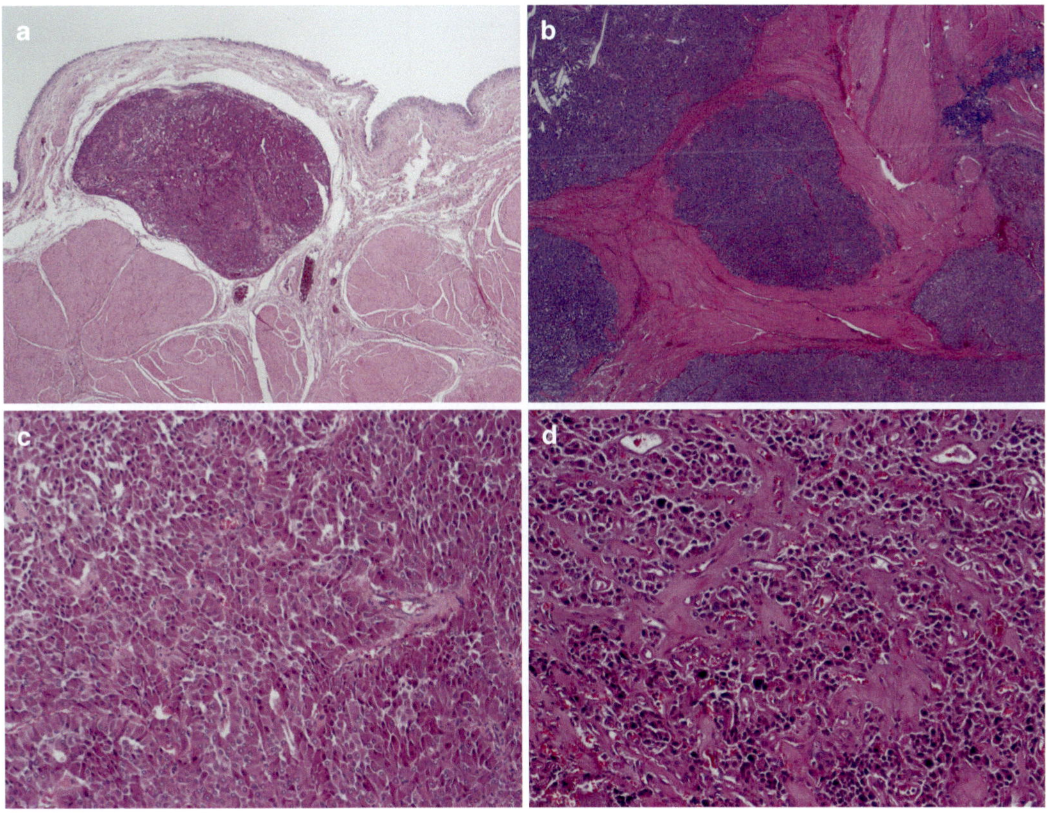

Fig. 9.5 (**a**) Primary urinary bladder paraganglioma forms a well-circumscribed submucosal nodule (hematoxylin and eosin, 20x). (**b**) Primary urinary bladder paraganglioma grows in the muscularis propria. As paraganglia are ubiquitously present in the urinary bladder wall, this should not be interpreted as muscle invasiveness (hematoxylin and eosin, 20x). (**c**) Primary urinary bladder paraganglioma shows polygonal cells with finely granular amphophilic cytoplasm and ovoid nuclei embedded in a richly vascularized stroma (hematoxylin and eosin, 100x). (**d**) Primary urinary bladder paraganglioma cells show nuclear atypia with nuclear pleomorphism and hyperchromasia (hematoxylin and eosin, 100x). (**e**) Primary urinary bladder paraganglioma shows nuclear staining with GATA3 (100x). (**f**) Primary urinary bladder paraganglioma shows cytoplasmic granular staining with synaptophysin (100x)

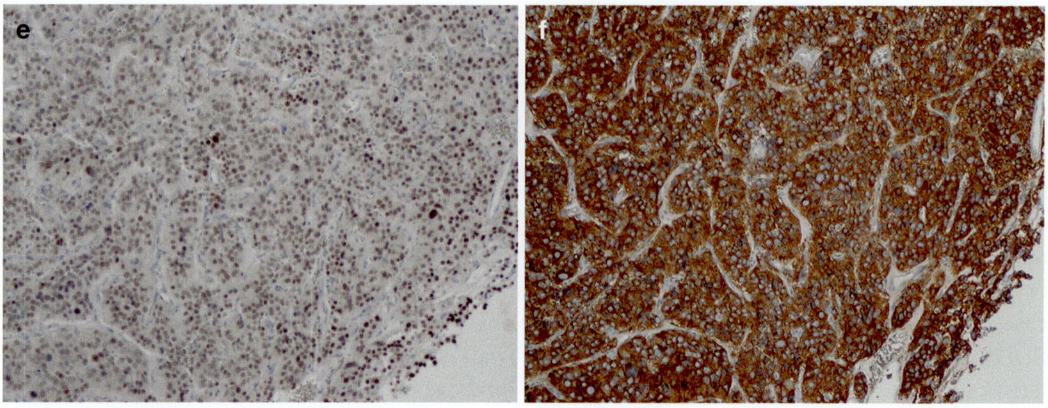

Fig. 9.5 (continued)

Histologically, paragangliomas show the characteristic "zellballen" morphology of paragangliomas elsewhere, with polygonal cells that have finely granular amphophilic cytoplasm and ovoid nuclei embedded in a richly vascularized fibrous stroma (Fig. 9.5c). Nuclear pleomorphism and hyperchromasia (Fig. 9.5d), occasional mitotic figures, and focal neuroblastic or ganglioneuromatous differentiation can be seen, but no correlation has been shown between these parameters and the malignant potential of the tumor [19, 67, 68, 74, 85, 86].

Although the diagnosis of paraganglioma can be readily rendered on hematoxylin- and eosin-stained sections, immunohistochemical stains may be needed for diagnosis in some cases. Bladder paraganglioma can have a histological resemblance to nested variant of urothelial carcinomas or urothelial carcinoma with neuroendocrine differentiation, especially on transurethral resection of bladder tumor (TURBT) specimens. In these cases, the presence of clusters of epithelioid tumor cells with intact normal-appearing urothelium should raise the possibility of paraganglioma. Additionally, cytokeratin and P63 positivity can be used to rule out paraganglioma, as paragangliomas are usually negative for cytokeratin and P63. On the other hand, GATA3, which is typically a urothelial marker, is positive in up to 89% of paraganglioma cases (Fig. 9.5e). This poses a potential pitfall of misdiagnosing paraganglioma as urothelial carcinoma based on GATA3 positivity [87–92].

Like other tumors of neuroendocrine origin, synaptophysin (Fig. 9.5f), chromogranin, and CD56 are positive in paraganglioma; S-100 and SOX10 highlight the sustentacular cells in paraganglioma, but not the polygonal cells, which helps in distinguishing paraganglioma from granular cell tumor of the bladder or melanoma [93]. The use of SDHB immunostain can be used to predict biological behavior. Subsequent mutational analysis can also be performed on cases that show loss of staining with SDHB immunostain [60, 82]. Also see "Paraganglioma" in Chap. 8, Mesenchymal Tumors.

Summary

Although NETs of the bladder are rare, proper recognition of NETs is clinically important, because SCNEC and LCNEC are highly malignant and require different treatment protocols than those for conventional urothelial carcinoma. Carcinoid tumors and paragangliomas, on the other hand, generally have benign and indolent clinical courses, though malignant behavior may sometimes be observed. To make a correct diagnosis of NETs, proper recognition of morphology with judicious immunohistochemical stain selection is required.

References

1. Moch H, Cubilla AL, Humphrey PA, Reuter VE, Ulbright TM. The 2016 WHO classification of tumours of the urinary system and male genital organs-part a: renal, penile, and testicular tumours. Eur Urol. 2016;70(1):93–105. https://doi.org/10.1016/j.eururo.2016.02.029.
2. Kouba E, Cheng L. Neuroendocrine tumors of the urinary bladder according to the 2016 World Health Organization classification: molecular and clinical characteristics. Endocr Pathol. 2016;27(3):188–99. https://doi.org/10.1007/s12022-016-9444-5.
3. Purnell S, Sidana A, Maruf M, Grant C, Agarwal PK. Genitourinary paraganglioma: demographic, pathologic, and clinical characteristics in the surveillance, epidemiology, and end results database (2000–2012). Urol Oncol. 2017;35(7):457.e9–457.e14. https://doi.org/10.1016/j.urolonc.2017.02.006.
4. Posfai B, Kuthi L, Varga L, et al. The colorful palette of neuroendocrine neoplasms in the genitourinary tract. Anticancer Res. 2018;38(6):3243–54. https://doi.org/10.21873/anticancers.12589.
5. Chen Y, Epstein JI. Primary carcinoid tumors of the urinary bladder and prostatic urethra: a clinicopathologic study of 6 cases. Am J Surg Pathol. 2011;35(3):442–6. https://doi.org/10.1097/PAS.0b013e318208f96a.
6. Mascolo M, Altieri V, Mignogna C, Napodano G, De Rosa G, Insabato L. Calcitonin-producing well-differentiated neuroendocrine carcinoma (carcinoid tumor) of the urinary bladder: case report. BMC Cancer. 2005;5:88. https://doi.org/10.1186/1471-2407-5-88.
7. Hemal AK, Singh I, Pawar R, Kumar M, Taneja P. Primary malignant bladder carcinoid— a diagnostic and management dilemma. Urology. 2000;55(6):949. https://doi.org/10.1016/S0090-4295(00)00470-2.
8. Sugihara A, Kajio K, Yoshimoto T, et al. Primary carcinoid tumor of the urinary bladder. Int Urol Nephrol. 2002;33(1):53–7. https://doi.org/10.1023/a:1014400818905.
9. Baydar DE, Tasar C. Carcinoid tumor in the urinary bladder: unreported features. Am J Surg Pathol. 2011;35(11):1754–7. https://doi.org/10.1097/PAS.0b013e31823455eb.
10. Zozumi M, Nakai M, Matsuda I, et al. Primary carcinoid tumor of the urinary bladder with prominent subnuclear eosinophilic granules. Pathol Res Pract. 2012;208(2):109–12. https://doi.org/10.1016/j.prp.2011.10.008.
11. Erdem GU, Özdemir NY, Demirci NS, Şahin S, Bozkaya Y, Zengin N. Small cell carcinoma of the urinary bladder: changing trends in the current literature. Curr Med Res Opin. 2016;32(6):1013–21. https://doi.org/10.1185/03007995.2016.1155982.
12. Sroussi M, Elaidi R, Fléchon A, et al. Neuroendocrine carcinoma of the urinary bladder: a large, Retrospective Study From the French Genito-Urinary Tumor Group. Clin Genitourin Cancer. Published online December 5, 2019. https://doi.org/10.1016/j.clgc.2019.11.014.
13. Sacco E, Pinto F, Sasso F, et al. Paraneoplastic syndromes in patients with urological malignancies. Urol Int. 2009;83(1):1–11. https://doi.org/10.1159/000224860.
14. Schneider NI, Zigeuner R, Langner C. Small cell carcinoma of the urinary bladder: a rare tumor with propensity for hepatic involvement. Am J Med Sci. 2013;345(2):155–7. https://doi.org/10.1097/MAJ.0b013e3182648759.
15. Perán Teruel M, Giménez Bachs JM, Martínez Ruiz J, et al. Neuroendocrine carcinoma of the urinary bladder. 15-year retrospective analysis. Arch Esp Urol. 2012;65(2):237–43.
16. Wang G, Xiao L, Zhang M, et al. Small cell carcinoma of the urinary bladder: a clinicopathologic and immunohistochemical analysis of 81 cases. Hum Pathol. 2018;79:57–65. https://doi.org/10.1016/j.humpath.2018.05.005.
17. Cheng L, Pan C-X, Yang XJ, et al. Small cell carcinoma of the urinary bladder: a clinicopathologic analysis of 64 patients. Cancer. 2004;101(5):957–62. https://doi.org/10.1002/cncr.20456.
18. Choong NWW, Quevedo JF, Kaur JS. Small cell carcinoma of the urinary bladder. The Mayo Clinic experience. Cancer. 2005;103(6):1172–8. https://doi.org/10.1002/cncr.20903.
19. Fine SW. Neuroendocrine lesions of the genitourinary tract. Adv Anat Pathol. 2007;14(4):286–96. https://doi.org/10.1097/PAP.0b013e3180ca8a89.
20. Smith J, Reidy-Lagunes D. The management of extrapulmonary poorly differentiated (high-grade) neuroendocrine carcinomas. Semin Oncol. 2013;40(1):100–8. https://doi.org/10.1053/j.seminoncol.2012.11.011.
21. Thompson S, Cioffi-Lavina M, Chapman-Fredricks J, Gomez-Fernandez C, Fernandez-Castro G, Jorda M. Distinction of high-grade neuroendocrine carcinoma/small cell carcinoma from conventional urothelial carcinoma of urinary bladder: an immunohistochemical approach. Appl Immunohistochem Mol Morphol. 2011;19(5):395–9. https://doi.org/10.1097/PAI.0b013e31820eca9a.
22. Pant-Purohit M, Lopez-Beltran A, Montironi R, MacLennan GT, Cheng L. Small cell carcinoma of the urinary bladder. Histol Histopathol. 2010;25(2):217–21. https://doi.org/10.14670/HH-25.217.
23. Vetterlein MW, Wankowicz SAM, Seisen T, et al. Neoadjuvant chemotherapy prior to radical cystectomy for muscle-invasive bladder cancer with variant histology. Cancer. 2017;123(22):4346–55. https://doi.org/10.1002/cncr.30907.
24. Niu Q, Lu Y, Xu S, et al. Clinicopathological characteristics and survival outcomes of bladder neuroendocrine carcinomas: a population-based study. Cancer Manag Res. 2018;10:4479–89. https://doi.org/10.2147/CMAR.S175286.
25. Kanagarajah P, Ayyathurai R, Saleem U, Manoharan M. Small cell carcinoma arising from

the bulbar urethra: a case report and literature review. Urol Int. 2012;88(4):477–9. https://doi.org/10.1159/000332154.
26. Acosta AM, Kajdacsy-Balla A. Primary neuroendocrine tumors of the ureter: a short review. Arch Pathol Lab Med. 2016;140(7):714–7. https://doi.org/10.5858/arpa.2015-0106-RS.
27. Kim TS, Seong DH, Ro JY. Small cell carcinoma of the ureter with squamous cell and transitional cell carcinomatous components associated with ureteral stone. J Korean Med Sci. 2001;16(6):796–800. https://doi.org/10.3346/jkms.2001.16.6.796.
28. Pompas-Veganzones N, Gonzalez-Peramato P, Sanchez-Carbayo M. The neuroendocrine component in bladder tumors. Curr Med Chem. 2014;21(9):1117–28.
29. Ploeg M, Aben KK, Hulsbergen-van de Kaa CA, Schoenberg MP, Witjes JA, Kiemeney LA. Clinical epidemiology of nonurothelial bladder cancer: analysis of the Netherlands Cancer registry. J Urol. 2010;183(3):915–20. https://doi.org/10.1016/j.juro.2009.11.018.
30. Grignon DJ, Ro JY, Ayala AG, et al. Small cell carcinoma of the urinary bladder. A clinicopathologic analysis of 22 cases. Cancer. 1992;69(2):527–36.
31. Abrahams NA, Moran C, Reyes AO, Siefker-Radtke A, Ayala AG. Small cell carcinoma of the bladder: a contemporary clinicopathological study of 51 cases. Histopathology. 2005;46(1):57–63. https://doi.org/10.1111/j.1365-2559.2004.01980.x.
32. Terracciano L, Richter J, Tornillo L, et al. Chromosomal imbalances in small cell carcinomas of the urinary bladder. J Pathol. 1999;189(2):230–5. https://doi.org/10.1002/(SICI)1096-9896(199910)189:2<230::AID-PATH407>3.0.CO;2-8.
33. Cheng L, Jones TD, McCarthy RP, et al. Molecular genetic evidence for a common clonal origin of urinary bladder small cell carcinoma and coexisting urothelial carcinoma. Am J Pathol. 2005;166(5):1533–9.
34. Chang MT, Penson A, Desai NB, et al. Small-cell carcinomas of the bladder and lung are characterized by a convergent but distinct pathogenesis. Clin Cancer Res. 2018;24(8):1965–73. https://doi.org/10.1158/1078-0432.CCR-17-2655.
35. Wang Y, Li Q, Wang J, et al. Small cell carcinoma of the bladder: the characteristics of molecular alterations, treatment, and follow-up. Med Oncol. 2019;36(12):98. https://doi.org/10.1007/s12032-019-1321-x.
36. Zheng X, Zhuge J, Bezerra SM, et al. High frequency of TERT promoter mutation in small cell carcinoma of bladder, but not in small cell carcinoma of other origins. J Hematol Oncol. 2014;7(1):47. https://doi.org/10.1186/s13045-014-0047-7.
37. Sjödahl G. Molecular subtype profiling of urothelial carcinoma using a subtype-specific immunohistochemistry panel. Methods Mol Biol. 1655;2018:53–64. https://doi.org/10.1007/978-1-4939-7234-0_5.
38. Kim IE, Amin A, Wang LJ, Cheng L, Perrino CM. Insulinoma-associated protein 1 (INSM1) expression in small cell neuroendocrine carcinoma of the urinary tract. Appl Immunohistochem Mol Morphol. Published online December 23, 2019. https://doi.org/10.1097/PAI.0000000000000824.
39. Lan MS, Breslin MB. Structure, expression, and biological function of INSM1 transcription factor in neuroendocrine differentiation. FASEB J. 2009;23:2024–33.
40. Soriano P, Navarro S, Gil M, Llombart-Bosch A. Small-cell carcinoma of the urinary bladder. A clinico-pathological study of ten cases. Virchows Arch. 2004;445(3):292–7. https://doi.org/10.1007/s00428-004-1041-1.
41. Blomjous CE, Vos W, Schipper NW, De Voogt HJ, Baak JP, Meijer CJ. Morphometric and flow cytometric analysis of small cell undifferentiated carcinoma of the bladder. J Clin Pathol. 1989;42(10):1032–9. https://doi.org/10.1136/jcp.42.10.1032.
42. Blomjous CE, Vos W, De Voogt HJ, Van der Valk P, Meijer CJ. Small cell carcinoma of the urinary bladder. A clinicopathologic, morphometric, immunohistochemical, and ultrastructural study of 18 cases. Cancer. 1989;64(6):1347–57. https://doi.org/10.1002/1097-0142(19890915)64:6<1347::aid-cncr2820640629>3.0.co;2-q.
43. Bezerra SM, Lotan TL, Faraj SF, et al. GATA3 expression in small cell carcinoma of bladder and prostate and its potential role in determining primary tumor origin. Hum Pathol. 2014;45(8):1682–7. https://doi.org/10.1016/j.humpath.2014.04.011.
44. Li W, Liang Y, Deavers MT, et al. Uroplakin II is a more sensitive immunohistochemical marker than uroplakin III in urothelial carcinoma and its variants. Am J Clin Pathol. 2014;142(6):864–71. https://doi.org/10.1309/AJCP1J0JPJBPSUXF.
45. Paner GP, Lopez-Beltran A, Sirohi D, Amin MB. Updates in the pathologic diagnosis and classification of epithelial neoplasms of urachal origin. Adv Anat Pathol. 2016;23(2):71–83. https://doi.org/10.1097/PAP.0000000000000110.
46. Fernández-Aceñero MJ, Córdova S, Manzarbeitia F, Medina C. Immunohistochemical profile of urothelial and small cell carcinomas of the bladder. Pathol Oncol Res. 2011;17(3):519–23. https://doi.org/10.1007/s12253-010-9341-z.
47. Iczkowski KA, Shanks JH, Bostwick DG. Loss of CD44 variant 6 expression differentiates small cell carcinoma of urinary bladder from urothelial (transitional cell) carcinoma. Histopathology. 1998;32(4):322–7. https://doi.org/10.1046/j.1365-2559.1998.00398.x.
48. Neşe N, Kumbaraci BS, Baydar DE, et al. Small cell carcinomas of the bladder highly express somatostatin receptor type 2A: impact on prognosis and treatment—a multicenter study of Urooncology society, Turkey. Appl Immunohistochem Mol Morphol. 2016;24(4):253–60. https://doi.org/10.1097/PAI.0000000000000188.

49. Gurel B, Ali TZ, Montgomery EA, et al. NKX3.1 as a marker of prostatic origin in metastatic tumors. Am J Surg Pathol. 2010;34(8):1097–105. https://doi.org/10.1097/PAS.0b013e3181e6cbf3.
50. Varinot J, Cussenot O, Roupret M, et al. HOXB13 is a sensitive and specific marker of prostate cells, useful in distinguishing between carcinomas of prostatic and urothelial origin. Virchows Arch. 2013;463(6):803–9. https://doi.org/10.1007/s00428-013-1495-0.
51. Akdeniz E, Bakirtas M, Bolat MS, Akdeniz S, Özer I. Pure large cell neuroendocrine carcinoma of the bladder without urological symptoms. Pan Afr Med J. 2018;30:134. https://doi.org/10.11604/pamj.2018.30.134.13437.
52. Martín IJP, Vilar DG, Aguado JM, et al. Large cell neuroendocrine carcinoma of the urinary bladder. Bibliographic review. Arch Esp Urol. 2011;64(2):105–13.
53. Watson GA, Ahmed Y, Picardo S, et al. Unusual Sites of High-Grade Neuroendocrine Carcinomas: A Case Series and Review of the Literature. Am J Case Rep. 2018;19:710–23. https://doi.org/10.12659/AJCR.908953.
54. Sari A, Ermete M, Sadullahoğlu C, Bal K, Bolükbaşi A. Large cell neuroendocrine carcinoma of urinary bladder; case presentation. Turk Patoloji Derg. 2013;29(2):138–42. https://doi.org/10.5146/tjpath.2013.01165.
55. Radović N, Turner R, Bacalja J. Primary "Pure" Large Cell Neuroendocrine Carcinoma of the Urinary Bladder: A Case Report and Review of the Literature. Clinical Genitourinary Cancer. 2015;13(5):e375–e377. https://doi.org/10.1016/j.clgc.2015.03.005.
56. Colarossi C, Pino P, Giuffrida D, et al. Large cell neuroendocrine carcinoma (LCNEC) of the urinary bladder: a case report. Diagn Pathol. 2013;8:19. https://doi.org/10.1186/1746-1596-8-19.
57. Liu C, Mo C-Q, Jiang S-J, Pan J-C, Qiu S-P, Wang D-H. Primary paraganglioma of seminal vesicle. Chin Med J. 2016;129(13):1627–8. https://doi.org/10.4103/0366-6999.184471.
58. Liu H-W, Liu L-R, Cao D-H, Wei Q. Paraganglioma in the renal pelvis. Kaohsiung J Med Sci. 2014;30(6):319–20. https://doi.org/10.1016/j.kjms.2013.04.007.
59. Awasthi NP, Kumari N, Krishnani N, Goel A. "Functional" paraganglioma of ureter: an unusual case. Indian J Pathol Microbiol. 2011;54(2):405–6. https://doi.org/10.4103/0377-4929.81631.
60. Alataki D, Triantafyllidis A, Gaal J, et al. A non-catecholamine-producing sympathetic paraganglioma of the spermatic cord: the importance of performing candidate gene mutation analysis. Virchows Arch. 2010;457(5):619–22. https://doi.org/10.1007/s00428-010-0966-9.
61. Yi C, Han L, Yang R, Yu J. Paraganglioma of the renal pelvis: a case report and review of literature. Tumori. 2017;103(Suppl. 1):e47–9. https://doi.org/10.5301/tj.5000677.
62. Kwon A-Y, Kang H, An HJ, et al. Spermatic cord paraganglioma with histologically malignant features. Urology. 2016;93:e7–8. https://doi.org/10.1016/j.urology.2016.03.014.
63. Alvarenga CA, Lopes JM, Vinagre J, et al. Paraganglioma of seminal vesicle and chromophobe renal cell carcinoma: a case report and literature review. Sao Paulo Med J. 2012;130(1):57–60.
64. Alberti C. Urology pertinent neuroendocrine tumors: focusing on renal pelvis, bladder, prostate located sympathetic functional paragangliomas. G Chir. 2016;37(2):55–60.
65. Cheng L, Leibovich BC, Cheville JC, et al. Paraganglioma of the urinary bladder: can biologic potential be predicted? Cancer. 2000;88(4):844–52. https://doi.org/10.1002/(sici)1097-0142(20000215)88:4<844::aid-cncr15>3.0.co;2-i.
66. Adraktas D, Caserta M, Tchelepi H. Paraganglioma of the urinary bladder. Ultrasound Q. 2014;30(3):233–5. https://doi.org/10.1097/RUQ.0000000000000113.
67. Liang J, Li H, Gao L, Yin L, Yin L, Zhang J. Bladder paraganglioma: clinicopathology and magnetic resonance imaging study of five patients. Urol J. 2016;13(2):2605–11.
68. Feng N, Li X, Gao H-D, Liu Z-L, Shi L-J, Liu W-Z. Urinary bladder malignant paraganglioma with vertebral metastasis: a case report with literature review. Chin J Cancer. 2013;32(11):624–8. https://doi.org/10.5732/cjc.012.10317.
69. Pichler R, Heidegger I, Klinglmair G, et al. Unrecognized paraganglioma of the urinary bladder as a cause for basilar-type migraine. Urol Int. 2014;92(4):482–7. https://doi.org/10.1159/000348829.
70. Hanji AM, Rohan VS, Patel JJ, Tankshali RA. Pheochromocytoma of the urinary bladder: a rare cause of severe hypertension. Saudi J Kidney Dis Transpl. 2012;23(4):813–6. https://doi.org/10.4103/1319-2442.98167.
71. Bagchi A, Dushaj K, Shrestha A, et al. Urinary bladder paraganglioma presenting as micturition-induced palpitations, dyspnea, and angina. Am J Case Rep. 2015;16:283–6. https://doi.org/10.12659/AJCR.891388.
72. She HL, Chan PH, Cheung SCW. Urinary bladder paraganglioma in a post-heart transplant patient. Ann Acad Med Singap. 2012;41(8):362–3.
73. Martucci VL, Lorenzo ZG, Weintraub M, et al. Association of urinary bladder paragangliomas with germline mutations in the SDHB and VHL genes. Urol Oncol. 2015;33(4):167.e13–20. https://doi.org/10.1016/j.urolonc.2014.11.017.
74. Ranaweera M, Chung E. Bladder paraganglioma: A report of case series and critical review of current literature. World J Clinic Cases. 2014;2(10):591. https://doi.org/10.12998/wjcc.v2.i10.591.
75. Rednam SP, Erez A, Druker H, et al. Von Hippel-Lindau and hereditary pheochromocytoma/paraganglioma syndromes: clinical features, genetics, and surveillance recommendations in childhood.

Clin Cancer Res. 2017;23(12):e68–75. https://doi.org/10.1158/1078-0432.CCR-17-0547.
76. Raygada M, Pasini B, Stratakis CA. Hereditary paragangliomas. Adv Otorhinolaryngol. 2011;70:99–106. https://doi.org/10.1159/000322484.
77. Wang H, Ye H, Guo A, et al. Bladder paraganglioma in adults: MR appearance in four patients. Eur J Radiol. 2011;80(3):e217–20. https://doi.org/10.1016/j.ejrad.2010.09.020.
78. Bosserman AJ, Dai D, Lu Y. Imaging characteristics of a bladder wall paraganglioma. Clin Nucl Med. 2019;44(1):66–7. https://doi.org/10.1097/RLU.0000000000002324.
79. Bishnoi K, Bora GS, Mavuduru RS, Devana SK, Singh SK, Mandal AK. Bladder paraganglioma: safe and feasible management with robot assisted surgery. J Robot Surg. 2016;10(3):275–8. https://doi.org/10.1007/s11701-016-0573-0.
80. Stigliano A, Lardo P, Cerquetti L, et al. Treatment responses to antiangiogenetic therapy and chemotherapy in nonsecreting paraganglioma (PGL4) of urinary bladder with SDHB mutation: a case report. Medicine (Baltimore). 2018;97(30):e10904. https://doi.org/10.1097/MD.0000000000010904.
81. Nayyar R, Singh P, Gupta NP. Robotic management of pheochromocytoma of the vesicoureteric junction. JSLS. 2010;14(2):309–12. https://doi.org/10.4293/108680810X12785289145042.
82. Park S, Kang SY, Kwon GY, et al. Clinicopathologic characteristics and mutational status of succinate dehydrogenase genes in paraganglioma of the urinary bladder: a multi-institutional Korean study. Arch Pathol Lab Med. 2017;141(5):671–7. https://doi.org/10.5858/arpa.2016-0403-OA.
83. Papathomas TG, de Krijger RR, Tischler AS. Paragangliomas: update on differential diagnostic considerations, composite tumors, and recent genetic developments. Semin Diagn Pathol. 2013;30(3):207–23. https://doi.org/10.1053/j.semdp.2013.06.006.
84. Maeda M, Funahashi Y, Katoh M, Fujita T, Tsuruta K, Gotoh M. Malignant bladder pheochromocytoma with SDHB genetic mutation. Aktuelle Urol. 2013;44(5):381–2. https://doi.org/10.1055/s-0033-1345147.
85. Beilan J, Lawton A, Hajdenberg J, Rosser CJ. Locally advanced paraganglioma of the urinary bladder: a case report. BMC Res Notes. 2013;6:156. https://doi.org/10.1186/1756-0500-6-156.
86. Iwamoto G, Kawahara T, Tanabe M, et al. Paraganglioma in the bladder: a case report. J Med Case Rep. 2017;11(1):306. https://doi.org/10.1186/s13256-017-1473-2.
87. Menon S, Goyal P, Suryawanshi P, et al. Paraganglioma of the urinary bladder: a clinicopathologic spectrum of a series of 14 cases emphasizing diagnostic dilemmas. Indian J Pathol Microbiol. 2014;57(1):19–23. https://doi.org/10.4103/0377-4929.130873.
88. Miettinen M, McCue PA, Sarlomo-Rikala M, et al. GATA3: a multispecific but potentially useful marker in surgical pathology: a systematic analysis of 2500 epithelial and nonepithelial tumors. Am J Surg Pathol. 2014;38(1):13–22. https://doi.org/10.1097/PAS.0b013e3182a0218f.
89. Nonaka D, Wang BY, Edmondson D, Beckett E, Sun C-CJ. A study of gata3 and phox2b expression in tumors of the autonomic nervous system. Am J Surg Pathol. 2013;37(8):1236–41. https://doi.org/10.1097/PAS.0b013e318289c765.
90. So JS, Epstein JI. GATA3 expression in paragangliomas: a pitfall potentially leading to misdiagnosis of urothelial carcinoma. Mod Pathol. 2013;26(10):1365–70. https://doi.org/10.1038/modpathol.2013.76.
91. Ghafoor A-U-R, Yousaf I, Pervez R, Khan RU, Mir K. Paraganglioma of urinary bladder: an unusual presentation. Pitfalls in diagnosis and treatment. J Pak Med Assoc. 2012;62(1):63–5.
92. Grignon DJ, Ro JY, Mackay B, et al. Paraganglioma of the urinary bladder: immunohistochemical, ultrastructural, and DNA flow cytometric studies. Hum Pathol. 1991;22(11):1162–9.
93. Ranaweera M, Chung E. Bladder paraganglioma: a report of case series and critical review of current literature. World J Clin Cases. 2014;2(10):591–5. https://doi.org/10.12998/wjcc.v2.i10.591.

Bladder Lymphoma and Leukemia

10

Jie Xu, Shaoying Li, and M. James You

Bladder Lymphomas

Lymphomas represent approximately 0.2% of all neoplasms of the bladder [1]. Most patients with bladder lymphomas present with nonspecific urinary symptoms, such as hematuria (most common), urinary frequency, dysuria, and lower abdominal and back pain [1–5]. Lymphomas most often involve retro-trigonal or lateral bladder [1, 6] and appear as a solitary, sometimes multifocal, submucosal mass on image studies, but their cystoscopic findings are not different compared to non-hematopoietic urothelial tumors [1]. Urine cytology is usually not diagnostic, and a tissue biopsy is required to reach a final diagnosis.

Bladder lymphomas can be either primary (without involving other organ sites) or secondary to systemic lymphomas. Primary bladder lymphomas are extremely rare, accounting for only 0.15–2% of all extranodal lymphomas [1, 7], which may be due to the shortage of lymphoid tissue in the bladder. Primary bladder lymphomas have a female predominance and are most commonly seen in middle-aged women [2, 4, 8, 9]. Marginal zone lymphoma of mucosa-associated lymphoid tissue (MALT lymphoma) is the most common primary bladder lymphoma [1–3, 9, 10]. MALT lymphoma is characterized by centrocyte-like lymphocytes (Fig. 10.1) accompanied with plasma cells and nonneoplastic germinal centers. In contrast to stomach and salivary gland MALT lymphoma, lymphoepithelial lesions were only found in a small subset of bladder MALT lymphoma cases and in the areas of cystitis cystica or cystitis glandularis [3, 9]. The rarity of lymphoepithelial lesions in bladder MALT lymphoma and their confinement to the areas of cystitis cystica or glandularis suggest that urothelial epithelium is resistant to invasion by lymphoma cells. The presence of lymphoepithelial lesions is not required for the diagnosis of bladder MALT lymphoma [9].

Some studies suggest that primary bladder lymphomas may be associated with chronic cystitis [1, 9, 11]. Since there is only scant lymphoid tissue in the normal bladder, it is possible that preexisting chronic inflammation of bladder can induce acquired MALT, which can lead to MALT lymphoma [9]. However, the history of chronic cystitis is only present in approximately 20% of patients with primary bladder lymphomas [4, 5]. Therefore, the relationship between chronic cystitis and primary bladder lymphomas is still uncertain. Primary bladder lymphomas are generally thought to be indolent with a favorable prognosis because they are confined to the bladder and respond well to chemotherapy [1–4].

J. Xu · S. Li · M. J. You (✉)
Department of Hematopathology, The University of Texas MD Anderson Cancer Center, Houston, TX, USA
e-mail: JXu9@mdanderson.org; sli6@mdanderson.org; mjamesyou@mdanderson.org

H. Zhou et al. (eds.), *Urinary Bladder Pathology*, https://doi.org/10.1007/978-3-030-71509-0_10

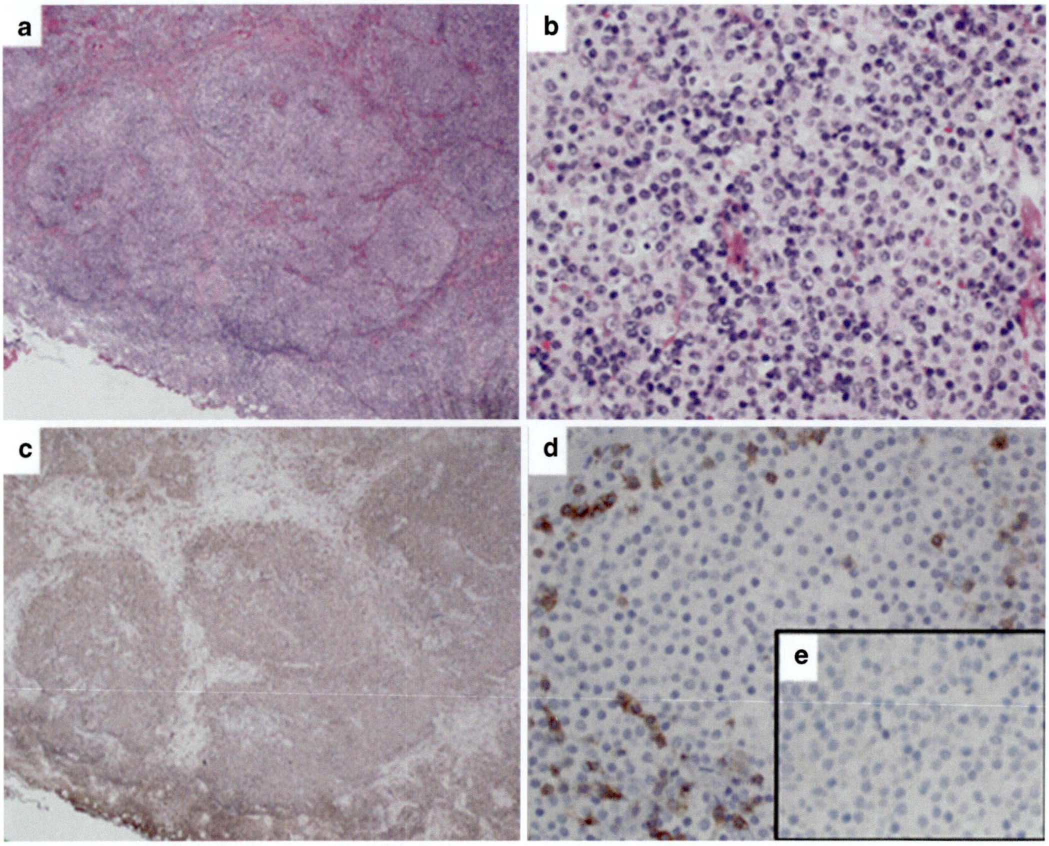

Fig. 10.1 MALT lymphoma in the bladder. (**a**) The MALT lymphoma has a nodular growth pattern. (**b**) The MALT lymphoma cells are predominantly small with slightly irregular nuclear contours and relatively abundant pale cytoplasm, presenting a monocytoid appearance. Occasional large cells resembling centroblasts or immunoblasts are present. (**c–e**) The MALT lymphoma cells are positive for CD20 (**c**) and negative for CD5 (**d**) and CD10 (**e**). CD5 (**d**) highlights background small T cells

Secondary bladder lymphomas are much more common and occur in 10–25% of patients with lymphomas, usually in patients with systemic lymphomas of advanced stage [1, 8, 12]. Thus, the prognosis of patients with secondary bladder lymphomas is usually poor. In our institution, chronic lymphocytic leukemia/small lymphocytic lymphoma (CLL/SLL) and diffuse large B-cell lymphoma (DLBCL) are the most common types of bladder lymphomas. Other subtypes of small B-cell lymphomas, such as follicular lymphoma (FL) and mantle cell lymphoma (MCL), are less frequently seen in the bladder [3]. Among the large cell lymphomas, high-grade B-cell lymphoma is not uncommon, but less frequently seen than DLBCL. Extreme rare cases of classic Hodgkin lymphoma [13], Burkitt lymphoma [14], and T-cell lymphomas have also been reported [1, 2, 15–18]. Anaplastic large cell lymphoma is the most commonly reported T-cell lymphoma involving the bladder.

CLL/SLL is the most common type of small B-cell lymphomas involving the bladder in our institution, although only a few cases have been reported in literature [19–21]. This is likely due to the fact that CLL/SLL is the most common leukemia of adults in Western countries [22]. Patients with CLL/SLL have an increased risk of developing subsequent neoplasms of epithelial and mesenchymal origins, likely due to the decreased immunity and B-cell dysfunction [23, 24]. Coexistence of CLL/SLL and urothelial carcinoma has been reported [24]. CLL/SLL is characterized by multiple lymphoid aggregates involving the bladder wall (Fig. 10.2). CLL/SLL lymphoma cells are small, with clumped chromatin and scant cytoplasm.

An important differential diagnosis of small B-cell lymphomas is MCL because it is thought to be very aggressive except for indolent variants (such as leukemic non-nodal MCL and in situ MCL). Classic MCL usually presents as a vaguely nodular proliferation of monotonous small lymphocytes (Fig. 10.3). MCL lymphoma cells show irregular nuclear contours resembling centrocytes, but their chromatins are somewhat more dispersed with inconspicuous nucleoli. Hyalinized blood vessels and scattered histiocytes are commonly seen in MCL. This diagnosis can be confirmed by the immunohistochemistry of cyclin D1 or SOX11.

In a reactive bladder, benign lymphoid follicles are often seen, which have preserved mantle zones and reactive germinal centers characterized by polarization (dark versus light zones) and tingible body macrophages. In contrast, the neoplastic follicles of FL generally have attenuated or absent mantle zones and lack both polarization and tangible body macrophages in the germinal centers (Fig. 10.4). FL cells are composed of centrocytes (small- to medium-sized, with irregular/cleaved nuclei, inconspicuous nucleoli) and centroblasts (large, with round or oval nuclei, vesicular chromatin, and one or more peripheral

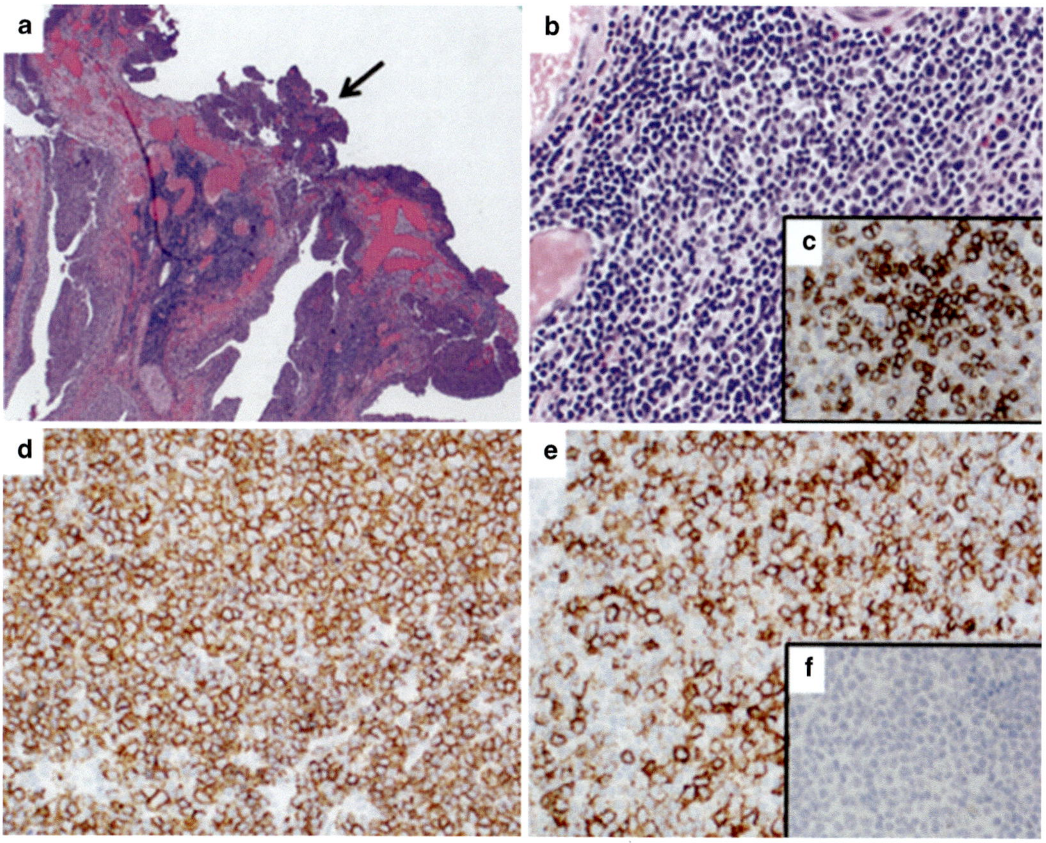

Fig. 10.2 Coexistence of urothelial carcinoma and CLL/SLL. (**a**) High-grade noninvasive papillary urothelial carcinoma is present (arrow). Multifocal lymphoid aggregates are also identified in the lamina propria, which is overlaid with urothelial carcinoma. (**b**) The lymphoid aggregates are comprised of predominantly small lymphocytes with scattered histiocytes. (**c–f**) The CLL/SLL cells are positive for CD5 (large subset, **c**), CD20 (**d**), and CD23 (**e**) and negative for cyclin D1 (**f**)

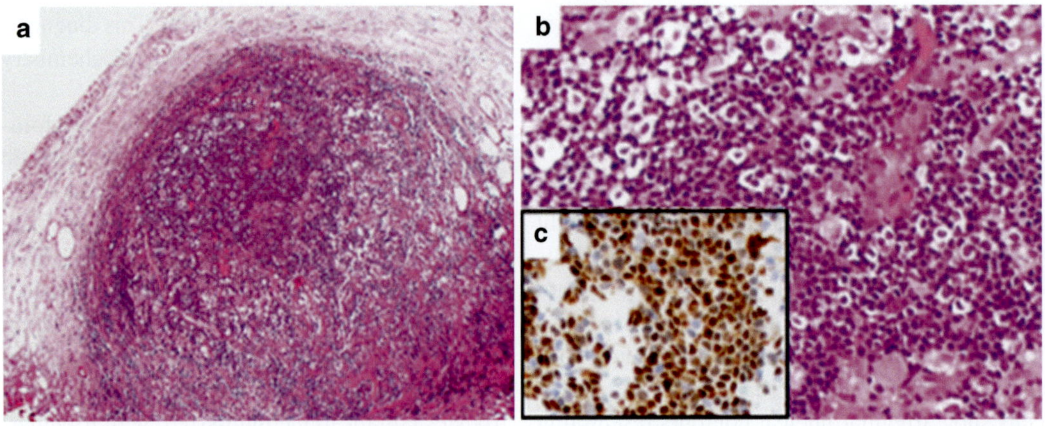

Fig. 10.3 MCL. (**a**) Underneath the urothelium are large lymphoid nodules rich in hyalinized blood vessels. Scattered histiocytes give a "starry sky" appearance. (**b** and **c**) MCL cells are monomorphic and small, with dense to somewhat dispersed chromatin and scant cytoplasm (**b**), and are strongly positive for cyclin D1 (**c**)

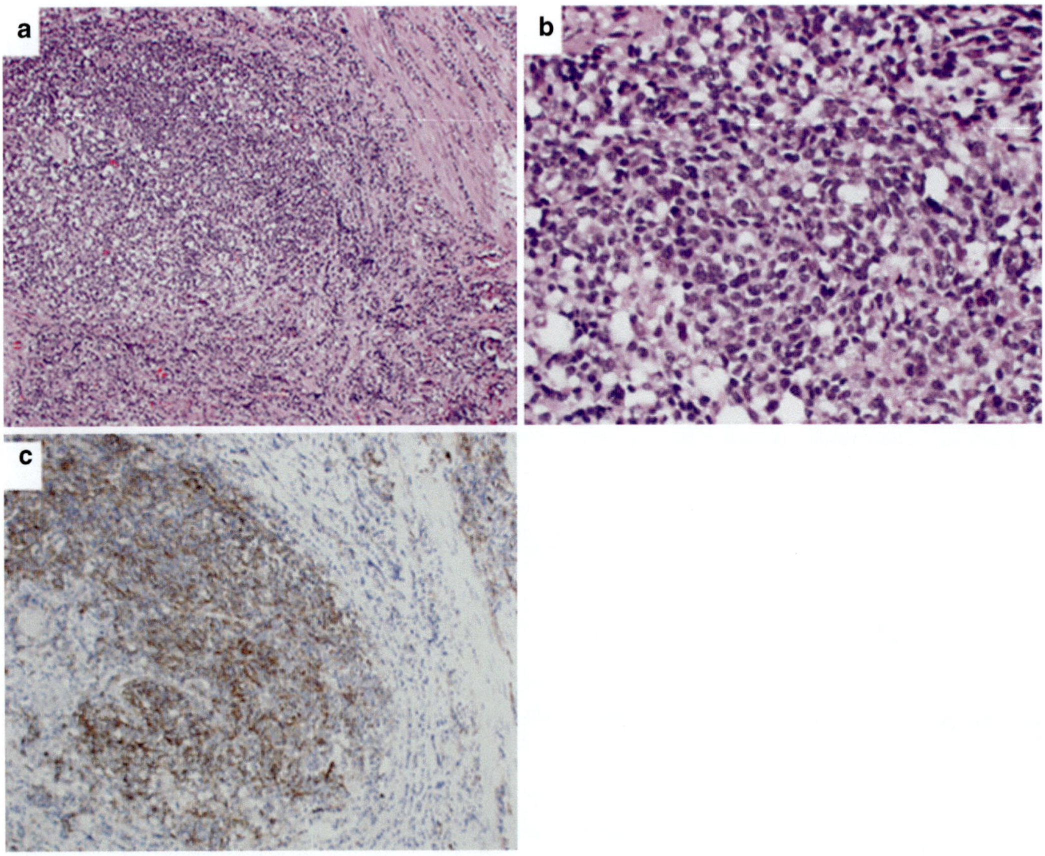

Fig. 10.4 FL. (**a**) Lymphoid nodules/follicles are identified in the bladder wall, adjacent to the muscularis propria (right upper corner). (**b**) The FL cells are predominantly centroblasts (>15/HPF), with a few admixed centrocytes, indicating high-grade follicular lymphoma. (**c**) The FL cells are positive for CD20. Other areas show diffuse large B-cell lymphoma (picture not shown), which is likely transformed from the follicular lymphoma

nucleoli). The grading of FL is based on the proportion of centroblasts (low grade if <15/HPF, high grade if >15/HPF) [22].

DLBCL is the most common type of large B-cell lymphomas involving the bladder [1, 3, 8]. The DLBCL can either be secondary involvement of a systemic diffuse large B-cell lymphoma or transformed from a low grade B-cell lymphomas (such as MALT lymphoma) of the bladder [1]. Histologic sections show diffuse proliferation of large lymphoma cells (Fig. 10.5). The DLBCL lymphoma cells usually have centroblastic morphology (oval to round, vesicular nuclei, two or more peripherally located nucleoli and scant cytoplasm), but sometimes they have immunoblastic morphology (a single centrally located nucleoli and more cytoplasm). The DLBCL is subclassified as either germinal center B-cell-like (GCB) or non-GCB subtype based on immunophenotype. The GCB subtype is generally thought to have better a prognosis than the non-GCB subtype [22]. It is important to perform FISH analysis for *MYC* rearrangement to rule out double or triple-hit lymphoma because some of them have the morphology of the DLBCL.

High-grade B-cell lymphomas are a group of aggressive mature B-cell lymphomas that have intermediate features between DLBCL and Burkitt lymphoma or appear blastoid (Fig. 10.6). High-grade B-cell lymphomas are classified into two categories: [1] high-grade B-cell lymphoma with *MYC* and *BCL2* and/or *BCL6* rearrangements (double- or triple-hit lymphoma) and [2] high-grade B-cell lymphoma NOS [22]. Patients with high-grade B-cell lymphoma have poor outcomes.

Acute Leukemia Involving the Bladder

In contrast to lymphoma infiltration, acute leukemia involving the bladder is less frequent. Acute leukemia in the bladder includes acute myeloid leukemia, B-lymphoblastic leukemia/lymphoma, or T-lymphoblastic leukemia/lymphoma, with acute myeloid leukemia being more often than the lymphoblastic leukemia. So far, only a few single cases and a small case series of the bladder infiltrated by acute leukemia have been reported, with myeloid cases being more often than lymphoid ones [25–28]. In the patients with acute myeloid leukemia, it is not surprising to see the blasts in the bladder's blood vessels (Fig. 10.7), which should not be considered as leukemic involvement of the bladder. The extravascular infiltration of myeloid blasts in the bladder is usually nondestructive and does not form tumor masses (Fig. 10.8). When they do form tumor masses effacing the normal bladder architecture, they are called myeloid sarcoma (Fig. 10.9) [25, 28]. The myeloid sarcoma is most commonly associated with acute myeloid leukemia, especially when there is a monocytic differentiation, but it can also be seen in patients with a history of a myeloproliferative neoplasm or myelodysplastic syndrome [22].

Differential Diagnosis of Bladder Lymphoma and Plasma Cell Neoplasms

Mimics of bladder lymphomas and plasma cell neoplasms include unusual variants of bladder cancer, such as lymphoepithelioma-like and plasmacytoid urothelial carcinoma variants [29, 30].

The lymphoepithelioma-like urothelial carcinoma is a rare variant of urothelial carcinoma that resembles undifferentiated carcinoma of the nasopharynx, but it is negative for EBV. The lymphoepithelioma-like urothelial carcinoma is composed of sheets of undifferentiated, pleomorphic cells with syncytial appearance. Admixed are background inflammatory cells, including T- and B-lymphocytes, plasma cells, histiocytes, and occasional neutrophils and eosinophils. In rare occasions, eosinophils may be prominent [29, 30].

Morphological features of epithelial component along with positive immunohistochemical stains by several cytokeratin markers (AE1/AE3 and CK7) and the co-expressions of p63 and GATA3 on the epithelia cells establish the diagnosis of lymphoepithelioma-like urothelial carcinoma. Lacking morphological atypia and

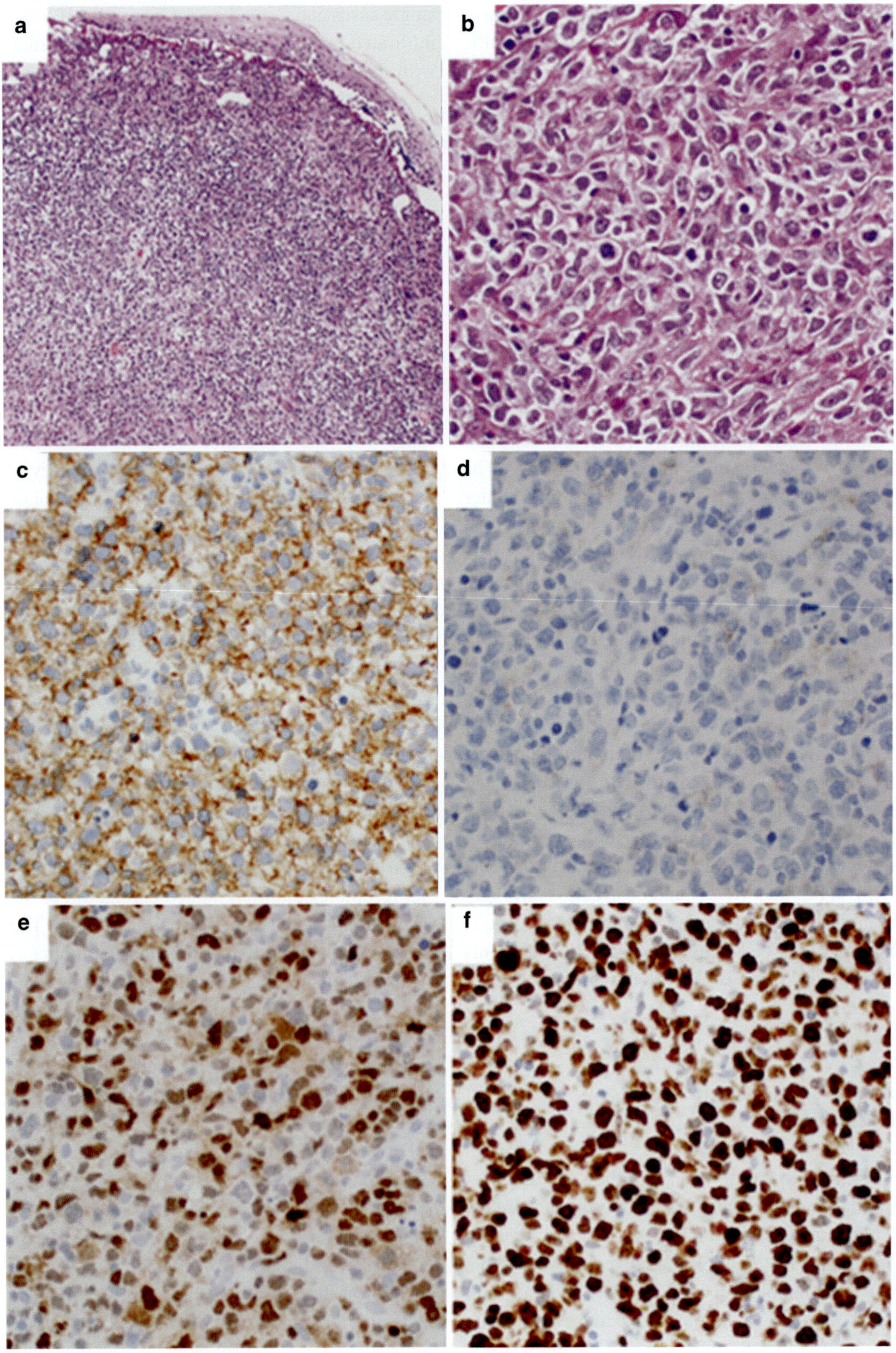
a
b
c
d
e
f

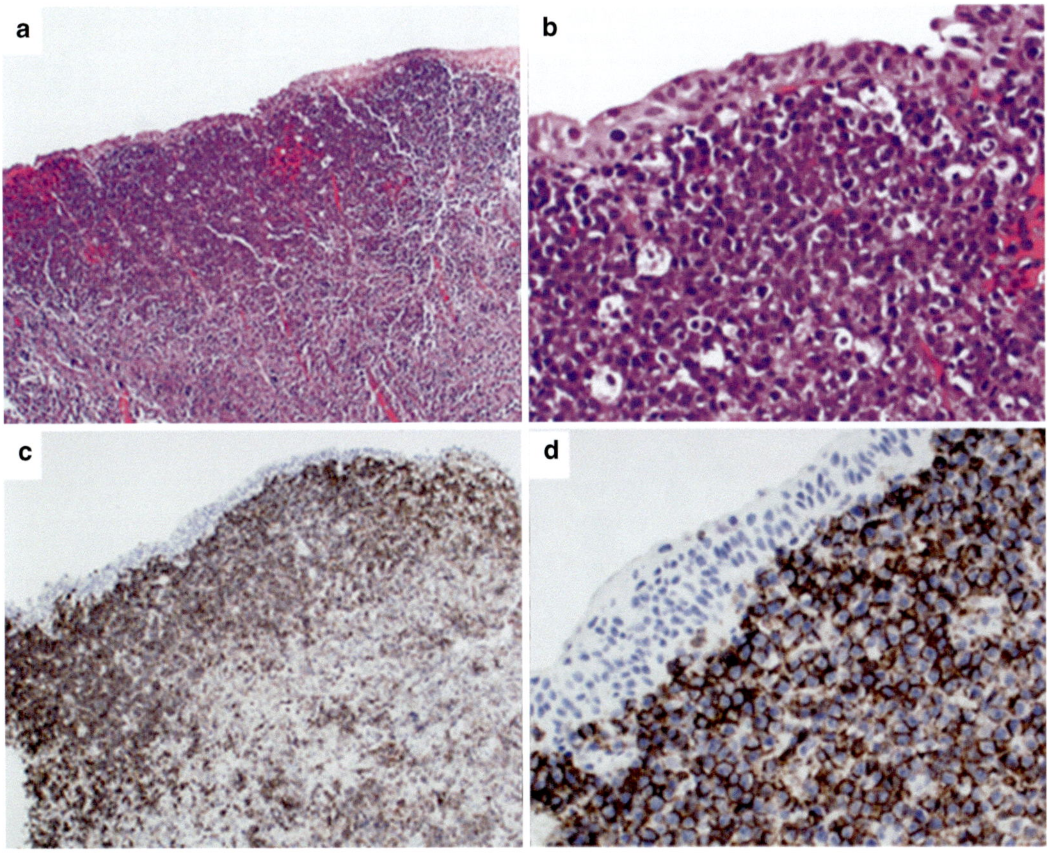

Fig. 10.6 High-grade B-cell lymphoma, NOS. (**a**) Diffuse lymphocytic infiltrate is identified beneath the urothelium. (**b**) The lymphoma cells are monotonous and medium-sized, with a blastoid appearance (round nuclei, fine chromatin, and small distinct nucleoli). A "starry sky" pattern is appreciated due to the scattered macrophages that have ingested apoptotic tumor cells. Mitoses are easily seen. (**c–d**) The lymphoma cells are positive for CD20. The lymphoma cells do not invade the overlying urothelium. FISH analysis is negative for *MYC* rearrangement (picture not shown), consistent with high-grade B-cell lymphoma NOS

Fig. 10.5 DLBCL, non-GCB immunophenotype. (**a**) The bladder urothelium (right upper corner) is unremarkable, but the tissue underlying the urothelium is extensively replaced by diffuse lymphoma cells. (**b**) The DLBCL cells are large, with fine chromatin, one to three small nucleoli and moderate to abundant amount of "clear" cytoplasm (likely due to retraction artifact). Mitosis and apoptotic debris are frequently seen. (**c–e**) The DLBCL cells are CD20+ (**c**), CD10- (**d**), BCL6+ (picture not shown), and MUM-1+ (E), consistent with non-GCB immunophenotype. (**f**) The DLBCL cell proliferation index by Ki67 is >95%. FISH analysis for *MYC* gene rearrangement is negative (picture not shown), excluding double- or triple-hit lymphomas

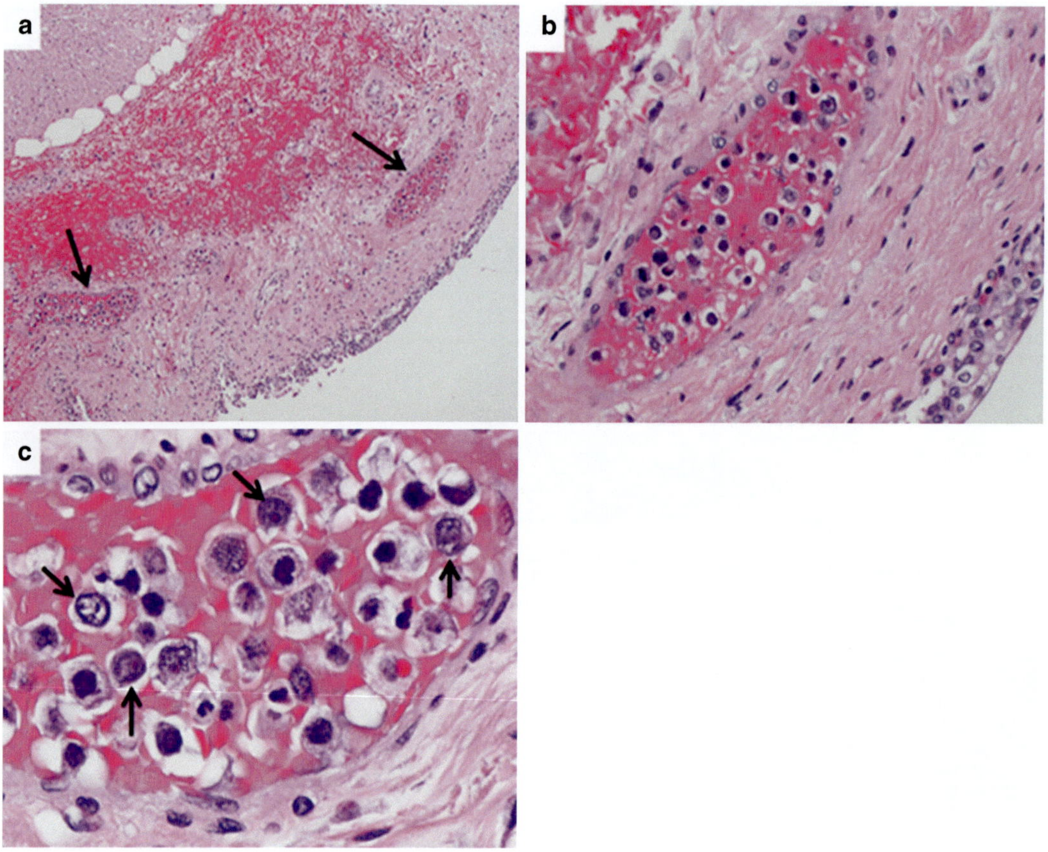

Fig. 10.7 Acute myeloid leukemia is only identified in the bladder's blood vessels. (**a**) At low power, the urothelium (right lower corner) is unremarkable, while the blood vessels (arrows) are expanded by cells. There is no extravascular blast infiltrate. (**b–c**) At high power, the blasts in the blood vessels are medium to large in size, with round to irregular nuclei, vesicular chromatin, and distinct nucleoli (arrows, **c**)

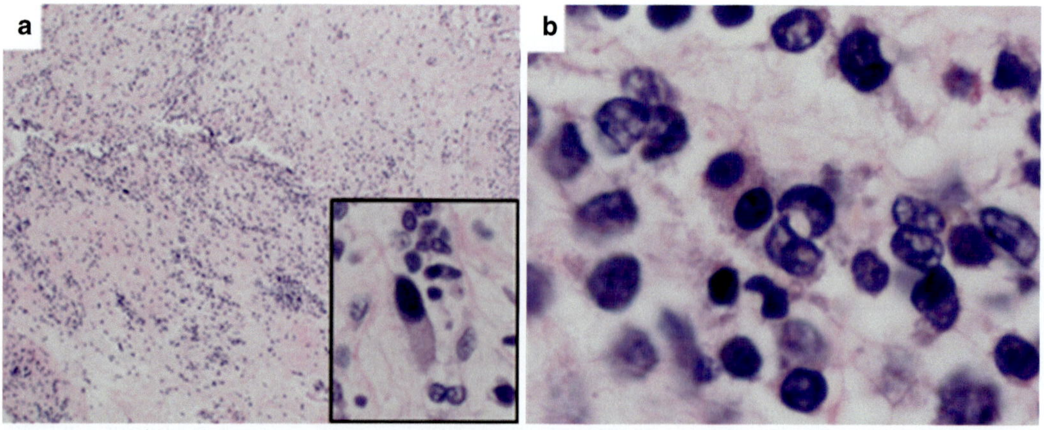

Fig. 10.8 Leukemic blasts infiltrating the bladder in a patient with history of acute myeloid leukemia. (**a**) Diffuse blasts are identified in the lamina propria of the bladder. Extramedullary hematopoiesis is seen (the insert shows a dysplastic megakaryocyte). (**b**) The blasts are intermediate to large in size, showing highly irregular nuclear contours, vesicular chromatin, and small nucleoli. (**c–d**) The blasts are negative for CD34 (**c**) but are positive for CD13 (subset)

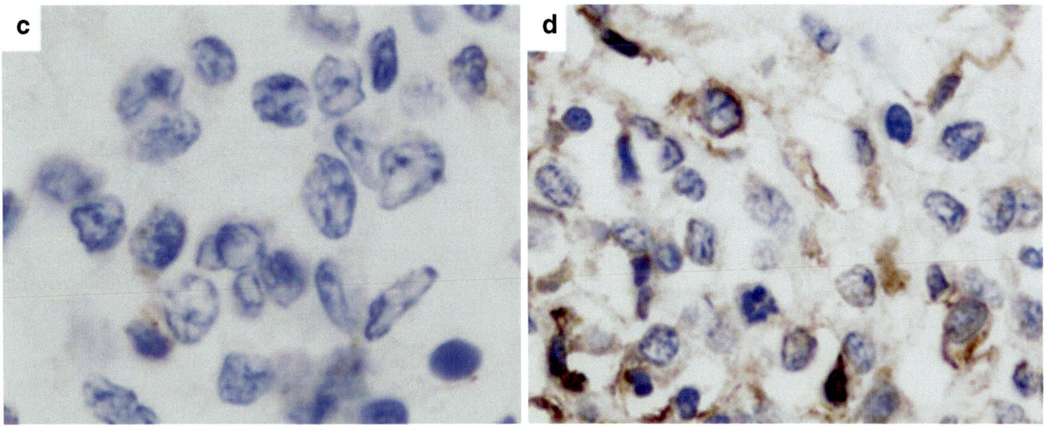

Fig. 10.8 (continued)

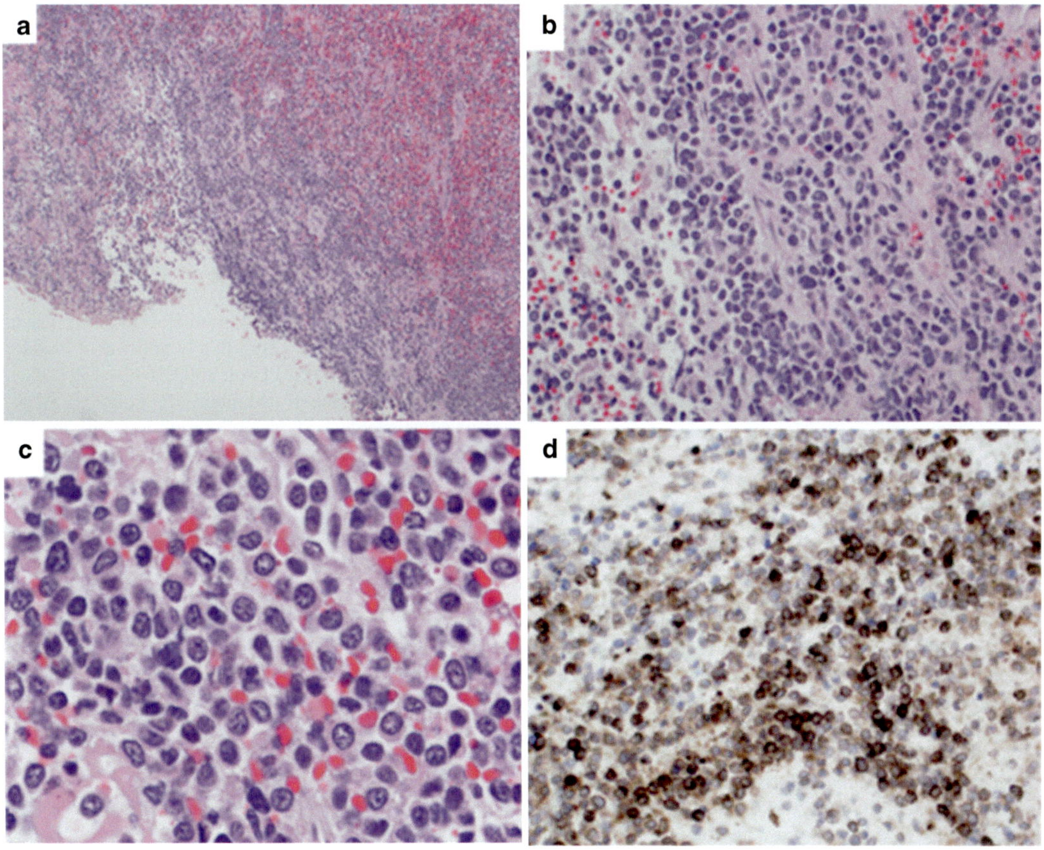

Fig. 10.9 Acute myeloid leukemia involving the bladder with multiple polypoid masses (myeloid sarcoma). (**a**) Diffuse leukemic blastic infiltrate in the bladder wall. (**b–c**) The blasts are medium-sized, showing round to irregular nuclear contours, vesicular chromatin, one or more small distinct nucleoli, and small to moderate amounts of cytoplasm. (**d**) The blasts are positive for CD34 (subset, variable)

immunophenotypic aberrancy in the background of lymphocytes exclude the diagnosis of lymphomas.

The plasmacytoid urothelial carcinoma is another rare, aggressive variant of urothelial carcinoma [31–33]. It is characterized by plasmacytoid cells with abundant eosinophilic cytoplasm, centrally or eccentrically located large nuclei, and small nucleoli. Some of the plasmacytoid urothelial carcinoma cells may show signet ring-like appearance. Approximately 50% of reported plasmacytoid urothelial carcinoma cases exhibit either urothelial carcinoma in situ or conventional urothelial carcinoma, which might be a hint for the correct diagnosis [29–33]. Immunohistochemical stains are also important in distinguishing the plasmacytoid urothelial carcinoma from a plasma cell neoplasm (plasmacytoma or plasma cell myeloma). The most commonly used plasma cell marker CD138 may not be helpful in this setting, as about one-third of the plasmacytoid urothelial carcinoma cells are positive for CD138. However, the neoplastic cells are positive for epithelial and urothelial lineage markers (CK7, CK20, p63, GATA3, and uroplakin III) but consistently negative for MUM1, a very useful marker in this setting which consistently expressed in plasma cell neoplasm and not in epithelial neoplasm [29, 30, 34].

References

1. Bates AW, Norton AJ, Baithun SI. Malignant lymphoma of the urinary bladder: a clinicopathological study of 11 cases. J Clin Pathol. 2000;53(6):458–61.
2. Hughes M, Morrison A, Jackson R. Primary bladder lymphoma: management and outcome of 12 patients with a review of the literature. Leuk Lymphoma. 2005;46(6):873–7.
3. Kempton CL, Kurtin PJ, Inwards DJ, Wollan P, Bostwick DG. Malignant lymphoma of the bladder: evidence from 36 cases that low-grade lymphoma of the MALT-type is the most common primary bladder lymphoma. Am J Surg Pathol. 1997;21(11):1324–33.
4. Ohsawa M, Aozasa K, Horiuchi K, Kanamaru A. Malignant lymphoma of bladder. Report of three cases and review of the literature. Cancer. 1993;72(6):1969–74.
5. Simpson RH, Bridger JE, Anthony PP, James KA, Jury I. Malignant lymphoma of the lower urinary tract. A clinicopathological study with review of the literature. Br J Urol. 1990;65(3):254–60.
6. Mahfoud T, Tanz R, Mesmoudi M, Khmamouche MR, El Khannoussi B, Ichou M, et al. Primary non-Hodgkin's lymphoma of the bladder: case report and literature review. Pan Afr Med J. 2013;15:136.
7. Wong-You-Cheong JJ, Woodward PJ, Manning MA, Sesterhenn IA. From the Archives of the AFIP: neoplasms of the urinary bladder: radiologic-pathologic correlation. Radiographics. 2006;26(2):553–80.
8. Venyo AK. Lymphoma of the urinary bladder. Adv Urol. 2014;2014:327917.
9. Al-Maghrabi J, Kamel-Reid S, Jewett M, Gospodarowicz M, Wells W, Banerjee D. Primary low-grade B-cell lymphoma of mucosa-associated lymphoid tissue type arising in the urinary bladder: report of 4 cases with molecular genetic analysis. Arch Pathol Lab Med. 2001;125(3):332–6.
10. Cohen DD, Lamarre C, Lamarre L, Fs FS. Primary low-grade B-cell lymphoma of the urinary bladder: case report and literature review. Can J Urol. 2002;9(6):1694–7.
11. Fernandez Acenero MJ, Martin Rodilla C, Lopez Garcia-Asenjo J, Coca Menchero S, Sanz EJ. Primary malignant lymphoma of the bladder. Report of three cases. Pathol Res Pract. 1996;192(2):160–3. discussion 4–5
12. Sufrin G, Keogh B, Moore RH, Murphy GP. Secondary involvement of the bladder in malignant lymphoma. J Urol. 1977;118(2):251–3.
13. Jones MW. Primary Hodgkin's disease of the urinary bladder. Br J Urol. 1989;63(4):438.
14. Mearini E, Zucchi A, Costantini E, Fornetti P, Tiacci E, Mearini L. Primary Burkitt's lymphoma of bladder in patient with AIDS. J Urol. 2002;167(3):1397–8.
15. Lobo J, Henrique R, Monteiro P, Lobo C. ALK-negative anaplastic large cell lymphoma with urinary bladder involvement diagnosed in urine cytology: a case report and literature review. Diagn Cytopathol. 2017;45(4):354–8.
16. Chen H, Li Y, Nand S, Quek ML, Kini AR, Barkan GA. Anaplastic large cell lymphoma involving the urinary bladder: a case report and review of the literature. Diagn Cytopathol. 2015;43(1):60–5.
17. Mourad WA, Khalil S, Radwi A, Peracha A, Ezzat A. Primary T-cell lymphoma of the urinary bladder. Am J Surg Pathol. 1998;22(3):373–7.
18. Pai SA, Naresh KN, Patil PU. Systemic anaplastic large cell lymphoma presenting as a bladder neoplasm. Leuk Lymphoma. 2004;45(4):841–3.
19. Desai V, Isharwal S, Pooli A, Lele S, Feloney M. Chronic lymphocytic leukemia of the bladder: an atypical etiology of gross hematuria. Ther Adv Urol. 2014;6(5):198–200.
20. Ramadan KM, Kyle A, McManus D, O'Rourke D, Cuthbert RJ. Urinary bladder infiltration with chronic B-lymphocytic leukemia: two cases with unusual presentation. Leuk Lymphoma. 2006;47(6):1184–7.
21. Carver JD, Calverley D, Shen P. Chronic lymphocytic leukemia/small lymphocytic lymphoma presenting

in urinary bladder without peripheral blood lymphocytosis: case report and literature review. Leuk Lymphoma. 2006;47(6):1163–5.
22. Swerdlow SH, Campo E, Pileri SA, Harris NL, Stein H, Siebert R, et al. The 2016 revision of the World Health Organization classification of lymphoid neoplasms. Blood. 2016;127(20):2375–90.
23. Tsimberidou AM, Wen S, McLaughlin P, O'Brien S, Wierda WG, Lerner S, et al. Other malignancies in chronic lymphocytic leukemia/small lymphocytic lymphoma. J Clin Oncol. 2009;27(6):904–10.
24. Gajendra S, Sharma R, Sahoo MK. Triple cancer: chronic lymphocytic leukemia with bladder and prostate carcinoma. Malays J Pathol. 2015;37(2):159–63.
25. Al-Quran SZ, Olivares A, Lin P, Stephens TW, Medeiros LJ, Abruzzo LV. Myeloid sarcoma of the urinary bladder and epididymis as a primary manifestation of acute myeloid leukemia with inv(16). Arch Pathol Lab Med. 2006;130(6):862–6.
26. Pham A, Steinberg A, Kwok B, Lopez A, Lim S, Lill M. Precursor T-Cell acute lymphoblastic leukemia/lymphoma with rare presentation in the urinary bladder. Hematol Rep. 2011;3(2):e18.
27. Chang CY, Chiou TJ, Hsieh YL, Cheng SN. Leukemic infiltration of the urinary bladder presenting as uncontrollable gross hematuria in a child with acute lymphoblastic leukemia. J Pediatr Hematol Oncol. 2003;25(9):735–9.
28. Delhi Kumar CG, Thilagavathy V, Arun BT. Granulocytic sarcoma of bladder in an 18-mo-old child with acute myeloid leukemia. Indian J Pediatr. 2014;81(10):1118–9.
29. Moch HHP, Ulbright TM, Reuter V. WHO classification of tumours of the urinary system and male genital organs. Lyon: International Agency for Research on Cancer; 2016.
30. Lopez-Beltran A, Henriques V, Montironi R, Cimadamore A, Raspollini MR, Cheng L. Variants and new entities of bladder cancer. Histopathology. 2019;74(1):77–96.
31. Keck B, Stoehr R, Wach S, Rogler A, Hofstaedter F, Lehmann J, et al. The plasmacytoid carcinoma of the bladder--rare variant of aggressive urothelial carcinoma. Int J Cancer. 2011;129(2):346–54.
32. Lopez-Beltran A, Requena MJ, Montironi R, Blanca A, Cheng L. Plasmacytoid urothelial carcinoma of the bladder. Hum Pathol. 2009;40(7):1023–8.
33. Amin MB, Trpkov K, Lopez-Beltran A, Grignon D. Members of the IIiDUPG. Best practices recommendations in the application of immunohistochemistry in the bladder lesions: report from the International Society of Urologic Pathology consensus conference. Am J Surg Pathol. 2014;38(8):e20–34.
34. Borhan WM, Cimino-Mathews AM, Montgomery EA, Epstein JI. Immunohistochemical differentiation of plasmacytoid urothelial carcinoma from secondary carcinoma involvement of the bladder. Am J Surg Pathol. 2017;41(11):1570–5.

Secondary Tumors in the Bladder

11

Miao Zhang

The urinary bladder may be involved secondarily by surrounding organs such as the prostate, colon, and cervix. Due to the proximity of the prostate and bladder, secondary involvement of the bladder by high-grade prostatic adenocarcinoma is not uncommon. The involvement is mostly by direct extension. Uncommonly, the bladder can be involved by metastasis from other primaries such as malignant melanoma, breast cancer, colon cancer, stomach cancer, and lung cancer. The bladder appears to be the second most common site to be involved in metastasis in the urinary tract following the kidney. The diagnosis is dependent on morphological features and clinical information.

Unlike primary bladder malignancies, which usually present with urinary symptoms, the metastatic involvement of bladder infrequently presents with any urinary symptoms. In one study, about 54% of the metastatic cancers of the bladder were located near the bladder neck and trigone area, in comparison to only 24% in primary cancers of the bladder [1].

Adenocarcinomas are the most frequent histological subtypes of metastatic cancers of the bladders, followed by squamous cell carcinomas and other subtypes like small cell carcinomas and clear cell carcinomas. Pure primary bladder adenocarcinomas are morphologically indistinguishable from metastatic adenocarcinomas. Therefore, a clinical history is the key in making the diagnosis. Because of the rarity of primary bladder adenocarcinomas, when such morphology is present, metastasis from other sites should be ruled out first.

Micropapillary carcinoma (MPC) can occur in the bladder, breast, ovary, and lung. While morphological features are quite similar, pathologists rely on immunohistochemical stains to distinguish these possible entities. Lotan et al. [2] found that immunostaining for uroplakin, CK20, TTF-1, estrogen receptor (ER), WT-1 and/or PAX8, and mammaglobin was the best panel for determining the most likely primary site of MPC. The best markers to identify urothelial MPC were uroplakin and CK20, whereas p63, high molecular weight cytokeratin, and thrombomodulin were less sensitive and specific. Lung MPC was uniformly TTF-1 positive. Breast MPC was ER positive, mammaglobin positive, and PAX8/WT-1 negative, while ovarian MPC was ER positive, mammaglobin negative, and PAX8/WT-1 positive. In the metastatic setting, or when MPC occurs without an associated in situ or conventional carcinoma component, staining for uroplakin, CK20, TTF-1, ER and WT-1, and/or PAX8, and mammaglobin is the best panel for accurately classifying the likely primary site of MPC. GATA3 is a good

M. Zhang (✉)
Department of Pathology, MD Anderson Cancer Center, Houston, TX, USA
e-mail: MZhang8@mdanderson.org

H. Zhou et al. (eds.), *Urinary Bladder Pathology*, https://doi.org/10.1007/978-3-030-71509-0_11

marker for determining the primary site of carcinoma in the bladder and breast.

Prostate Cancer High-grade prostatic adenocarcinoma can have overlapping morphological features with high-grade urothelial carcinoma; however, even high-grade prostate cancers retain their characteristic cytologic features, such as cellular uniformity, prominent nucleolus, and rare or no mitoses. In general, it is not a problem to differentiate prostate carcinoma from urothelial carcinoma. Prostatic adenocarcinoma involves the bladder mostly by direct extension through prostatic urethra, causing obstruction. Although most patients are at high stages with extensive high-grade prostatic adenocarcinoma and treatment, rarely, it can present as a primary mass lesion in the bladder without a prior diagnosis of primary prostatic adenocarcinoma. It may pose a diagnostic difficulty, as ductal-type adenocarcinomas (Fig. 11.1) or acinar-type adenocarcinomas with pseudopapillary areas mimic papillary urothelial carcinoma [3]. Immunohistochemical positivity for NKX3.1 and negativity for GATA-3 should help to distinguish prostatic from urothelial primary. It is worth noting that after extensive treatment, tumor glands losing immunoreactivity for PSA do not exclude prostate primary. Careful review of clinical history and serum PSA level is also key.

Breast Cancer Breast cancer involving the bladder is rare with only 50 cases reported in the literature (2.5% of all secondary neoplasm). The first report of bladder metastasis from breast cancer was in 1980 [4]. In most cases, breast cancer has already become widespread at the time of diagnosis; however, in some rare cases, only bladder metastasis is detected [5]. Clinically, patients present with lower abdominal pain and hematuria. Imaging studies show irregular thickening of the bladder wall. Invasive lobular breast carcinoma metastatic to urinary bladder occurs more frequently compared to its ductal counterpart [6]. Histologically, signet ring cell morphology of individual cells, eosinophilic cytoplasm, and rounded eccentrically located nuclei are typical features of lobular carcinoma (Fig. 11.2). In addition, signet ring cells with intraluminal targetoid mucin droplet are a very helpful finding to favor a breast primary. Immunohistochemical markers such as ER, PR, mammaglobin, and GCDFP-15 can be helpful in distinguishing bladder primary from metastatic breast primary. GATA-3 is not helpful, as it is positive in both breast and bladder primaries. Attention to clinical history is very helpful. It is critical to recognize breast carcinoma in the bladder, given the therapy implications. Bladder metastasis from breast cancer is often advanced at the time of diagnosis. The prognosis is very poor and most patients die within 1 year. However, some cases with a survival of 5 years or more have also been reported [7].

Renal Cell Carcinoma Metastatic renal cell carcinoma (RCC) to the urinary bladder is rare. When this occurs, it might complicate the diagnosis. Morphologically, RCC can be confused with transitional cell carcinomas (TCCs), especially those exhibiting clear cell features, and

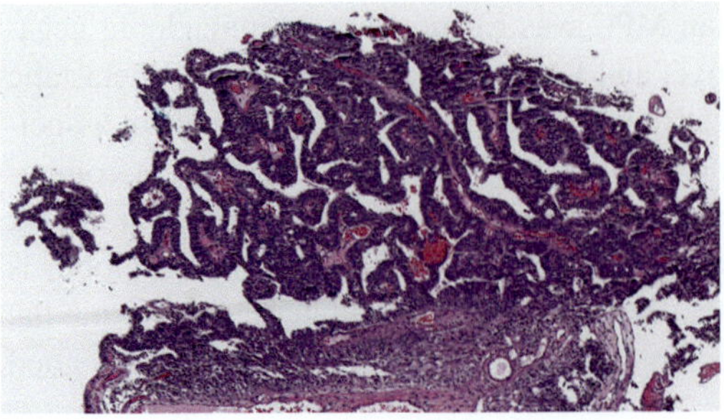

Fig. 11.1 Prostatic ductal adenocarcinoma involving the bladder

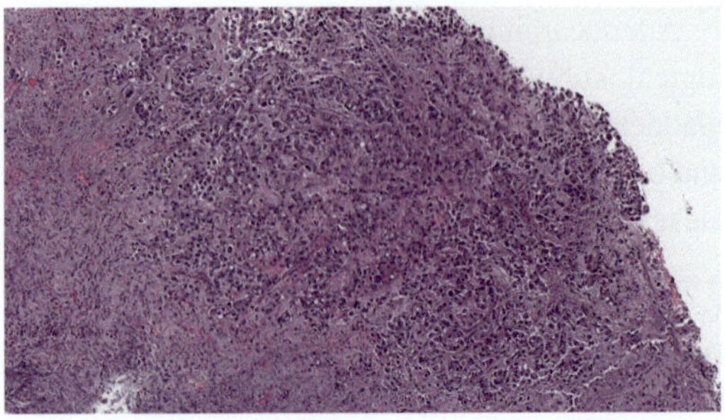

Fig. 11.2 Metastatic breast cancer involving ulcerated bladder mucosa

with other bladder tumors, such as paragangliomas and metastatic melanomas [8]. Reported metastatic RCC subtypes include clear cell RCC (most common), papillary RCC, and chromophobe RCC. Clinically, patients present with hematuria or urinary retention or obstruction. Although most patients have histories of RCC, in rare cases, patients presented with metastatic clear cell RCC to the bladder and were subsequently found to have renal masses. Cystoscopy examination shows fungating or nodular mass lesions and some as "not typical appearance of bladder tumor." These tumors may be located at the bladder neck, trigone, dome, posterior wall, and posterior wall near dome and base. Histologically, most tumors are clear cell RCCs (Fig. 11.3), and some are associated with sarcomatoid carcinoma; papillary RCC have also been reported and very rarely chromophobe RCCs [9]. In general, there is histological fidelity between the primary and metastatic tumors in the bladder in terms of cell type and grade. Metastatic tumors in the bladder may undermine the urothelium, float in the lumen or ulcerate the surface. The one reported case of chromophobe RCC showed pagetoid spread to preexisting urothelial papilloma. Most cases of clear cell RCC are readily identifiable on the H&E sections. Immunohistochemical studies are that of typical RCCs, which show PAX-8 positivity and AMACR and CK7 positivity of papillary RCCs. GATA-3 is negative in all reported cases.

Because of the rarity of metastatic RCC involving the bladder, misdiagnosis is not uncommonly seen. Some were misdiagnosed as papillary urothelial carcinoma and some as prostatic adenocarcinoma or urachal adenocarcinoma. Management of metastatic RCC involving the bladder is not standardized. Surgical interventions such as transurethral resection and partial or radical cystectomy have been used. Although implicating a poor prognosis, long-term survival has been reported [10].

Gynecological Malignancies Metastatic cervical and ovarian cancers are the most common gynecological malignancies involving the bladder in women [11]. Metastatic high-grade serous carcinoma (Fig. 11.4) is a common finding and morphologically deceptive as these tumors can mimic papillary urothelial carcinoma. Female gender and a clinical history of gynecological cancer should raise suspicion. Immunohistochemical study for PAX8 is useful when considering gynecological origin.

Squamous cell carcinoma (SCC) of the cervix (Fig. 11.5) can be morphologically indistinguish-

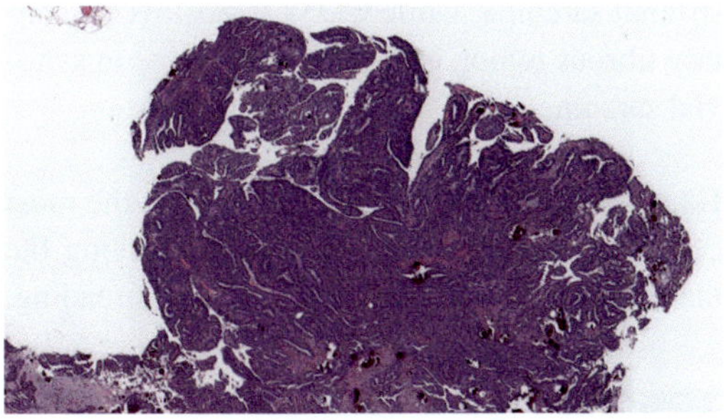

Fig. 11.4 Metastatic high-grade serous carcinoma involving the bladder wall

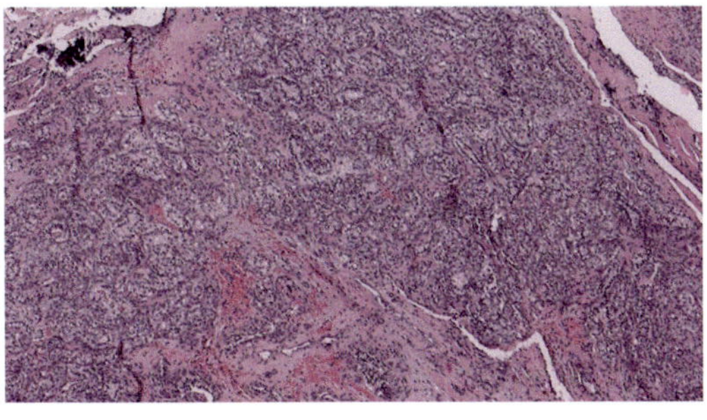

Fig. 11.3 Metastatic clear cell renal cell carcinoma involving the bladder

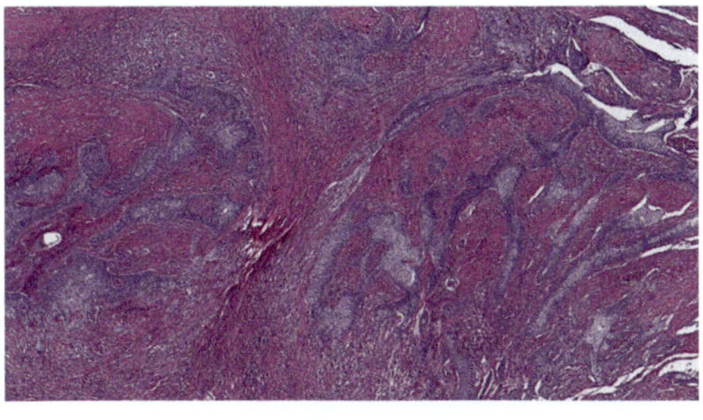

Fig. 11.5 Metastatic cervical squamous cell carcinoma involving the bladder wall

able from urothelial carcinoma with squamous differentiation or primary squamous cell carcinoma of the bladder. Imaging and clinical information are most useful. The demographic distribution of cervical SCC is quite different from bladder SCC, as cervical SCC happens in younger women. Ancillary study such as in situ hybridization study for high-risk HPV can be used too, as positivity for high-risk HPV is rarely seen in high-grade urothelial carcinomas (<20%) [12]. Immunohistochemical study for p16, however, is less helpful, as positivity can be seen in up to 80% of high-grade urothelial carcinomas [12, 13].

Primary uterine carcinomas such as endometrial neuroendocrine tumor and endometrial stromal sarcoma are rare and were also reported to involve the urinary bladder [14]. Main differential diagnoses with endometrial stromal sarcoma are soft tissue mesenchymal tumors of the bladder including solitary fibrous tumor, synovial sarcoma, and large nested variant of urothelial carcinoma. Immunohistochemical studies for CD10, ER, and PR are positive in endometrial stromal sarcoma, while CD34 is positive in solitary fibrous tumor, and TLE1 is positive in synovial sarcoma.

Gastrointestinal Cancer The colon is the most common primary site secondarily involving the bladder (Fig. 11.6), mostly by direct spreading. The most common distant site of origin is the stomach (4.3% of all secondary neoplasms). Other reported cases from the gastrointestinal tract include metastatic rectal adenocarcinoma, appendiceal adenocarcinoma, ileal carcinoid tumor, and gastrointestinal stromal tumor (Fig. 11.7) [7, 15]. The metastatic foci are mass forming, and biopsy material showed typical histological and immunohistochemical features concordant with the primary tumors.

Malignant Melanoma Of the malignancies arising from the skin, melanomas appear to be the most common involving the bladder, morphologically mimicking urothelial carcinoma in situ in some cases, though the presence of pigment helps with the diagnosis (Fig. 11.8). Various cuta-

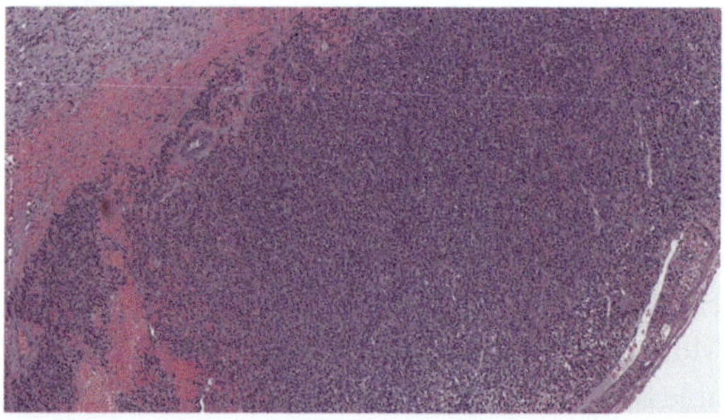

Fig. 11.7 Metastatic epithelioid gastrointestinal stromal tumor involving bladder serosa

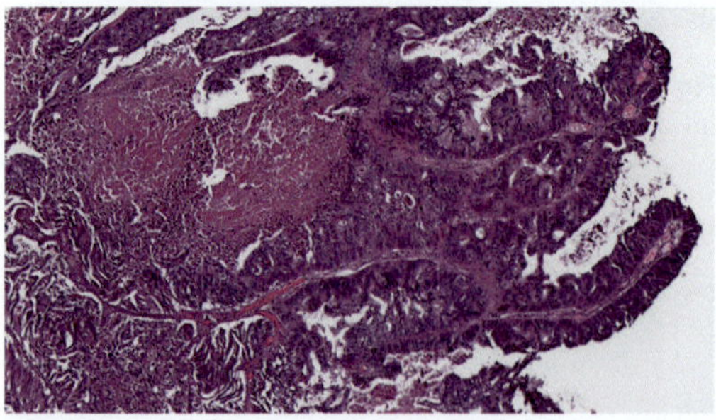

Fig. 11.6 Metastatic colonic adenocarcinoma involving the bladder

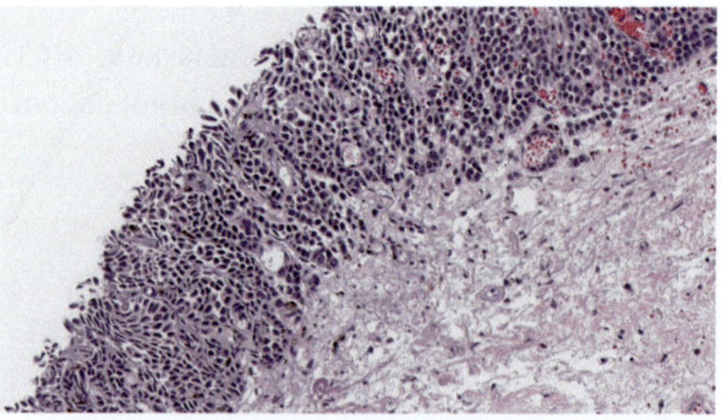

Fig. 11.8 Metastatic melanoma involving bladder mucosa, mimicking urothelial carcinoma in situ

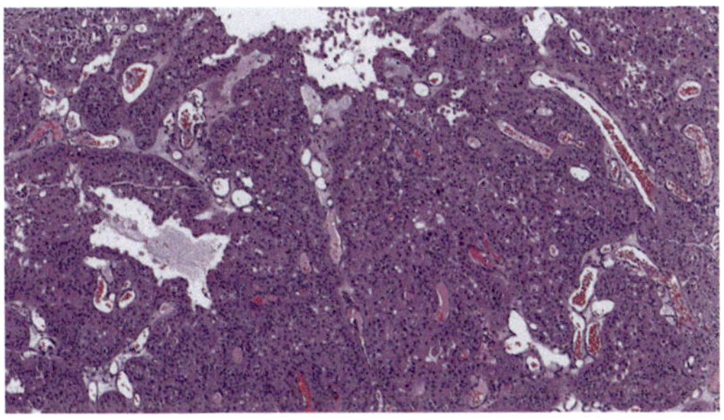

Fig. 11.9 Metastatic thyroid hurtle cell carcinoma involving the bladder

neous primary sites were reported, including cases of vulvar melanoma [16]. Metastasized melanomas involving the urinary bladder are almost always accompanied by distant metastasis to other sites.

Lung Primary lung squamous cell carcinoma, adenocarcinoma, and neuroendocrine tumor have all been reported to metastasize to the bladder (2.8% of all secondary malignancy). Metastatic lung squamous cell carcinoma possesses extreme diagnostic difficulties as primary urothelial carcinoma bears the same immunohistochemical features as lung squamous cell carcinomas. Not surprisingly, clinical correlation is crucial in making the distinction between primary and metastasis.

Other rare primary sites such as the pancreas, gallbladder, thyroid (Fig. 11.9), testis, liver, bone, and tongue have all been reported to involve the urinary bladder [16].

Conclusion The diagnosis of metastasis based on the histologic appearance involving the bladder is often difficult and poses a significant challenge to the clinicians and pathologists. The bladder is not a common site for metastasis of cancer and often goes undiagnosed in the clinical follow-up of patients with cancer. Primary bladder adenocarcinomas are rare, and when encountered, a metastasis from other sites should be considered and ruled out.

References

1. Roberts DI. Secondary neoplasms of the genitourinary tract. Br J Ruol. 1978;50:68.
2. Lotan TL, Ye H, Melamed J, Wu XR, Shih LM, Epstein JI. Immunohistochemical panel to identify the primary site of invasive micropapillary carcinoma. Am J Surg Pathol. 2009;33(7):1037–41.
3. Gordetsky J, Epstein JI. Pseudopapillary features in prostatic adenocarcinoma mimicking urothelial carcinoma: a diagnostic pitfall. Am J Surg Pathol. 2014;38(7):941–5.
4. Haid M, et al. Urinary bladder metastases from breast carcinoma. Cancer. 1980;46(1):229–32.
5. Zagha RM, Hamawy KJ. Solitary breast cancer metastasis to the bladder: an unusual occurrence. Urol Oncol. 2007;25(3):236–9.
6. Yoneyama K, et al. Bladder metastasis from primary breast cancer: a case report. Surgical Case Reports. 2018;4(1):73.
7. Xiao GQ, et al. Metastatic tumors to the urinary bladder: clinicopathologic study of 11 cases. Int J Surg Pathol. 2012;20(4):342–8.
8. Sim SJ, Ro JY, Ordonez NG, Park YW, Kee KH, Ayala AG. Metastatic renal cell carcinoma to the bladder: a clinicopathologic and immunohistochemical study. Mod Pathol. 1999;12(4):351–5.
9. Zhang M, et al. Metastatic renal cell carcinoma to the urinary bladder: a report of 11 cases. Am J Surg Pathol. 2014;38(11):1516–21.
10. Raviv S, et al. Long-term survival after "drop metastases" of renal cell carcinoma to the bladder. Urology. 2002;60(4):697.
11. Feldman A, et al. Secondary malignancies of the bladder: avoiding the diagnostic pitfall. Int J Surg Pathol. 2018;26(2):120–5.
12. Alexander RE, et al. p16 expression is not associated with human papillomavirus in urinary bladder squamous cell carcinoma. Mod Pathol. 2012;25(11):1526–33.
13. Nakazawa K, et al. p16(INK4a) expression analysis as an ancillary tool for cytologic diagnosis of urothelial carcinoma. Am J Clin Pathol. 2009;132(5):776–84.
14. Tian W, et al. Endometrial stromal sarcoma involving the urinary bladder: a study of 6 cases. Am J Surg Pathol. 2014;38(7):982–9.
15. Farhat MH, et al. Secondary adenocarcinoma of the urinary bladder from a primary gastric cancer. J Med Liban. 2007;55(3):162–4.
16. Bates AW, Baithun SI. Secondary neoplasms of the bladder are histological mimics of nontransitional cell primary tumours: clinicopathological and histological features of 282 cases. Histopathology. 2000;36(1):32–40.

12 Urine Cytology

Haijun Zhou

Introduction

Urine cytology is the microscopic examination of cells that exfoliate from the urinary tract. Urine cytology was first developed by Papanicolau [1] and is now the most common morphological test used to evaluate a wide variety of benign and malignant diseases that originate from the urothelium overlying the kidney, ureter, bladder, and urethra [2–4].

The detection of hematuria by urinalysis is typically the initial presentation of urothelial carcinoma. Urine cytology is usually performed in patients with microscopic or gross hematuria, and the goal is to detect high-grade urothelial carcinoma at an early stage (non-muscle invasive high-grade urothelial carcinoma and carcinoma in situ) [5]. Dyscohesive high-grade urothelial carcinoma cells exfoliated into urine can be detected microscopically without a tissue biopsy. Urine cytology is also an essential modality for patients undergoing surveillance for a previously diagnosed bladder neoplasm, although this may present diagnostic challenges due to the effects of prior treatment. Other indications for urinary tract cytology include follow-up for patients with atypical cytology caused by either neoplastic or benign conditions.

The urine specimen generally consists of voided urine and instrumental urine, i.e., brushing or washing (barbotage) specimens. Although urine cytology has high specificity (84.0% to 100.0%) for detecting high-grade invasive and/or in situ urothelial carcinoma, it is limited by its low sensitivity (ranging from 28.0% to 97% with a median of 48.0%) [6, 7] due to nontargeted sampling and overlapping cytomorphology shared with many benign or reactive conditions, particularly for low-grade urothelial neoplasms [8, 9].

In conjunction with urine cytology, urologists may perform cystoscopy and upper urinary tract (UUT) imaging studies for possible gross lesions. With cystoscopy, papillary lesions, bladder calculi, and bladder diverticula can be visualized. Papillary lesions and suspicious erythematous mucosa changes can be biopsied for histology diagnosis. Imaging studies, including computerized tomography (CT) urograms and retrograde pyelograms, will help detect renal pelvis and ureter lesions. Grossly identified or suspicious lesions will be biopsied or brushed for histological and cytological evaluation.

There are two recently published international classifications: The Paris System for Reporting Urinary Cytology (2013) and the International Consultation on Urologic Disease–European Association of Urology (2015) [10, 11]. Unlike in cervical cytology, there has not been a wide-

H. Zhou (✉)
Department of Pathology and Genomic Medicine, Weill Medical College of Cornell University/Houston Methodist Hospital, Houston, TX, USA
e-mail: hzhou@houstonmethodist.org

H. Zhou et al. (eds.), *Urinary Bladder Pathology*, https://doi.org/10.1007/978-3-030-71509-0_12

spread acceptance and use of any single reporting system for urine cytology studies as uniform terminology and criteria for urine cytology reporting have not been established among pathologists [12]. This chapter will not address the strengths and weaknesses of each classification system but will rather focus on the diagnostic features of urine cytology.

Because of the intrinsic limitations of urine cytology, ancillary tests have been developed to help monitor patients undergoing surveillance to assure that there is no residual or recurrent disease and to detect high-grade tumors when cytology or biopsy specimens are limited or suboptimal.

This chapter discusses the spectrum of urine cytological abnormalities, diagnostic pitfalls, and the clinical use of ancillary studies in the practice of urine cytology from the perspective of the cytopathologist.

Specimen Type

Urine specimens include voided urine, catheterized urine, bladder washings (barbotage), bladder brushings, ureteral and renal pelvic brushings and washings, and neobladder urine from an ileal conduit [13, 14].

Voided urine specimens are the most commonly submitted urine specimens to the cytology lab. Specimens collected from voided urine are noninvasive and easy to procure. The disadvantages of voided urine include low cellularity, degenerative changes, and vaginal contamination from female patients, which may pose certain diagnostic challenges.

Instrumented urine specimens include catheterized urine, bladder washings (barbotage or irrigation), and UUT washings and brushings. These types of specimens have relatively high cellularity and good preservation. However, instrumented specimens require caution because they may produce artifactually clustered urothelium, papillary cell clusters, and increased basal cells that will lead to "atypical" or false-positive diagnosis [15].

Post-cystectomy ileal conduit/neobladder specimens contain acute inflammation, columnar cells from ileal mucosa, and bacterial colonies. The nature of this type of specimen makes the detection of true recurrent neoplastic conditions difficult, and the positive predictive value of ileal conduit specimens is low [16].

Specimen Adequacy

The cytological criteria of adequacy for urine specimens are not well defined due to the existence of many pre-analytic variables, including collection type, cellularity, specimen volume, and cytomorphological findings. The cytomorphological presence of any atypical, suspicious, or malignant findings makes a specimen intrinsically adequate regardless of collection type, cellularity, or specimen volume. An unsatisfactory or inadequate specimen is one that is poorly cellular, predominantly degenerated, and/or completely obscured by inflammatory cells, blood, lubricants, debris, crystals, bacteria, spermatozoa, etc. [17]. Urine specimen volume only affects the adequacy of voided urine specimens because instrumental urine specimens have artificial volume. Low volume indicates undersampling of the voided urine and is arbitrarily linked to the finding of a lack of malignancy. One study suggests that a cut-off of 30 mL is an adequate volume of voided urine [18]. An adequate instrumented urine specimen is suggested to have at least 20 urothelial cells in 10 high-power fields using the ThinPrep method [19].

The determination of adequacy is important enough to warrant repeated sampling in order to avoid missing high-grade malignancy. However, rendering meaningful interpretation in the correct clinical setting is important in order to avoid unnecessary repeated sampling. Urine specimen processing methods commonly include cytospin, membrane filtration, and ThinPrep and SurePath liquid preparations, and all produce satisfactory results.

Reporting and Classification

Unlike in cervical cytology, there has not been a universally accepted single reporting system for urine cytology. Several published reporting and classification systems for urine cytology have their own strengths and weaknesses. The Paris System for Reporting Urinary Cytology (The Paris System) was created to decrease the use of the atypical category and to emphasize the risk of high-grade urothelial carcinoma rather than low-grade urothelial carcinoma. Prospective and retrospective studies have shown that The Paris System improves the diagnostic performance [20–22].

The diagnostic categories in The Paris System are (1) nondiagnostic/unsatisfactory; (2) negative for high-grade urothelial carcinoma (NHGUC); (3) atypical urothelial cells (AUC); (4) suspicious for high-grade urothelial carcinoma (SHGUC); (5) high-grade urothelial carcinoma (HGUC); (6) low-grade urothelial neoplasm (LGUN); and (7) others: primary and secondary malignancies and miscellaneous lesions. Each category has its correspondent risk of malignancy and recommended clinical response. Explanatory notes as to the diagnostic categories are useful supplements to cytology reports.

Normal Components of Urinary Sediment

Normal urine has few urothelial cells in a clean background without inflammatory cells. Normal cellular components of a urine specimen include superficial urothelial cells (umbrella cells), intermediate urothelial cells, basal cells, squamous cells, columnar cells, renal tubular cells, and red blood cells, spermatozoa, and seminal vesicle cells.

Benign superficial and intermediate urothelial cells are the most common cellular elements in urine specimens. They are variable in size, ranging from 20 μm in diameter for intermediate cells up to 100 μm for the typical umbrella or superficial cells. Urothelial cells have round-to-oval nuclei and delicate cytoplasm. Binucleate and multinucleate cells are common for superficial urothelial cells, with a low nucleus to cytoplasm ratio (Fig. 12.1). Basal urothelial cells are more commonly observed in instrumented specimens. Basal urothelial cells are smaller than intermediate cells with small nuclei in relatively uniformed size, with finely granular and evenly distributed chromatin. Benign clusters or fragments of urothelial cells are often seen, particularly in instrumented urine, and the benign cytomorphology of the cells forming the group fulfills The Paris System criteria for negative.

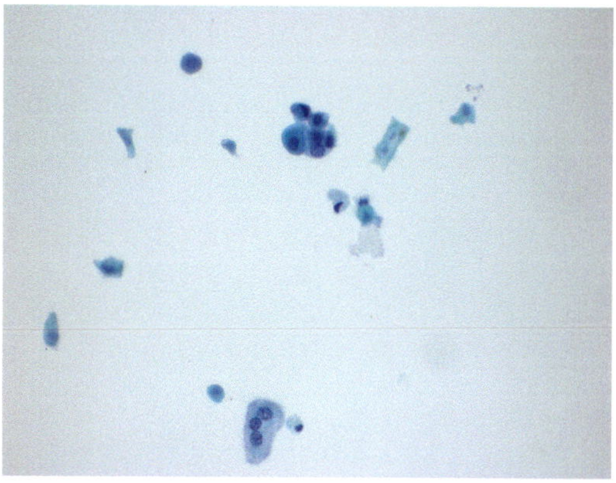

Fig. 12.1 Normal urothelial intermediate and superficial cells with low nuclear to cytoplasmic ratio and abundant delicate cytoplasm. The nucleus is round with a smooth contour and fine chromatin and conspicuous nucleoli. Note the superficial cell (umbrella cell) has multinucleation (ThinPrep Papanicolaou stain; 40X)

Superficial squamous cells are rarely seen in males but are more commonly seen in females. Squamous cells originate in the urethral squamous epithelium and in the trigone of the urinary bladder. Voided urine sediment may also contain squamous cells that originated in the female genital tract (Fig. 12.2).

Columnar urothelial cells are common and exhibit as single cells or small groups with well-preserved polarization. Sometimes, mucus-secreting columnar epithelial cells with peripheral nuclei and distended clear cytoplasm may be

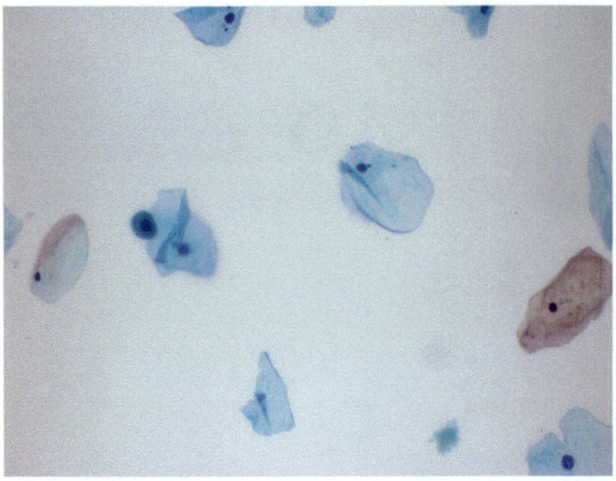

Fig. 12.2 Normal urine with urothelial intermediate cells and keratinizing squamous cells. The background is clean (ThinPrep Papanicolaou stain; 40X)

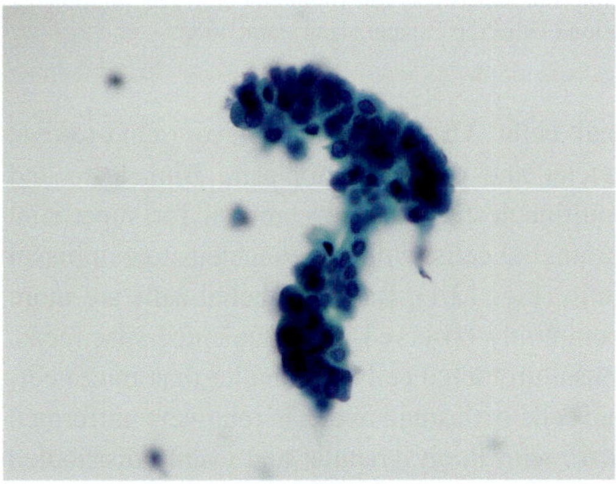

Fig. 12.3 Benign urine with a cluster of columnar cells seen in glandularis cystica. The cluster of columnar cells forms a three-dimensional structure with the preservation of a glandular architecture (ThinPrep Papanicolaou stain; 40X)

seen. Columnar cells are often seen from cystitis cystica or cystitis glandularis (Fig. 12.3). Glandular cells from urachal remnant, nephrogenic metaplasia, or Müllerian rest (endometriosis or endocervicosis) may sometimes also be seen.

Sloughed renal tubular cells may be found in urine specimens. Proximal/distal tubular cells in urine are singly displaced and easily identified by their large size (20 to 60 μm in diameter) with irregular and coarsely granular basophilic cytoplasm. Their nuclei are small and only slightly larger than erythrocytes. In urine specimens, they may be intact preserved cells or appear as "ghost" or necrotic forms that retain their size and cytoplasmic characteristics. Renal collecting duct cells are small (12 to 18 μm in diameter) with a single, slightly eccentric nucleus, coarse and evenly distributed chromatin, and a uniform basophilic cytoplasm and distinct borders.

Other benign cells in males may include seminal vesicle cells and spermatozoa on occasion, usually after prostatic massage [23]. Erythrocytes are a frequent component, particularly in patients with clinical evidence of hematuria [3].

Inflammatory, Infectious, and Reactive Changes

Inflammatory Cells, Bacteria, and Fungi

The presence of large numbers of neutrophils, macrophages, and lymphocytes indicates inflammation. Bacterial cystitis may be acute or chronic; most bacterial cystitis is caused by coliforms and other gram-negative rods. Urine specimens that form acute cystitis contain numerous exfoliated urothelial cells, necrotic material, and inflammatory cells, with a predominance of neutrophils. In chronic cystitis, the urine usually contains a background of chronic inflammation with macrophages and erythrocytes [3]. Urothelial cells may be abundant and poorly preserved, occasionally forming small clusters.

Bacillus Calmette-Guérin (BCG) treatment on patients with non-muscle invasive urothelial carcinoma can cause similar changes seen in tuberculous cystitis. Inflammatory cells, granuloma formation, necrosis, multinucleated Langhans-type giant cells, and reactive atypia of urothelial cells are present. Ziehl-Neelsen staining may reveal acid-fast bacilli but is not required in patients with a history of BCG therapy. True tuberculous cystitis is not common and may be seen in AIDS patients.

Fungi, particularly *Candida albicans*, may be seen in pregnant women, diabetics, immunocompromised patients and those undergoing chemotherapy for cancer. Other fungi are uncommon, although fungus of the species *Alternaria* is a common laboratory contaminant [24].

Degenerative Changes and Necrosis

Degenerative changes are very common in urine cytology. The cell cytoplasm starts to become granular and vacuolated, and some contain spherical eosinophilic inclusions (Melamed-Wolinska bodies) in degenerating cells [25]. Slight nuclear enlargement and hyperchromasia may be seen, but the contours of the nuclei are usually regular without the coarse granularity seen in cancer cells. Necrotic urothelial cells have nuclear pyknosis and marked cytoplasmic vacuolization. Of note, marked necrosis and inflammation can also be seen in necrotic tumors, particularly high-grade urothelial carcinoma and squamous cell carcinoma.

Viral Infection

BK polyomavirus infection is common and may cause hemorrhagic cystitis and nephritis in patients with stem cell or renal transplantations. Polyomavirus plays a significant role in urine cytology because of its "decoy" cells mimicking cancer [26]. Decoy cells exhibit a high N:C ratio and eccentric nucleus, features shared with high-grade urothelial carcinoma [27]. However, the large, homogenous, amorphous ground glass-like intranuclear inclusions and a condensed rim of chromatin differentiate decoy cells from cancer cells [28]. Other features of polyomavirus-infected cells include a reticular chromatin pattern and decoy cells that show a typical eccentric cytoplasm resembling the tail of a comet (comet cells). Cytomegalovirus (CMV) and herpes viral infections with their characteristic cytomorphological features may occasionally be encountered in urine cytology.

Rarely, parasites may be observed in urine cytology. The most common is *Schistosoma haematobium*, which may be associated with squamous cell carcinoma [29].

Lithiasis

Patients with calculi commonly have abnormal cytologic findings in voided urine [30]. The presence of stones can cause numerous large, smooth-bordered clusters and papillary fragments of benign urothelial cells (Fig. 12.4). These changes overlap with the features of low-grade urothelial carcinoma and thus may cause a major diagnostic pitfall in urine cytology interpretation. Significant atypia of urothelial cells due to lithiasis is uncommon, and the clinical history of lithiasis is helpful for accurate cytology evaluation.

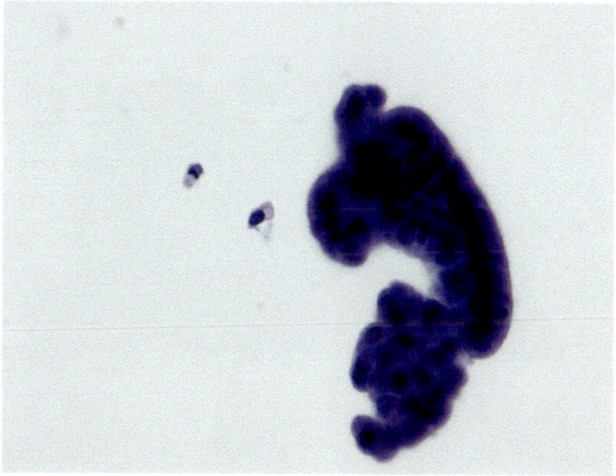

Fig. 12.4 Benign reactive urothelial cells in lithiasis patient urine. The papillary fragments of those benign reactive urothelial cells caused by stone share some features of low-grade urothelial carcinoma (ThinPrep Papanicolaou stain; 60X)

Reactive changes associated with infection may be misinterpreted as atypical or even suspicious/malignant. The reactive non-neoplastic changes involving the urothelium should be classified as negative or atypia of unknown significance in The Paris System.

Low-Grade Urothelial Neoplasia

Low-grade urothelial neoplasia is a combined cytologic term which accounts for urine findings from low-grade papillary urothelial neoplasm (low malignant potential, low-grade papillary carcinoma and papilloma) and flat low-grade intraurothelial neoplasia, in keeping with the 2004 WHO/ISUP terminology.

The presence of three-dimensional cellular papillary clusters with fibrovascular cores is the required diagnostic feature for low-grade urothelial neoplasm in The Paris System [31].

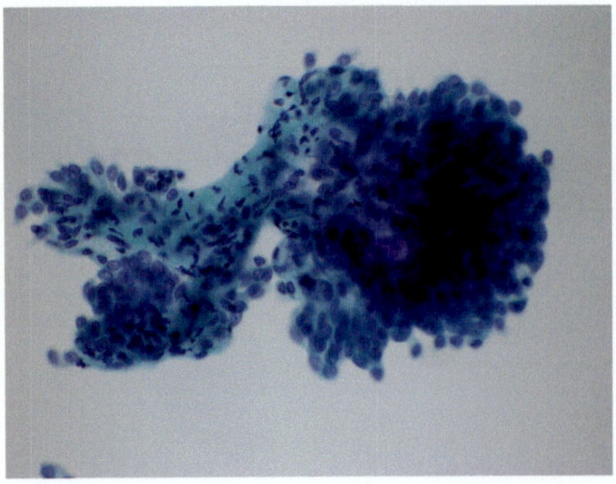

Fig. 12.5 A three-dimensional cellular papillary cluster with fibrovascular core is shown from a biopsy diagnosis of a low-grade urothelial carcinoma. No high-grade cytologic atypia is seen (ThinPrep Papanicolaou stain; 40X)

Meanwhile, the high-grade cytologic atypia should not be present [11] (Fig. 12.5).

Urine cytology has low sensitivity (21% to 53%) for detecting low-grade urothelial tumors, and this low sensitivity is a major cause of false-negative results in urine cytology [9]. Pathologists should not attempt to differentiate low-grade papillary urothelial carcinoma from papillary urothelial neoplasm of low malignant potential or papilloma in urine cytology specimens [32].

Diagnostic pitfalls include differentiating between urothelial cell clusters arranged in a papillary configuration from those shed from normal benign urothelium after instrumentation, or irritation by calculi (Fig. 12.4) or inflammation [30, 33]. Benign cell clusters have smooth borders at the edge lined by a densely stained cytoplasm. Spontaneously shed complex clusters with morphologically benign urothelial cells in voided urine may suggest a papillary tumor when clinical trauma is excluded.

Ancillary techniques that may be valuable for separating benign and neoplastic urothelial cells include FISH, immunocytochemical tests, and DNA ploidy analysis [34–36].

Atypical and Suspicious Cases

The atypical category poses one of the greatest challenges in urine cytology interpretation, with a range of 11% to 33% variable incidence in several large published series [36–38].

Reported diagnostic criteria for the atypical category in The Paris System include a major required criterion that the N/C ratio is greater than 0.5 in well-preserved cells and that at least one of the three minor criteria be met: nuclear hyperchromasia, nuclear membrane irregularity, and/or irregular/coarse/clumped chromatin [31]. Meeting all of these criteria would upgrade the diagnosis to the suspicious category.

The rate of diagnosis in the atypical category should be as low as possible, and it should not be overused by pathologists as a wastebasket category. It is critical for clinicians to undertake follow-up of these patients; therefore, efficient communication with urologists is important when confronted with this sometimes inevitable diagnosis.

The "suspicious" urine cytology category should be restrictively used and only applies to situations in which the abnormal urothelial cells are insufficient to categorize as high-grade urothelial carcinoma in The Paris System. The predictive value of the suspicious category for high-grade carcinoma found is 79% [39].

High-Grade Urothelial Carcinoma

Diagnosing and monitoring high-grade urothelial carcinoma is a central role for urine cytology. There are five criteria in The Paris System for a diagnosis of high-grade urothelial carcinoma: at least five to ten abnormal cells, an elevated N:C ratio of 0.7 or greater, moderate to severe nuclear hyperchromasia, marked nuclear membrane irregularity, and coarse/clumped chromatin (Fig. 12.6).

The background of the urine samples can be clean with free of necrotic debris and lacks

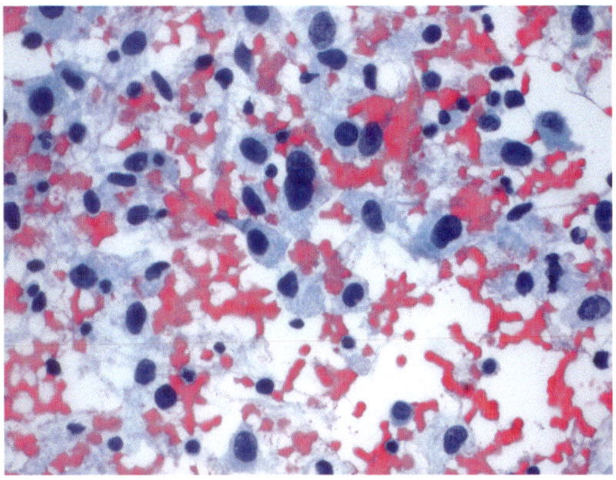

Fig. 12.6 Dyscohesive, singly dispersed, and highly atypical urothelial cells with markedly increased nuclear to cytoplasmic ratio, hyperchromasia, and irregular nuclear outline (ThinPrep Papanicolaou stain; 40X)

inflammation or with necrotic tumor diathesis and prominent inflammation. Multinucleate cancer cells and prominent nucleoli and mitotic figures are often readily identified [40].

Tumor cells may be poorly preserved and degenerated, particularly when there is inflammation or necrosis. In this scenario, cellular changes such as vacuolated cytoplasm, nonspecific eosinophilic cytoplasmic inclusions, and pyknotic nuclei are present predominately. In most cases, atypical urothelial cells may be observed, typically in small amounts, alerting the urologist of the need for follow-up cystoscopic examination.

The reporting of cytologic features of urothelial carcinoma variants is limited. High-grade papillary tumors usually do not shed large fragments, and the dominant cytologic finding may be the presence of single cancer cells or small tumor groups without large papillary configuration. The micropapillary variant shares similar features with conventional urothelial carcinoma in urine specimens [41]. The plasmacytoid variant may show plasmacytoid tumor cells in urine specimens which must be differentiated from multiple myeloma or signet ring cell adenocarcinoma [42].

Of note, the cytological diagnosis of high-grade urothelial carcinoma includes carcinoma in situ and invasive carcinoma. Positive void urine cytology diagnosis of high-grade urothelial carcinoma will be followed with cystoscopy and biopsy. Instrumented urine specimens are commonly accompanied with concurrent biopsy. Thus, real-time histology-cytology correlation may be achieved.

Non-urothelial Primary and Metastatic Malignancy in Urine Cytology

Primary Non-urothelial Tumor

Non-urothelial bladder tumors account for less than 5% of all bladder tumors. They are rarely present in urine cytology and pose a diagnostic challenge [43, 44].

Squamous cell carcinoma is the most common non-urothelial carcinoma of the urinary bladder, and it is more prevalent in North Africa and the Middle East where *Schistosoma haematobium* infection is endemic [29]. Urinary squamous cell carcinoma is usually well to moderately differentiated with abundant keratinization. Cytologic features are similar to those seen in other organ systems, i.e., large polygonal tumor cells with a keratinized cytoplasm, sharp cell borders, and atypical hyperchromatic nuclei. Tadpole cells, squamous pearls, or tumor nests may be present (Fig. 12.7). The cytologic diagnosis of squamous cell carcinoma cannot exclude urothelial carci-

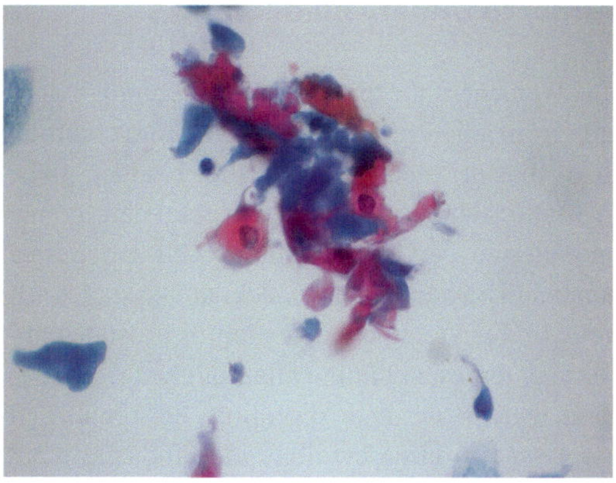

Fig. 12.7 Keratinizing squamous cell carcinoma displays large polygonal tumor cells with orangeophilic cytoplasm and atypical hyperchromatic nuclei. Tadpole cells and necrotic squamous tumor cells are present (ThinPrep Papanicolaou stain; 40X)

noma with divergent squamous differentiation. The diagnosis of pure squamous cell carcinoma should be based on resection specimens.

Adenocarcinoma of the bladder can arise either from the urothelium or from urachal remnants with similar histologic features. Variable enteric, mucinous, signet ring-type, and clear cell-type adenocarcinoma cells may be detected in urine cytology. Cytomorphologic exclusion of urothelial carcinoma with glandular differentiation is difficult. Meanwhile, it is important to rule out secondary involvement from a colorectal primary [45].

Rarely, neuroendocrine carcinoma such as small cell carcinoma can be detected in urine cytology specimens. In small cell carcinoma, the singly dispersed tumor cells with high N:C ratio with nuclear molding due to scant cytoplasm, no or inconspicuous nucleolus and hyperchromatic nuclei are seen [46]. Ancillary cell block preparation with neuroendocrine marker immunohistochemical studies is important for a definitive diagnosis if specimen volume is adequate.

Urinary mesenchymal sarcoma, hematologic malignancy, and melanoma can also be seen in urine cytology. In these settings, cytology interpretation should be incorporated with biopsy and other necessary ancillary studies.

Direct Extension and Metastatic Tumor to Urinary Bladder

Involvement of the bladder by direct tumor extension from adjacent organs is much more common than distant metastasis to the bladder [47]. Prostatic adenocarcinoma, colorectal carcinoma, and uterine cervical squamous cell carcinoma can readily extend to the bladder at late stages. Of note, urine cytological detection of prostate cancer may represent tumor cells sloughed from urethral extension, and detection of renal cell carcinoma in urine cytology may indicate renal pelvic extension of renal cell carcinoma instead of distant metastasis to the bladder. Voided urine contamination associated with uterine tumors is a pitfall which may potentially over-stage the primary uterine carcinoma (Fig. 12.8) because genital tract contamination is common in voided urine specimens from female patients.

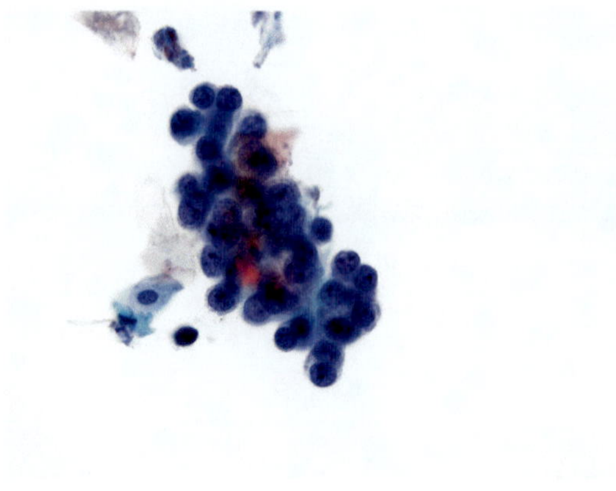

Fig. 12.8 High-grade uterine adenocarcinoma cells present in a void urine specimen as genital tract contamination. The high N:C ratio, nuclear hyperchromasia, and prominent nuclei can also be seen in high-grade urothelial carcinoma (ThinPrep Papanicolaou stain; 40X)

Ancillary Tests

Ancillary tests have been developed to supplement the detection of urothelial carcinoma in urine because urine cytology alone has low sensitivity. Ancillary tests can be used in primary screening as well as surveillance, especially when the tissue specimen is limited or suboptimal and cytology or even histological diagnosis falls into the undetermined category. There are several FDA-approved assays, and many other tests are currently in development.

UroVysion is one of the most well-established FDA-approved multitarget multicolor FISH assays for the primary detection and surveillance of urothelial carcinoma. This assay utilizes centromeric fluorescent-denatured chromosomal enumeration probes for chromosome 3, 7, and 17 to detect copy number increase and the locus-specific identifier probe for 9p21 to detect homozygous deletion. The overall sensitivity and specificity are reported to be 72% and 83%, respectively [48]. The combined use of urine cytology and FISH improves the performance of the urine test, particularly for the undetermined category [49, 50]. False-positive UroVysion results can occasionally be seen in reactive conditions such as irritative bladder, radiotherapy, cystitis and urolithiasis, and high-titer BK virus infection [51, 52].

ImmunoCyt/uCyt test is another FDA-approved immunocytochemical assay that can be used for the surveillance of urothelial carcinoma. The test uses three monoclonal antibodies (M344, LDQ10, and 19A211) to detect mucin-like antigen and the high molecular form of carcinoembryonic antigen with different fluorescent signals. The sensitivity and specificity are 78–90% and 77–87%, respectively [53]. The test detects both low-grade and high-grade tumors [54, 55].

NMP22 is a nuclear matrix protein and its level can increase 25-fold or greater in patients with bladder cancer [6]. The FDA-approved NMP22 ELISA and NMP22 Bladder-Check can be performed at a laboratory or physician's office for surveillance or primary screening of bladder cancer [53]. The overall sensitivity and specificity are 62–75% and 70–83%, respectively [53].

BTA stat and BTA TRAK are FDA-approved tests that detect complement factor H-related protein in urine. BTA stat is an immunoassay, whereas BTA TRAK is a standard ELISA. The sensitivity and specificity of BTA stat for detection of urothelial carcinoma are 54–75% and 64–82%, respectively [53]. The sensitivity and specificity of BTA TRAK for detection of urothelial carcinoma are 58–69% and 73–81%, respectively [53].

The abovementioned ancillary tests are all FDA-approved. UroVysion and ImmunoCyt/uCyt tests are slide-based assays that can correlate directly with cytomorphology. NMP22 and BTA stat/TRAK are slide-free assays that can be used as a point-of-care test with acellular, low-volume specimens [56]. Other non-FDA-approved assays are also available with variable sensitivities and specificities, such as the Sienna test (anti-Htert), ProExC, CellDetect, Cxbladder Assay, and UroSEEK [56].

Conclusion

Urine cytology is a key component in the practice of bladder pathology and plays a fundamental role in bladder cancer screening and surveillance. Numerous benign conditions with diagnostic pitfalls complicate the accurate interpretation of urine cytology. Minimizing the usage of the atypical category and triaging patients correctly for next-step management is essential for urine cytology. The diagnostic accuracy of urine cytology can be improved with ancillary tests. Recognizing primary or secondary non-urothelial malignancies in urine cytology within the appropriate clinical setting is critical in daily practice.

References

1. Papanicolaou GN, Marshall VF. Urine sediment smears as a diagnostic procedure in cancers of the urinary tract. Science. 1945;101(2629):519–20.
2. Ooms EC, Veldhuizen RW. Cytological criteria and diagnostic terminology in urinary cytology. Cytopathology. 1993;4(1):51–4.
3. Fracchia JA, Motta J, Miller LS, Armenakas NA, Schumann GB, Greenberg RA. Evaluation of asymptomatic microhematuria. Urology. 1995;46(4):484–9.
4. Potts SA, Thomas PA, Cohen MB, Raab SS. Diagnostic accuracy and key cytologic features of high-grade transitional cell carcinoma in the upper urinary tract. Mod Pathol. 1997;10(7):657–62.
5. Smith ZL, Christodouleas JP, Keefe SM, Malkowicz SB, Guzzo TJ. Bladder preservation in the treatment of muscle-invasive bladder cancer (MIBC): a review of the literature and a practical approach to therapy. BJU Int. 2013;112(1):13–25.
6. Têtu B. Diagnosis of urothelial carcinoma from urine. Mod Pathol. 2009;22 Suppl 2:S53–9.
7. Nasuti JF, Gomella LG, Ismial M, Bibbo M. Utility of the BTA stat test kit for bladder cancer screening. Diagn Cytopathol. 1999;21(1):27–9.
8. Zhang ML, Rosenthal DL, VandenBussche CJ. The cytomorphological features of low-grade urothelial neoplasms vary by specimen type. Cancer Cytopathol. 2016;124(8):552–64.
9. McCroskey Z, Pambuccian SE, Kleitherms S, Antic T, Cohen MB, Barkan GA, et al. Accuracy and interobserver variability of the cytologic diagnosis of low-grade urothelial carcinoma in instrumented urinary tract cytology specimens. Am J Clin Pathol. 2015;144(6):902–8.

10. Amin MB, Smith SC, Reuter VE, Epstein JI, Grignon DJ, Hansel DE, et al. Update for the practicing pathologist: The International Consultation On Urologic Disease-European association of urology consultation on bladder cancer. Mod Pathol. 2015;28(5):612–30.
11. Barkan GA, Wojcik EM, Nayar R, Savic-Prince S, Quek ML, Kurtycz DF, et al. The Paris System for Reporting Urinary Cytology: The Quest to Develop a Standardized Terminology. Acta Cytol. 2016;60(3):185-97. Barkan GA, Wojcik EM, Nayar R, Savic-Prince S, Quek ML, Kurtycz DF, et al. The Paris System for Reporting Urinary Cytology: The Quest to Develop a Standardized Terminology. Acta Cytol. 2016;60(3):185–97.
12. Owens CL, Vandenbussche CJ, Burroughs FH, Rosenthal DL. A review of reporting systems and terminology for urine cytology. Cancer Cytopathol. 2013;121(1):9–14.
13. Matzkin H, Moinuddin SM, Soloway MS. Value of urine cytology versus bladder washing in bladder cancer. Urology. 1992;39(3):201–3.
14. Bian Y, Ehya H, Bagley DH. Cytologic diagnosis of upper urinary tract neoplasms by ureteroscopic sampling. Acta Cytol. 1995;39(4):733–40.
15. Reynolds JP, Voss JS, Kipp BR, Karnes RJ, Nassar A, Clayton AC, et al. Comparison of urine cytology and fluorescence in situ hybridization in upper urothelial tract samples. Cancer Cytopathol. 2014;122(6):459–67.
16. Yoshimine S, Kikuchi E, Matsumoto K, Ide H, Miyajima A, Nakagawa K, et al. The clinical significance of urine cytology after a radical cystectomy for urothelial cancer. Int J Urol. 2010;17(6):527–32.
17. Layfield LJ, Elsheikh TM, Fili A, Nayar R, Shidham V. Review of the state of the art and recommendations of the Papanicolaou Society of Cytopathology for urinary cytology procedures and reporting : the Papanicolaou Society of Cytopathology Practice Guidelines Task Force. Diagn Cytopathol. 2004;30(1):24–30.
18. VandenBussche CJ, Rosenthal DL, Olson MT. Adequacy in voided urine cytology specimens: The role of volume and a repeat void upon predictive values for high-grade urothelial carcinoma. Cancer Cytopathol. 2016;124(3):174–80.
19. Prather J, Arville B, Chatt G, Pambuccian SE, Wojcik EM, Quek ML, et al. Evidence-based adequacy criteria for urinary bladder barbotage cytology. J Am Soc Cytopathol. 2015;4(2):57–62.
20. Cowan ML, Rosenthal DL, VandenBussche CJ. Improved risk stratification for patients with high-grade urothelial carcinoma following application of the Paris System for Reporting Urinary Cytology. Cancer Cytopathol. 2017;125(6):427–34.
21. Cowan ML, VandenBussche CJ. The Paris System for Reporting Urinary Cytology: early review of the literature reveals successes and rare shortcomings. J Am Soc Cytopathol. 2018;7(4):185–94.
22. Wang Y, Auger M, Kanber Y, Caglar D, Brimo F. Implementing The Paris System for Reporting Urinary Cytology results in a decrease in the rate of the "atypical" category and an increase in its prediction of subsequent high-grade urothelial carcinoma. Cancer Cytopathol. 2018;126(3):207–14.
23. Gutmann EJ. Seminal vesicle cell in a spontaneously voided urine. Diagn Cytopathol. 2006;34(12):824–5.
24. Koss LG. Errors and pitfalls in cytology of the lower urinary tract. Monogr Pathol. 1997(39):60–74.
25. Rashidi B, Tongson-Ignacio JE. Melamed-Wolinska bodies in urine cytology an interesting aggregate in a degenerated urothelial cell. Diagn Cytopathol. 2011;39(2):117.
26. Crabbe JG. "Comet" or "decoy" cells found in urinary sediment smears. Acta Cytol. 1971;15(3):303–5.
27. Boon ME, van Keep JP, Kok LP. Polyomavirus infection versus high-grade bladder carcinoma. The importance of cytologic and comparative morphometric studies of plastic-embedded voided urine sediments. Acta Cytol. 1989;33(6):887–93.
28. Herawi M, Parwani AV, Chan T, Ali SZ, Epstein JI. Polyoma virus-associated cellular changes in the urine and bladder biopsy samples: a cytohistologic correlation. Am J Surg Pathol. 2006;30(3):345–50.
29. Khaled H. Schistosomiasis and cancer in egypt: review. J Adv Res. 2013;4(5):461–6.
30. Highman W, Wilson E. Urine cytology in patients with calculi. J Clin Pathol. 1982;35(3):350–6.
31. Rosenthal DL WE, Kurtycz DF. The Paris System for Reporting Urinary Cytology. 1st ed.: Springer; 2015.
32. Renshaw AA, Nappi D, Weinberg DS. Cytology of grade 1 papillary transitional cell carcinoma. A comparison of cytologic, architectural and morphometric criteria in cystoscopically obtained urine. Acta Cytol. 1996;40(4):676–82.
33. Kannan V, Bose S. Low grade transitional cell carcinoma and instrument artifact. A challenge in urinary cytology. Acta Cytol. 1993;37(6):899–902.
34. Bubendorf L, Grilli B, Sauter G, Mihatsch MJ, Gasser TC, Dalquen P. Multiprobe FISH for enhanced detection of bladder cancer in voided urine specimens and bladder washings. Am J Clin Pathol. 2001;116(1):79–86.
35. Cajulis RS, Haines GK, 3rd, Frias-Hidvegi D, McVary K, Bacus JW. Cytology, flow cytometry, image analysis, and interphase cytogenetics by fluorescence in situ hybridization in the diagnosis of transitional cell carcinoma in bladder washes: a comparative study. Diagn Cytopathol. 1995;13(3):214–23; discussion 24.
36. Lodde M, Mian C, Negri G, Berner L, Maffei N, Lusuardi L, et al. Role of uCyt+ in the detection and surveillance of urothelial carcinoma. Urology. 2003;61(1):243–7.
37. Muus Ubago J, Mehta V, Wojcik EM, Barkan GA. Evaluation of atypical urine cytology progression to malignancy. Cancer Cytopathol. 2013;121(7):387–91.
38. Virk RK, Abro S, de Ubago JMM, Pambuccian SE, Quek ML, Wojcik EM, et al. The value of the UroVysion® FISH assay in the risk-stratification of patients with "atypical urothelial cells" in urinary cytology specimens. Diagn Cytopathol. 2017;45(6):481–500.

39. Ton Nu TN, Kassouf W, Ahmadi-Kaliji B, Charbonneau M, Auger M, Brimo F. The value of the "suspicious for urothelial carcinoma" cytology category: a correlative study of 4 years including 337 patients. Cancer Cytopathol. 2014;122(11):796–803.
40. Shenoy UA, Colby TV, Schumann GB. Reliability of urinary cytodiagnosis in urothelial neoplasms. Cancer. 1985;56(8):2041–5.
41. Heymann JJ, Saqi A, Turk AT, Crapanzano J. Micropapillary urothelial carcinoma: Cytologic features in a retrospective series of urine specimens. Cytojournal. 2013;10:4.
42. Molek KR, Seili-Bekafigo I, Štemberger C, Jonjić N, Đordević G, Duletić-Načinović A. Plasmacytoid urothelial carcinoma--diagnostic challenge in cytology. Diagn Cytopathol. 2013;41(4):369-73.
43. Dahm P, Gschwend JE. Malignant non-urothelial neoplasms of the urinary bladder: a review. Eur Urol. 2003;44(6):672–81.
44. Chalasani V, Chin JL, Izawa JI. Histologic variants of urothelial bladder cancer and nonurothelial histology in bladder cancer. Can Urol Assoc J. 2009;3(6 Suppl 4):S193–8.
45. Zhong M, Gersbach E, Rohan SM, Yang XJ. Primary adenocarcinoma of the urinary bladder: differential diagnosis and clinical relevance. Arch Pathol Lab Med. 2013;137(3):371–81.
46. Alijo Serrano F, Sánchez-Mora N, Angel Arranz J, Hernández C, Alvarez-Fernández E. Large cell and small cell neuroendocrine bladder carcinoma: immunohistochemical and outcome study in a single institution. Am J Clin Pathol. 2007;128(5):733–9.
47. Velcheti V, Govindan R. Metastatic cancer involving bladder: a review. Can J Urol. 2007;14(1):3443–8.
48. Hajdinjak T. UroVysion FISH test for detecting urothelial cancers: meta-analysis of diagnostic accuracy and comparison with urinary cytology testing. Urol Oncol. 2008;26(6):646–51.
49. Daniely M, Rona R, Kaplan T, Olsfanger S, Elboim L, Zilberstien Y, et al. Combined analysis of morphology and fluorescence in situ hybridization significantly increases accuracy of bladder cancer detection in voided urine samples. Urology. 2005;66(6):1354–9.
50. Skacel M, Fahmy M, Brainard JA, Pettay JD, Biscotti CV, Liou LS, et al. Multitarget fluorescence in situ hybridization assay detects transitional cell carcinoma in the majority of patients with bladder cancer and atypical or negative urine cytology. J Urol. 2003;169(6):2101–5.
51. Tapia C, Glatz K, Obermann EC, Grilli B, Barascud A, Herzog M, et al. Evaluation of chromosomal aberrations in patients with benign conditions and reactive changes in urinary cytology. Cancer Cytopathol. 2011;119(6):404–10.
52. Kipp BR, Sebo TJ, Griffin MD, Ihrke JM, Halling KC. Analysis of polyomavirus-infected renal transplant recipients' urine specimens: correlation of routine urine cytology, fluorescence in situ hybridization, and digital image analysis. Am J Clin Pathol. 2005;124(6):854–61.
53. Chou R, Gore JL, Buckley D, Fu R, Gustafson K, Griffin JC, et al. Urinary Biomarkers for Diagnosis of Bladder Cancer: A Systematic Review and Meta-analysis. Ann Intern Med. 2015;163(12):922–31.
54. Black PC, Brown GA, Dinney CP. Molecular markers of urothelial cancer and their use in the monitoring of superficial urothelial cancer. J Clin Oncol. 2006;24(35):5528–35.
55. Comploj E, Mian C, Ambrosini-Spaltro A, Dechet C, Palermo S, Trenti E, et al. uCyt+/ImmunoCyt and cytology in the detection of urothelial carcinoma: an update on 7422 analyses. Cancer Cytopathol. 2013;121(7):392–7.
56. Allison DB, VandenBussche CJ. A Review of Urine Ancillary Tests in the Era of the Paris System. Acta Cytol. 2020;64(1-2):182–92.

Diagnostic Values of Immunohistochemistry in Bladder Cancer

13

Qihui "Jim" Zhai and Fang-Ming Deng

General Considerations

Immunohistochemistry (IHC) has been used as a valuable tool in our surgical pathology practice for more than 50 years. Since then more and more biomarkers have been developed, introduced, and applied in our daily practice. This tool has revolutionized the field of surgical pathology and offered relatively objective parameters and evidence-based support for our diagnoses, prognoses, and potentially therapeutic correlation.

There are always new biomarkers published in the literature; and they typically generate much excitement with an initial report of high specificity. However, as more studies are performed with more sensitive detection systems, its specificity usually decreases. In our practice, we do not introduce all the new antibodies that become popular, unless they can offer new information that is not available by current well-established ones in the lab.

With recent advances in molecular studies of urinary bladder cancers, many new diagnostic markers have been identified and reported in the literature. Like any other organ, application of IHC in bladder pathology should follow the same general considerations. In this chapter, we will discuss the utilities of IHC with focus on the practical pearls and pitfalls in some commonly seen diagnostic challenges instead of reviewing all the established and new markers.

When Do We Need to Request IHC?

There is no clear-cut guideline regarding when IHC should be used. Each pathologist may have a different threshold, because of a different level of confidence secondary to various backgrounds and experiences. When and how to use this tool is more like a combination of science and art. Personally, we request immunostains when we feel the features are not typical for a certain entity, and different interpretations may be rendered if this case is shown to different pathologists. Another important parameter for us is the clinical implications, as we want the patients to be managed with solid evidence.

In most of the cases, the routine hematoxylin-eosin (H&E) stain demonstrates typical features that make us confident about the diagnosis of bladder cancer, and immunostains are not needed. However, for a subset of cases, the histology is not typical and presents some overlapping features between two or even more possible

Q. "J". Zhai
Lab Medicine and Pathology, Mayo Clinic Florida, Jacksonville, FL, USA
e-mail: zhai.qihui@mayo.edu

F.-M. Deng (✉)
Department of Pathology, New York University Langone Health, New York, NY, USA
e-mail: fang-ming.deng@nyumc.org

H. Zhou et al. (eds.), *Urinary Bladder Pathology*, https://doi.org/10.1007/978-3-030-71509-0_13

diagnoses. At this time, ancillary tests may offer additional evidence for an accurate diagnosis.

We frequently hear "H&E stain trumps the immunostains." Our personal view is that it is usually true; however, it is individually case based. Most of the time, the immunostains should confirm what we think based on the H&E sections. Only rarely should it be "I am glad I ordered the immunostains," a sign that the immunostains offered some additional information that we did not feel confident or were not in favor of it with only on the H&E sections. Even more rarely, we wish we never requested those immunostains, which further muddied the water, and we do not know what to do with all the immunostains in a certain case. A too generous and casual use of IHC without justification could generate more confusion to us rather than providing help, because the different expressions of biomarkers may point us in different directions.

What Panel Do We Need to Pick?

IHC is considered an ancillary test which can support, but not replace, careful morphological evaluation. The practical approach is to form a short list of differential diagnoses based on the histology of the lesion. Look into the clinical setting and understand the clinical impacts of our possible diagnoses. A panel of biomarkers that are complimentary to each other among the differential diagnoses should be used to increase the diagnostic accuracy.

To choose the proper panel of immunostains, we need a strong basic, constant study, innovative and creative thinking, and enjoyment of proper selection (BEST approach). Also, 3C practice (consultation, communication, and collaboration) is commonly required.

Because of the biological nature of a tumor and technical issues associated with the IHC procedures, none of the IHC markers is 100% specific and 100% sensitive in any lesions, including bladder lesions. We must use these markers with justification and caution. Usually we should not rely on one single immunostain, to avoid a false-positive or false-negative result.

How to Interpret the Results?

We need to be aware of the approximate sensitivity and specificity for each biomarker that is used in the panel. Sensitivity and specificity for any given antibody is relative, and so far we do not have absolutely specific and sensitive antibodies. There are at least four issues need to be considered for immunostaining interpretation:

1. What cellular compartment is stained: nuclear, cytoplasmic, membranous, or both nuclear and cytoplasmic.
2. When the marker stains cytoplasm, check whether it is membranous, granular cytoplasmic, or fibrillar cytoplasmic.
3. Check whether the tumor cells stain or entrapped normal cell stain.
4. Check the degree of staining: strong or weak or diffuse or focal.

The signal location is fundamental in our immunostain interpretation. There are three possible signal locations, namely, nuclear, membranous, and cytoplasmic. Also possible is the combination of different locations. It is extremely important to remember the expression pattern for each marker. GATA 3, PAX2/8, and p63 are nuclear patterns. Cytokeratin and racemase are both cytoplasmic markers, but cytokeratin should be fibrillar stain and racemase granular stain. Uroplakin is membranous expression. Some markers may present combined staining patterns, such as S-100, which manifests both cytoplasmic and nuclear immunoreactivity.

How to define a positive stain is essential. The lesional area must be present and recognized, and the targeted cells have to be positive or negative; not all brown stain is necessarily positive. Ideally, non-lesional normal or benign tissue is present to control the immunostained slides. The cells of interest in the immunostained slides may be hard to appreciate when evaluated by hematoxylin counter stain only. Therefore, H&E sections should be reviewed and compared with the immunostains to make sure that we are interpreting the lesional tissue in the right areas.

The Economics of the IHC

Economy should not be the primary consideration when we handle a difficult case. Cost-effectiveness can be achieved by careful planning. Sometimes a phone call with related physicians can save much time and the number of immunostains. Clinical history and imaging results will help shorten the list of our differential diagnosis; subsequently we can use fewer immunostains. Under the new economic-medical climate, efficient utility is extremely important to sustain the lab and practice.

Practical Approach in Specific Diagnostic Dilemmas

There are many diagnostic dilemmas with overlapping histologic features, and yet they are clinically relevant. Now we use some frequently encountered diagnostic dilemmas in bladder pathology to discuss the histologic features, complimentary immunostain panel, signal location, interpretation skills, and clinical implications.

Flat Urothelial Lesions

This group of lesions includes urothelial carcinoma (UC) in situ, dysplasia, proliferation of uncertain malignant potential, and reactive atypia [1]. To separate them from each other is extremely important and not always easy. Several markers are valuable in this setting (Fig. 13.1 and Table 13.1).

CK20 is a marker often applied in the evaluation of flat lesions of bladder. The key is how to interpret its expression pattern. In normal and benign reactive urothelium, CK20 is restricted to the surface umbrella cells. In contrast, CK20 is positive in the full urothelial thickness of dysplastic urothelium or in situ carcinoma (CIS) [2–4]. CK20 cannot separate dysplasia from UC in situ, which relies on histologic evaluation.

P53 is often used in this setting. In normal and reactive urothelium, p53 is usually of scattered and weak nuclear expression. In dysplastic urothelium and CIS, p53 is often diffusely and strongly expressed [2, 3].

Ki-67, a marker for proliferation index, is usually high with whole layer distribution while low and limited to basal and suprabasal layers of normal urothelium [3, 4].

CD44 is also reported to be useful, with an inversed expression pattern with CK20. Namely, it is positive with a membranous pattern in the benign basal and suprabasal cell layers [2]. This membranous expression of CD44 is lost in CIS, particularly the pagetoid type of CIS. It is not hard to understand why some pathologists like to use the combination of these two complimentary markers together to evaluate flat urothelial lesions.

AMACR is another maker that can be used to differentiate reactive atypia from CIS, which is usually positive in CIS while negative in benign reactive urothelium. Comparing with CK20, AMACR was less sensitive and more specific with the same caveat of less staining intensity [5, 6].

Cocktails containing two or three antibodies have been applied on the same slide, offering different color detection and complimentary expression patterns [7, 8].

It should be kept in mind that the IHC in the differential diagnosis of flat urothelial lesion is limited, such as CK20 can be totally lost in CIS and only ~50% CIS has P53 mutation and shows abnormal P53 expression by IHC. Ki-67 labeling can be increased in reactive urothelium, such as inflamed urothelium.

Histologic Variants of Infiltrating UC

This is a very important topic; Chap. 6, "Morphological Variants of Invasive Urothelial Carcinoma," is completely dedicated to the details, including histologic features, immunoprofile, and clinical significance.

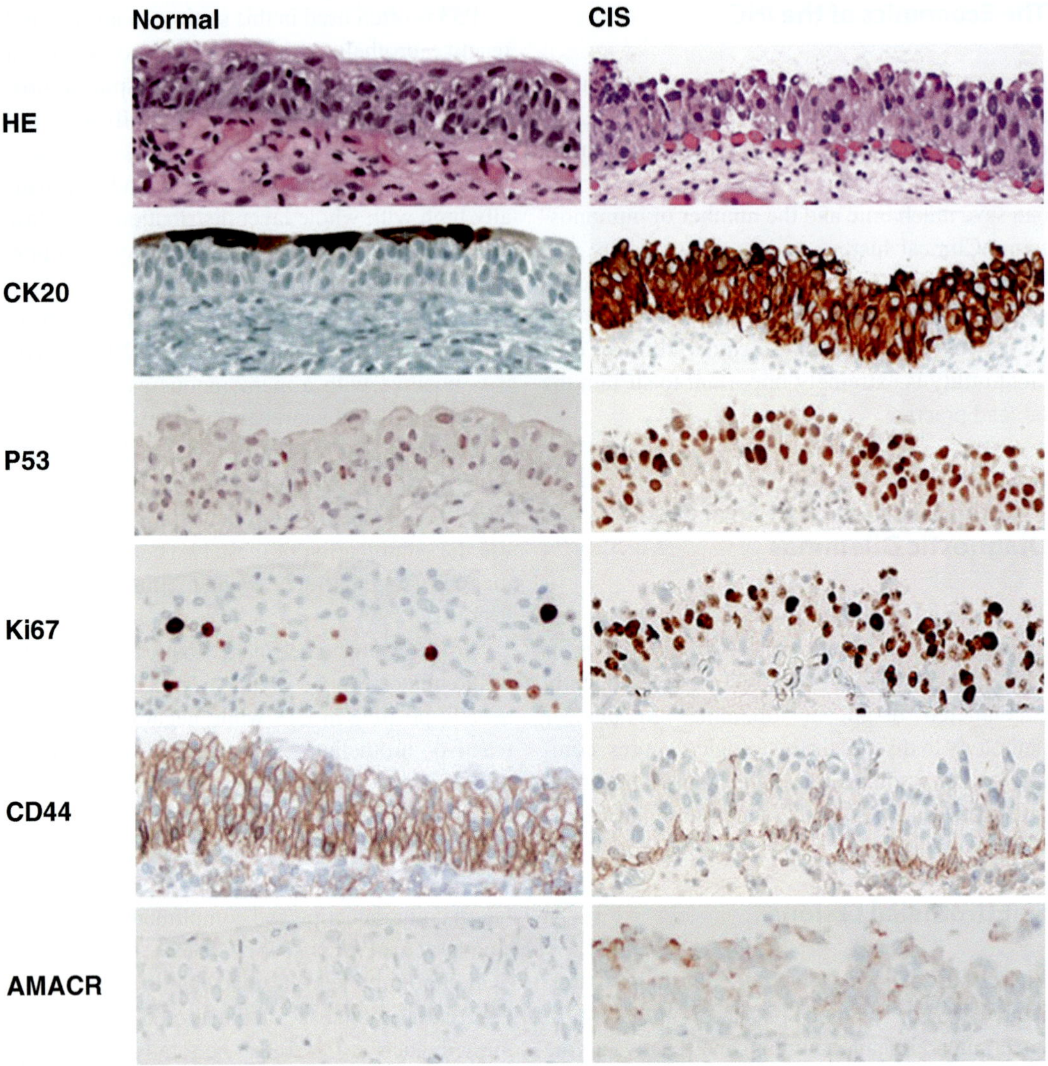

Fig. 13.1 IHC panel for differentiation of benign urothelium from urothelial carcinoma in situ

Table 13.1 IHC panel for differentiation of reactive urothelium from urothelial carcinoma in situ

	Normal	Reactive	Carcinoma in situ
CK20	+ (limited to surface umbrella layer)	–	+ (transurothelial), ~70%
P53	+ (scattered, weak)	+ (scattered, weak)	+ (strong and diffuse)
CD44	+ (limited to the basal)	+ (transurothelial)	– (or limited to basal +)
Ki-67	Low	Moderate to high	High
AMACR	+ (transurothelial), ~70%	–	–

Assess the Depth of an Invasive Urothelial Carcinoma on the Biopsy and Transurethral Resection Specimens

In bladder biopsy or transurethral resection of prostate (TURP) specimens, the depth of invasion of infiltrating UC is critical for the clinician to design the most appropriate subsequent therapeutic approach, cystectomy, or more conservative procedure. Most of the time, we can handle these cases with confidence based on H&E sections alone; however, in difficult cases IHC may offer additional evidence to support our H&E impression.

Smoothelin is reported to be specifically immunoreactive with the contractile muscle bundles, which are muscularis propria (MP); therefore, it is used to distinguish muscularis propria from muscularis mucosae (MM) [9–11]. A diffuse and strong staining pattern is specific and can be considered as MP; on the other hand, a weak and blush pattern is usually considered as MM (Fig. 13.2). However, MP can be weakly stained; therefore, strong and diffuse stain is only useful in this situation. Occasionally smoothelin immunostain can be difficult to interpret; and pitfalls should be kept in mind [12]. If this is the case, smoothelin is not reliable.

Careful lab validation with different conditions/protocols and personal experience are very important. As with any other markers, smoothelin will not solve all the problematic cases. Occasionally, we are not confident whether the muscle bundles represent hyperplastic MM or true MP. It is critical that we communicate with the urologist and comment that we are not sure based on the pathological features. The urologist can either proceed with the imaging findings or perform a very close follow-up and/or re-biopsy of a deeper portion to obtain a more straightforward diagnosis.

Most clinicians including urologists, medical oncologists, and radiation oncologists use muscle involving urothelial carcinoma as interchangeable with urothelial carcinoma involving the MP. So, it is not recommended to use invasive urothelial carcinoma involving muscle bundles in our pathology report; we need to clearly specify it is MM or MP or not sure for MM or MP. Potential misunderstanding should be avoided in this setting, because the clinical implications are dramatic. Patient may undergo an unnecessary cystectomy based on a vague terminology.

Establish the Urothelial Lineage and Rule Out Metastasis

GATA3

GATA3 was described a few years ago, which was considered most specific for urothelial

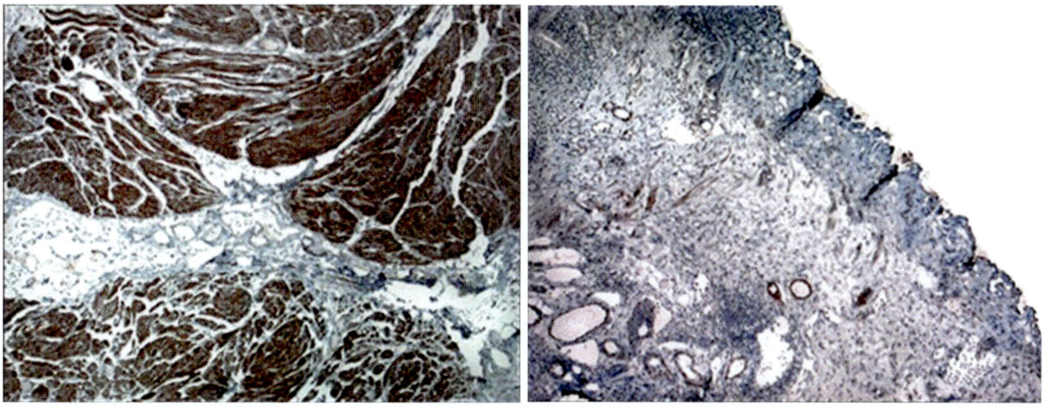

Fig. 13.2 Smoothelin to differentiate muscularis propria from muscularis mucosae

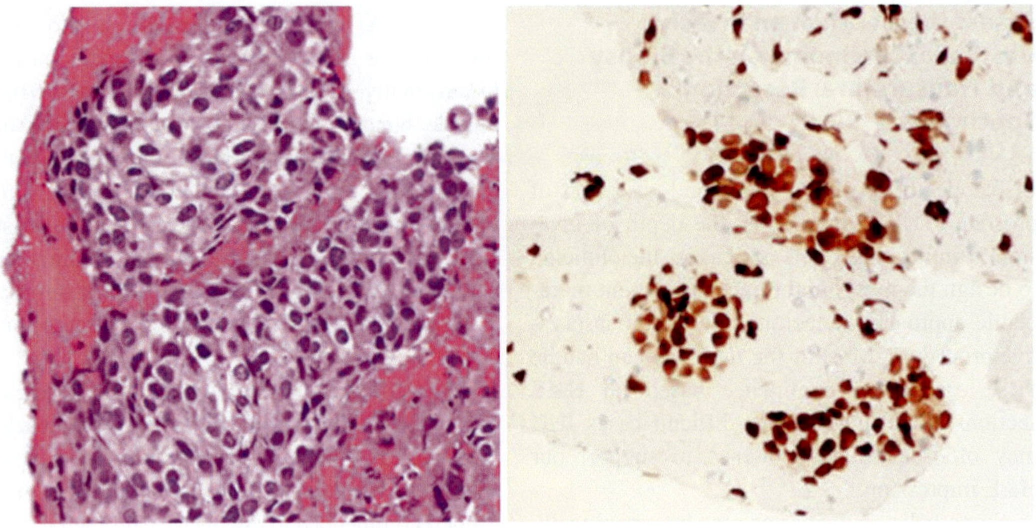

Fig. 13.3 A small biopsy of urothelial carcinoma with GATA3 reactivity

differentiation [13]. GATA3 has higher sensitivity than p63 and CK20 on high-grade urothelial carcinoma, as high-grade (HG) UC usually partially or even totally lose p63 or CK20, while most of these cases retain the expression of GATA3 (14 and Fig. 13.3). Like most immunohistochemical markers, its sensitivity increased, and its specificity declined significantly in the subsequent literature. However, it is still a valuable nuclear marker, particularly when used along with a well-designed panel based on the histology. We should be aware that GATA3 is positive in most of breast carcinomas and many other tumor types [15]. Clinical history and additional urothelial and breast cancer markers might be needed, if GATA3 is positive in metastatic carcinoma cells.

Uroplakin II

Uroplakins are a group of transmembrane proteins that are urothelial specific and differentiation-dependent markers and have been shown to be highly specific but with low to moderate sensitivity for urothelial carcinoma [16]. Hoang et al. published their data in 2013 and concluded "The mouse monoclonal uroplakin II antibody (BC21) demonstrated superior sensitivity and specificity in urothelial carcinoma, compared with uroplakin III (BC17 and AU1), suggesting its advantages in the differential diagnosis of urothelial carcinoma and in the detection of tumors of unknown origin" [17].

p63

p63 is a highly sensitive nuclear marker of squamous and urothelial cell neoplasms [18]. However, p63 is not specific; it also stains the myoepithelial cells in the prostate and breast with a rim of nuclear positive myoepithelial cells indicating a noninvasive process. p63 can be used to differentiate between urothelial and prostate carcinomas; it has a similar sensitivity but greater specificity than HMWCK 34βE12 because of nuclear staining which minimizes the nonspecific staining inherent in cytoplasmic stains. However, a special precaution is recommended, since a subset of prostate cancers can be p63 positive. It also needs to be kept in mind that p63 can significantly decrease in high stage and HGUC and virtually absent in micropapillary UC [19].

S100P

S100P or so-called "placental" S100 is another promising marker derived from gene expression-based studies that has been used to confirm urothelial histogenesis, which is a member of the S100 family of calcium-binding proteins [20]. It was initially believed as relatively urothelial specific, while immunopositivity for S100P has been documented with significant prevalence in several cancers, including significant prevalence of immunopositivity in tumors of the pancreas, breast, colon, lung, desmoplastic melanomas, and ovarian mucinous neoplasms. Notwithstanding this finding, this marker may be of significant value in supporting urothelial differentiation based on its high degree of sensitivity and proven performance in several clinical scenarios [21].

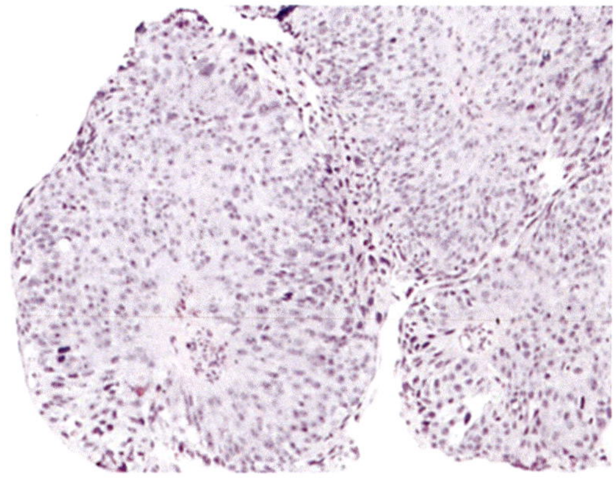

Fig. 13.4 High-grade prostate cancer mimics urothelial carcinoma

Distinction of High-Grade Prostate Adenocarcinoma from Urothelial Carcinoma

Neoplasms within the prostate and urinary bladder can be primary or result from metastasis or direct extension from adjacent organs. Primary prostate adenocarcinoma can extend up to the urinary bladder, and primary urothelial carcinomas arising either in the urinary bladder or in the urethra can invade into the prostate. The clinical management and prognosis are different for prostate adenocarcinoma and urothelial carcinoma. Hormone therapy is often used to manage patients with advanced prostate adenocarcinoma; chemotherapy is often selected to treat patients with high-stage UC.

Well-differentiated lower-grade UCs and prostate adenocarcinomas can easily be distinguished by histology, and these low-grade tumors do not usually create differential diagnostic problems, but high-grade/poorly differentiated urothelial carcinomas can mimic prostate adenocarcinoma, especially those of Gleason patterns 4 and 5 (score 8, 9, and 10). High-grade adenocarcinoma with solid and papillary growth pattern can mimic high-grade urothelial carcinoma (Fig. 13.4). The possibility of overlapping histologic features, especially in the limited material available from a biopsy specimen, may make it a challenging exercise to accurately distinguish between urothelial and prostate adenocarcinoma. Here we outline a few major morphologic characters on H&E sections and then focus on discussing the utilization of IHC to separate these two different entities.

Morphologic Characteristics on H&E Sections

High-grade urothelial carcinomas usually show a nesting architecture, squamous differentiation, higher degrees of nuclear pleomorphism, and brisker mitotic activity, compared to poorly differentiated prostate adenocarcinomas which typically show much less nuclear pleomorphism (relatively uniform cells), more prominent nucleoli arranged in infiltrating cords and focal cribriform glands, and lastly, even though high grade, few or no mitoses (Fig. 13.4). However, the morphologic characteristics of the two tumors may overlap, and therefore immunostains may be required to distinguish them.

Commonly Used Immunohistochemical Markers

Numerous immunomarkers expressed on prostatic and urothelial cells have been extensively studied for differentiating between urothelial and prostate adenocarcinomas, including prostate specific antigen (PSA), prostate-specific acid phosphatase (PSAP), prostate-specific membrane antigen (PSMA), prostein (P501s), NKX3.1, cytokeratins (CK7, CK20, and high molecular weight cytokeratins through antibody 34βE12 or CK5/6), uroplakin, thrombomodulin, p63, carcinoembryonic antigen (CEA), GATA3, and many others. [22–25] Different studies delineate the use of different markers for distinguishing between the two neoplasms, and in our practice we have found that NKX3.1, PSA, PSAP, P501S, thrombomodulin, and 34βE12 are useful markers for this purpose. Other useful markers including GATA3, p63, and Uroplakin II have been discussed in the previous section.

Thrombomodulin and uroplakin are relatively specific for UCs, compared to prostate adenocarcinomas. However, uroplakin has been mentioned to be inconsistent in staining UCs. Thrombomodulin is expressed in UCs though it has a sensitivity ranging from 49 to 91%. This wide variation in sensitivity for thrombomodulin has been ascribed to the varying cutoffs used by different studies with high sensitivity being from studies with any degree of positivity versus lower sensitivities in studies using higher degrees of cutoff for positivity. Whatever the degree of cut-off for positivity, thrombomodulin was not expressed in prostate adenocarcinomas, and therefore it can be used in distinguishing prostate adenocarcinoma from UC [26].

NKX3.1 The homeobox protein NKX3.1 is a transcription factor and tumor suppressor. NKX3.1 has been shown to be highly specific for prostatic origin. Prostate adenocarcinoma and lobular carcinoma of the breast are the only cancers that have been shown to express it. NKX3.1 was expressed from 92% to 97% of high-grade prostatic adenocarcinomas. NKX3.1 proved to be specific and sensitive when differentiating high-grade prostatic adenocarcinomas from poorly differentiated UCs [27–30] (Fig. 13.5).

PSA and PSMA are markers of prostatic epithelium that have been useful in identifying carcinoma of uncertain origin. PSA is expressed in prostate glandular tissue and also in other tissues like breast and salivary gland neoplasms and also anal glands. It is a highly sensitive marker; however, its sensitivity decreases with increasing Gleason score. PSA has a sensitivity ranging from 73% to 97% for poorly differentiated prostate adenocarcinomas. PSMA is like PSA, with a high specificity and a sensitivity of 95–97% in poorly differentiated prostate adenocarcinomas. Since high-grade prostate adenocarcinomas, particularly castration-resistant prostate adenocarcinoma, may be negative for PSA or PSAP, the absence of these markers does not completely exclude a prostatic origin [30–33].

Recent study shows PSMA and NKX3.1 are more sensitive markers than PSA for metastatic prostate adenocarcinoma to the bone following decalcification. We recommend use of PSMA and NKX3.1, rather than PSA, as the IHC markers to confirm metastatic prostate adenocarcinoma to the bone [34].

ERG A nuclear marker ERG (ETS avian erythroblastosis virus E26 oncogene homology) has recently generated interest. Its expression in prostate depends on the TMPRSS2-ERG fusion

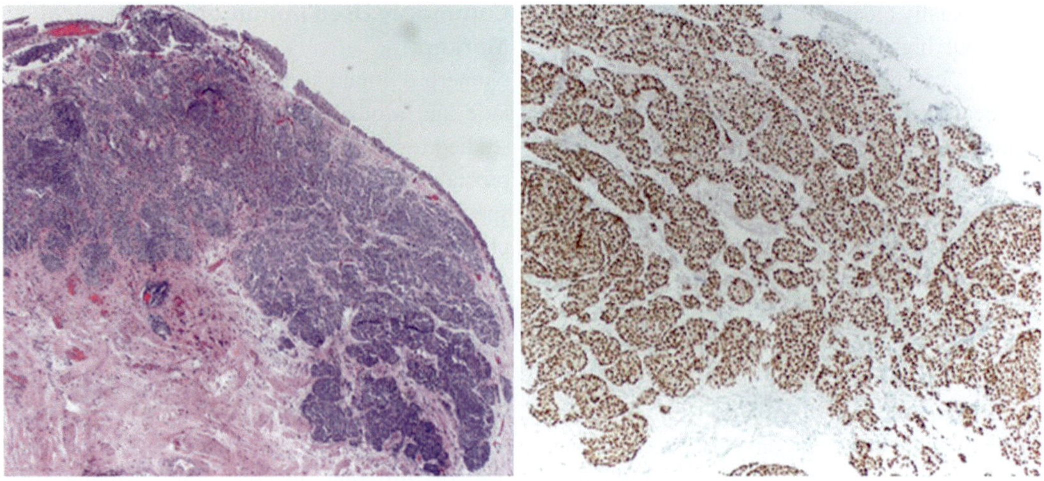

Fig. 13.5 NKX3.1 highlights high-grade prostate adenocarcinoma involving bladder neck

status, which ranges from 2% to 49% sensitivity depending on population studies. It is highly specific for prostate adenocarcinoma and is very helpful when positive in a tumor with the differential diagnoses of UC and prostate cancer. However, ERG has low sensitivity, and high-grade prostate adenocarcinoma, particularly castration-resistant prostate adenocarcinoma, is more likely to be negative [35, 36].

HMWCK Antibody Clone 34βE12 is a specific marker for prostatic glandular basal cells that is directed against cytokeratins CK1, CK5/6, CK10, and CK14. It also stains the urothelium and has a sensitivity ranging from 65% to 100% for UCs, with the variation in sensitivity attributed to be possibly from the antigen retrieval method. With microwave heat retrieval, there was diffuse positivity in all cases of HGUCs as compared to enzyme retrieval methods which showed patchy staining and diffuse positivity only in 65% of UCs. HMWCK in contrast is expressed in up to 11% of prostate adenocarcinomas and has a specificity of 89–97% for UCs. Since prostate cancer can rarely express HMWCK, a precaution is required.

Selection of Immunostain Panel

As we have discussed earlier, the principle of selecting markers should include a complementary panel with speculated positive and negative profile (Table 13.2).

Pitfalls

A very small percent of high-grade prostate adenocarcinomas may lose the expression of PSA; on the other hand, very rarely p63, a marker for UC, can be positive in prostate adenocarcinoma [37]. Therefore, the interpretation of immunostains in this small proportion of cases requires even more caution, and a constellation of features should be used.

Table 13.2 IHC panel for differentiation of urothelial carcinoma from prostate adenocarcinoma

	Urothelial Ca	Prostate Ca
Uroplakin	+	–
GATA3	+	–
P63	+	–
HMWK	+	–
NKX3.1	–	+
PSA	–	+
PSMA	–	+
P501S	–	+
PSAP	–	+

UCs arising from the prostate and direct extension from the urinary bladder share the very same histologic features and immunoprofile. Careful clinical examination of the bladder is essential, and it is directly related to the tumor staging.

A useful algorithmic approach based on our practice is to stain with two or more complementary immunostains that are available in the laboratory, including NKX3.1, PSA, PSMA, P501S, or PSAP and GATA3, HMWK, p63. If it still unresolved, then stain with other markers as needed. Very rarely is the tumor unresolved after these markers.

Nephrogenic Adenoma and Its Mimickers

Nephrogenic adenoma (NA) is a relatively frequent lesion of the urinary tract, which occurs predominantly in the bladder, as well as in the renal pelvis, ureter, and urethra, with a male to female incidence ratio of 2:1. The term nephrogenic metaplasia can be used interchangeably with NA.

Irritative bladder symptoms, occasionally with hematuria, are the usual chief complaints. A well-established association between NA and mucosal trauma (i.e., nephrolithiasis, bladder reconstruction, catheterization, chronic inflammation, intravesical BCG therapy, urinary tract infection, and radiation) led to the once widely accepted conclusion that NA results from a metaplastic response. However, relatively recent studies have shown an association of NA with renal transplant and immunosuppression, and these lesions likely represent an implantation of renal tubular epithelium into a disturbed urothelial mucosa [38].

Cystoscopically, NA is seen as single or multiple papillary, polypoid, mulberry-like, or shaggy exophytic lesions in the background of an inflamed urothelial mucosa (Fig. 13.6).

Several histologic patterns for NA have been described, including tubular, cystic, polypoid, solid, and very recently flat and their combinations [41]. The epithelium lining these structures is composed of a single- or multi-cellular layer of eosinophilic cuboidal and hobnail cells. Often, the tubules are small and lined by only one cell layer with luminal blue mucin compressing a nucleus, resembling a signet ring cell. However, the presence of prominent basement membrane around these tubules is a useful diagnostic feature for this entity. As for the stroma, it is usually edematous and accompanied by a mixed inflammatory cell infiltrate.

The lining cells of NA are positive for different types of keratin, which have limited value in separating this entity with other malignant tumors, since the latter are of epithelial differentiation as well. However, there are two markers that can be used to diagnose NA.

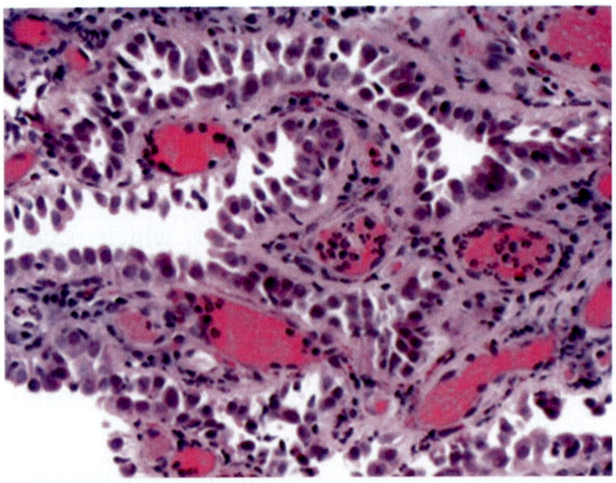

Fig. 13.6 Nephrogenic adenoma mimics urothelial carcinoma or prostate adenocarcinoma

AMACR: Most NAs (58–78%) are immunoreactive for Alpha-methylacyl-CoA racemase (AMACR), a molecule that is expressed in prostate adenocarcinoma [39] (Fig. 13.7).

PAX2 or PAX-8 is a renal transcription factor that is relatively specific for renal tubular epithelium. We and others reported 100% staining with PAX2 in a series of 39 examples of NA and 100% positive for PAX8 in 15/15 flat pattern nephrogenic adenoma [40, 41] (Fig. 13.7).

Diagnostic Dilemmas

NA is a benign lesion, with some features mimicking malignant tumors. The major differential diagnoses are those of malignant lesions including clear cell adenocarcinoma, urothelial papillary carcinoma, and prostate adenocarcinoma. The necessity to distinguish NA from the above mimickers cannot be overstated since there are significant differences in management and patient outcome. Whereas patients with NA generally require no further intervention, those with a diagnosis of carcinoma typically undergo transurethral resection, partial or complete cystectomy, and/or adjuvant chemoradiation.

NA vs. Clear Cell Adenocarcinoma of the Bladder

NA is a reactive process and the clustered tubules are most frequently confined to the lamina propria in an inflammatory background. The basement membranes around these tubules are usually

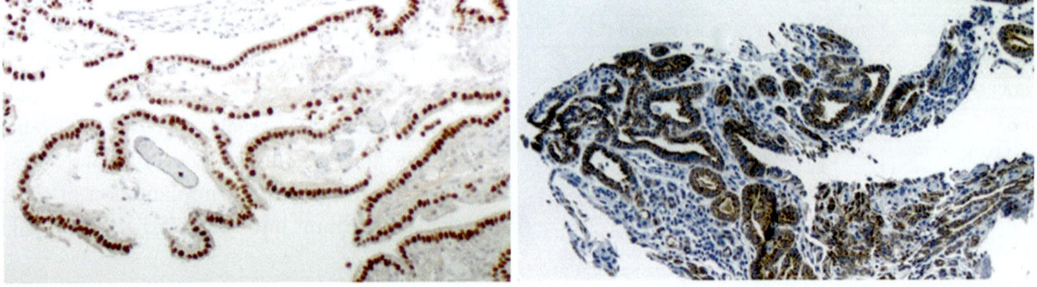

Fig. 13.7 Positive stains of PAX-8 and AMACR in nephrogenic adenoma

well formed, and mitoses are very rare. On the other hand, clear cell adenocarcinoma, like most of the malignant tumors, demonstrates larger size and aggressive histologic features including stromal invasion, anaplastic cytology, high mitotic index, and tumor necrosis.

p53 and Ki-67 are useful in separating these two entities. Clear cell adenocarcinoma shows strong and diffuse p53 nuclear staining, whereas NA shows weak and focal staining. Ki-67 activity is found to be between 10% and 80% in clear cell adenocarcinoma and less than 5% in NA.

Hepatocyte nuclear factor-1β (HNF-1β) is another good but not definitive discriminatory marker in differentiating clear cell adenocarcinomas from NAs. All cases of clear cell adenocarcinomas of the bladder/urethra (n = 18) are positive for HNF-1β, while most of the NAs are negative for HNF-1β [42].

PAX8 is not helpful to differentiate the two lesions because both are immunoreactive for this antibody.

NA vs. Prostate Adenocarcinoma

In male patients, most NAs are found in the bladder neck region and adjacent urethra, which is a frequent site of surgical manipulation in patients with prostate and bladder pathology [43]. The most important diagnostic dilemma when encountering NA in urethral biopsies or TURP from male patients is to distinguish this lesion from prostate adenocarcinoma. It is not uncommon to observe the tubules of NA encroaching deeply into the periurethral stroma of the prostate. Such cases may possibly be misinterpreted as prostate adenocarcinoma.

NA should demonstrate negative staining for NKX3.1, PSA, and PSAP. Prostate adenocarcinoma should stain positively for these markers. Additionally, NA is positive for PAX2/PAX8, whereas prostate adenocarcinoma is negative for both.

AMACR is positive in both NA and prostate adenocarcinoma; immunostains alone can be a potential trap and misleading. Awareness of this pitfall is critical to separate these two lesions; one is benign and the other is malignant.

NA vs. Papillary Urothelial Carcinoma

NA and papillary UC can overlap due to the presence of cellular atypia and papillary growth pattern with fibrovascular cores, which are seen in both entities. Sometimes, there may be a clinical history of papillary UC, and a re-biopsy is performed. We should be cautious not to jump to the conclusion of a recurrence of papillary UC, when we see papillary structures with cytologic atypia. The most important difference is the cell layer: papillary urothelial carcinoma has multiple cell layers, but papillary NA is lined usually by single cell layer.

NA is positive for PAX-2/PAX8, but negative for GATA3 and p63. Conversely UC is positive for GATA3 and p63 and negative for PAX2/PAX8. Again, this complementary panel should be very useful in handling most of the cases within this problematic scenario.

Rarely NA may be associated with various tumors including urothelial neoplasms, prostate or bladder adenocarcinoma, or squamous cell carcinoma of the bladder.

The message is that we should not ignore the associated pathology.

Immunostains for Neuroendocrine Tumors of the Bladder

We have a dedicated chapter for neuroendocrine tumors including small cell carcinoma, carcinoid, and large cell carcinoma with neuroendocrine differentiation. Chapter 9, "Neuroendocrine Tumors of the Urinary Bladder," has concentrated on this important topic.

Distinction of Primary Adenocarcinoma of the Bladder from Secondary Adenocarcinoma Involving the Bladder

If adenocarcinoma is found in the bladder, the key issue for clinical management is whether this is a primary or secondary adenocarcinoma, including metastatic and direct tumor extension from other pelvic organs such as the colon, cervix, or uterus. The treatment of choice for primary adenocarcinoma of the bladder is radical cystectomy or cystoprostatectomy (for male patient). In the case of secondary bladder adenocarcinoma, finding the primary site and administering systemic treatment to control tumor spread will be the focus.

The histologic spectrum of primary urinary bladder adenocarcinoma is wide and should be handled with care. Common histologic patterns are enteric type, which closely resembles colorectal adenocarcinoma histologically and immunohistochemically (CDX2+, CK20+, GATA3-, P63-, CK7-), and non-enteric type, which displays variable histologic and immunohistochemical features, distinct from a colon primary.

If it is enteric type, clinical work-up is necessary to rule out a colonic primary. Coexisting urothelial dysplasia, carcinoma in situ, or invasive urothelial carcinoma strongly favors a primary bladder adenocarcinoma.

Immunostains have limited value in separating primary bladder adenocarcinoma from colorectal adenocarcinoma metastasis or direct extension to the bladder. β-catenin is reported to be the most helpful marker in this setting. More than 90% of colorectal adenocarcinomas demonstrate a strong nuclear positivity, while more than 90% of the primary urinary bladder adenocarcinomas express beta-catenin with a strong membranous pattern [44, 45].

Metastatic Carcinoma of the Urinary Bladder

Usually a clinical history of other primary carcinoma such as breast, colon, and kidney will make us think about the possibility of a metastasis involving the urinary bladder. However, any unusual histology should alert us of the possibility of metastasis to bladder. Communication with the treating physician and a small panel of immunostains can be useful.

We have discussed GATA3, uroplakin II, and p63, and these markers can be used as evidence of urothelial differentiation, although they are not 100% specific. Of note, GATA3 can be positive in UC, breast cancer, and many other tumors, which should caution us to take advantage of additional tools and information in making the final diagnosis.

Again, clinical history and associated urothelial dysplasia or urothelial CIS can be very valuable for the final accurate diagnosis.

Immunohistochemistry in Separating Spindle Cell Neoplasms of the Bladder

The first consideration should be sarcomatoid urothelial carcinoma; we usually are able to appreciate somewhere on the slide a component of conventional urothelial carcinoma or squamous or adenocarcinoma component. An epithelial marker is necessary to confirm this impression. However, in limited specimens without typical areas of recognizable carcinoma, we may need to use immunostains to work up the lesion (Table 13.3).

Immunohistochemistry in Prognosis and Molecular Classification

At present, there is no marker or panel of IHC markers that can be recommended for routine clinical use to prognosticate the clinical behavior

Table 13.3 IHC panel for differentiation of bladder spindle cell lesions

	AE1/3	p63	HMWCK or CK5/6	ALK-1	SMA	Desmin	Myogenin or MyoD1
Sarcomatoid UC	+	+/−	+/−	−	−/+	−	−
IMT	+	−	−	+	+	+/−	−
Leiomyosarcoma	−	−	−	−	+	+	−
Rhabdomyosarcoma	−	−	−	−/+	+	+	+

or to select therapy for urothelial carcinoma, although the need to improve and personalize therapy for this disease is pressing [16]. Predictive biomarkers that are able to forecast and stratify patient response to novel and emerging targeted therapies are also currently sought. Several markers, in varying stages of validation, which have been reported for various prognostic or predictive roles, are briefly described below.

CK20, CD44, Uroplakin, CK14, GATA3, and CK5/6

Recent integrated genomic and protein analysis studies have been used to delineate urothelial carcinoma subgroups. It may help to define subsets of patients who will response and achieve higher survival rates. IHC analysis using limited markers (CK5/6, CD44, CK14, GATA3 and CK20, uroplakin) can fairly subtype urothelial carcinoma into luminal and basal groups [46].

PD-L1

The introduction of immune checkpoint blockade therapy has transformed the management of advanced bladder cancer. The prognostic value of programed death-ligand 1 (PD-L1) in UC has been assessed in several studies, while the results remain controversial and heterogeneous. Despite its limitations, PD-L1 immunohistochemistry may serve as a predictive biomarker of anti-PD-L1/PD1 therapy. Three antibody clones for PD-L1 (SP263, 22C3, and SP142) are considered predictive assays to identify UC patients who are more likely to respond to anti-PD-1/PD-L1 inhibitors, durvalumab, pembrolizumab, and atezolizumab, respectively. Various studies have shown overall good analytical comparability of PD-L1 companion assays and indicate that all three clones are potentially useful in the evaluation of PD-L1 expression in UC [47].

Other promising markers including Ki-67 have potential utility for predicting disease recurrence in noninvasive UC, p53 may have a role in prognostication of progression in muscle invasive disease, and Her2, EGFR, and VEGF may have a role in selection of appropriate therapy [16].

Summary

A few messages need to be emphasized: use the histologic features to formulate a short list of differential diagnoses; and select a panel of immunomarkers which will be expected to be complimentary among the possible entities. Be aware of the staining patterns (expression locations) of each antibody that are applied in the case, taking the clinical history, histology, immunoprofile, and clinical consequences into consideration to render an accurate final diagnosis confidently.

References

1. Moch H, Humphrey PA, Ulbright TM, Reuter VE. WHO classification of tumors of the urinary system and male genital organs. 4th ed. Lyon: IARC Press; 2016.
2. McKenney JK, Desai S, Cohen C, Amin MB. Discriminatory immunohistochemical staining of urothelial carcinoma in situ and non-neoplastic urothelium. An analysis of cytokeratin 20, P53, and CD44 antigens. Am J Surg Pathol. 2001;25(8):1074–8.
3. Mallofre C, Castillo M, Morente V, Sole M. Immunohistochemical expression of CK20, P53, and Ki-67 as objective markers of urothelial dysplasia. Mod Pathol. 2003;16:187–91.
4. Kunju LP, Lee CT, Montie J, Shah RB. Utility of cytokeratin 20 and Ki-67 as objective markers of urothelial dysplasia. Pathol Int. 2005;55(5):248–54.
5. Alston ELJ, Zynger DL. Does the addition of AMACR to CK20 help to diagnose challenging cases of urothelial carcinoma in situ? Diagn Pathol. 2019;14(1):91.
6. Neal DJ, Amin MB, Smith SC. CK20 versus AMACR and p53 immunostains in evaluation of Urothelial Carcinoma in Situ and Reactive Atypia. Diagn Pathol. 2020;15:61. https://doi.org/10.1186/s13000-020-00984-2.
7. Aron M, Luthringer DJ, Mckenney JK, Hansel DE, Westfall DE, Parakh R, et al. Utility of a triple antibody cocktail intraurothelial neoplasm-3 (IUN-3-CK20/CD44s/p53) and α-methylacyl-CoA racemase (AMACR) in the distinction of urothelial carcinoma in situ (CIS) and reactive urothelial atypia. Am J Surg Pathol. 2013;37(12):1815–23.
8. Brent Arville, Emily O'Rourke, Fai Chung, Mahul Amin, Shikha Bose. Evaluation of a triple combination of cytokeratin 20, p53 and CD44 for improving detection of urothelial carcinoma in urine cytology specimens. Cytojournal. 2013, 10:25.
9. Paner GP, Shen SS, Lapetino S, Venkataraman G, Barkan GA, Quek ML, Ro JY. Amin diagnostic utility

of antibody to smoothelin in the distinction of muscularis propria from muscularis mucosae of the urinary bladder: a potential ancillary tool in the pathologic staging of invasive urothelial carcinoma. Am J Surg Pathol. 2009;33(1):91–8.
10. Bovio IM, Al-Quran SZ, Rosser CJ, Algood CB, Drew PA, Allan RW. Smoothelin immunohistochemistry is a useful adjunct for assessing muscularis propria invasion in bladder carcinoma. Histopathology. 2010;56(7):951–6.
11. Hansel DE, Paner GP, Nese N, Amin MB. Limited smoothelin expression the muscularis propria: validation in bladder diverticula. Human Pathol. 2011;42(11):1770–6.
12. Miyamoto H, Sharma RB, Illei PB, Epstein JI. Pitfalls in the use of smoothelin to identify muscularis propria invasion by urothelial carcinoma. Am J Surg Pathol. 2010;34(3):418–22.
13. Liu H, Shi J, Wilkerson ML, Lin F. Immunohistochemical evaluation of GATA3 expression in tumors and normal tissues: a useful immunomarker for breast and urothelial carcinomas. Am J Clin Pathol. 2012;138(1):57–64.
14. Verduin L, Mentrikoski MJ, Heitz CT, Wick MR. The utility of GATA3 in the diagnosis of urothelial carcinoma with variant morphologic patterns. Appl Immunohistochem Mol Morphol. 2016;24(7):509–13.
15. Clark BZ, Beriwal S, Dabbs DJ, Bhargava R. Semiquantitative GATA-3 immunoreactivity in breast, bladder, gynecologic tract, and other cytokeratin 7-positive carcinomas. Am J Clin Pathol. 2014;142(1):64–71.
16. Amin MB, Trpkov K, Lopez-Beltran A, Grignon D, et al. Best practices recommendations in the application of immunohistochemistry in the bladder lesions: report from the International Society of Urologic Pathology consensus conference. Am J Surg Pathol. 2014;38(8):e20–34.
17. Hoang L, Tacha DE, Qi W, Yu C, Bremer RE, Chu J, Haas TS, Cheng L. A newly developed uroplakin II antibody with increased sensitivity in urothelial carcinoma of the bladder. Arch Pathol Lab Med. 2014;138:943–9.
18. Chuang AY, DeMarzo AM, Veltri RW, Sharma RB, Bieberich CJ, Epstein JI. Immunohistochemical differentiation of high-grade prostate carcinoma from urothelial carcinoma. Am J Surg Pathol. 2007;31(8):1246–55.
19. Lin X, Zhu B, Villa C, Zhong M, Kundu S, Rohan S, Yang XJ. The utility of p63, p40, and GATA-binding protein 3 immunohistochemistry in diagnosing micropapillary urothelial carcinoma. Hum Pathol. 2014;45(9):1824–9.
20. Higgins JPT, Kaygusuz G, Wang L, et al. Placental S100 (S100P) and GATA3: markers for transitional epithelium and urothelial carcinoma discovered by complementary DNA microarray. Am J Surg Pathol. 2007;31:673–80.
21. Suryavanshi M, Sanz-Ortega J, Sirohi D, et al. S100P as a marker for urothelial histogenesis: a critical review and comparison with novel and traditional urothelial immunohistochemical markers. Adv Anat Pathol. 2017;24(3):151–60.
22. Paner GP, Luthringer DJ, Amin MB. Best practice in diagnostic immunohistochemistry: prostate carcinoma and its mimics in needle core biopsies. Arch Pathol Lab Med. 2008;132(9):1388–96. Review
23. Mai KT, Collins JP, Veinot JP. Prostatic adenocarcinoma with urothelial (transitional cell) carcinoma features. Appl Immunohistochem Mol Morphol. 2002;10(3):231–6.
24. Chuang AY, DeMarzo AM, Veltri RW, Sharma RB, Bieberich CJ, Epstein JI. Immunohistochemical differentiation of high-grade prostate carcinoma from urothelial carcinoma. Am J Surg Pathol. 2007;31(8):1246–55.
25. Genega EM, Hutchinson B, Reuter VE, Gaudin PB. Immunophenotype of high-grade prostatic adenocarcinoma and urothelial carcinoma. Mod Pathol. 2000;13(11):1186–91.
26. Parker DC, Folpe AL, Bell J, et al. Potential utility of uroplakin III, thrombomodulin, high molecular weight cytokeratin, and cytokeratin 20 in noninvasive, invasive, and metastatic urothelial (transitional cell) carcinomas. Am J Surg Pathol. 2003;27(1):1–10.
27. GurelB ATZ, Montgomery EA, et al. NKX3.1 as a marker of prostatic origin in metastatic tumors. Am J Surg Pathol. 2010;34(8):1097–105.
28. Kalos M, Askaa J, Hylander BL, et al. Prostein expression is highly restricted to normal and malignant prostate tissues. Prostate. 2004;60(3):246–56.
29. Oh WJ, Chungm AM, Kim JS, et al. Differential immunohistochemical profiles for distinguishing prostate carcinoma and urothelial carcinoma. J Pathol Transl Med. 2016;50(5):345–54.
30. Epstein JI, Egevad L, Humphrey PA, Montironi R. Members of the ISUP Immunohistochemistry in Diagnostic Urologic Pathology Group. Best practices recommendations in the application of immunohistochemistry in the prostate: report from the International Society of Urologic Pathology consensus conference. Am J Surg Pathol. 2014;38(8):e6–e19.
31. Goldstein NS. Immunophenotypic characterization of 225 prostate adenocarcinomas with intermediate or high Gleason scores. Am J Clin Pathol. 2002;117(3):471–7.
32. Mhawech P, Uchida T, Pelte MF. Immunohistochemical profile of high-grade urothelial bladder carcinoma and prostate adenocarcinoma. Hum Pathol. 2002;33(11):1136–40.
33. Varma M, Morgan M, Jasani B, Tamboli P, Amin MB. Polyclonal anti-PSA is more sensitive but less specific than monoclonal anti-PSA: implications for diagnostic prostatic pathology. Am J Clin Pathol. 2002;118(2):202–7.

34. Huang H, Guma SR, Melamed J, Zhou M, Lee P, Deng FM. NKX3.1 and PSMA are sensitive diagnostic markers for prostatic carcinoma in bone metastasis after decalcification of specimens. Am J Clin Exp Urol. 2018;6(5):182–8.
35. Shah RB. Clinical applications of novel ERG immunohistochemistry in prostate cancer diagnosis and management. Adv Anat Pathol. 2013;20(2):117–24.
36. Brooks JD, Wei W, Hawley S, et al. Evaluation of ERG and SPINK1 by Immunohistochemical staining and Clinicopathological outcomes in a multi-institutional radical prostatectomy cohort of 1067 patients. PLoS One. 2015;10(7):e0132343.
37. Parsons JK, Gage WR, Nelson WG, De Marzo AM. p63 protein expression is rare in prostate adenocarcinoma: implications for cancer diagnosis and carcinogenesis. Urology. 2001;58(4):619–24.
38. Mazal PR, et al. Derivation of nephrogenic adenomas from renal tubular cells in kidney-transplant recipients. N Engl J Med. 2002;347(9):653–9.
39. Gupta A, Wang HL, Policarpio-Nicolas ML, et al. Expression of alpha-methylacyl-coenzyme a racemase in nephrogenic adenoma. Am J Surg Pathol. 2004;28(9):1224–9.
40. Tong GX, Melamed J, Mansukhani M, et al. PAX2: a reliable marker for nephrogenic adenoma. Mod Pathol. 2006;19(3):356–63.
41. Piña-Oviedo S, Shen SS, Truong LD, Ayala AG, Ro JY. Flat pattern of nephrogenic adenoma: previously unrecognized pattern unveiled using PAX2 and PAX8 immunohistochemistry. Mod Pathol. 2013;26(6):792–8.
42. Brimo F, Herawi M, Sharma R, Netto GJ, Epstein JI, Illei PB. Hepatocyte nuclear factor-1β expression in clear cell adenocarcinomas of the bladder and urethra: diagnostic utility and implications for histogenesis. Hum Pathol. 2011;42(11):1613–9.
43. Malpica A, Ro JY, Troncoso P, Ordoñez NG, Amin MB, Ayala AG. Nephrogenic adenoma of the prostatic urethra involving the prostate gland: a clinicopathologic and immunohistochemical study of eight cases. Hum Pathol. 1994;25(4):390–5.
44. Wang HL, Lu DW, Yerian LM, et al. Immunohistochemical distinction between primary adenocarcinoma of the bladder and secondary colorectal adenocarcinoma. Am J Surg Pathol. 2001;25(11):1380–7.
45. Rao Q, Williamson SR, Lopez-Beltran A, et al. Distinguishing primary adenocarcinoma of the urinary bladder from secondary involvement by colorectal adenocarcinoma: extended immunohistochemical profiles emphasizing novel markers. Mod Pathol. 2013;26(5):725–32.
46. Choi W, Porten S, Kim S, et al. Identification of distinct basal and luminal subtypes of muscle-invasive bladder cancer with different sensitivities to frontline chemotherapy. Cancer Cell. 2014;25(2):152–65.
47. Rijnders M, van der Veldt AAM, Zuiverloon TCM, et al. PD-L1 antibody comparison in Urothelial carcinoma. Eur Urol. 2019;75(3):538–40.

Molecular Pathology

14

Dilek Ertoy Baydar

Mutational Frame

Development and progression of bladder UC occur mainly through genomic modifications affecting almost all chromosomes. All types of genetic changes that include aneusomies, epigenetic alterations, activating or silencing mutations, amplifications, and deletions are commonly seen in this disease [1, 2].

Numerical Chromosomal Alterations

The most frequently detected copy number aberrations in UC are on chromosomes 1, 8, 9, 10, 11, 13, and 14 [3]. These changes offer the necessary setting of genetic instability that in turn allows for the accumulation of succeeding genetic defects. Although most non-muscle invasive bladder cancer (NMIBC) are diploid or near diploid, loss of specific regions is common and associated with higher recurrence [4–6]. A study comparing genetic deviations between Ta and T1 tumors has found that losses of 9q (54%), 9p (39%), and Y (28%) and gain of 1q (14%) were more prevalent in Ta tumors, whereas deletions at 2q (36%), 8p (32%), and 11p (21%) and gains at 1q (54%), 8q (32%), 3p, 3q, 5p, 6p, and 10p (18% each) were more common in T1 neoplasia [6]. Notably, loss of 9q has also been shown in normal surface epithelium adjacent to tumor. Loss of 9q appears to be an early marker of local genomic instability and may act in the initiation of bladder cancer [5, 7]. NOTCH1 and TSC1 are the candidate tumor suppressor genes on chromosome 9q that may factor in the cancer pathogenesis. Gains of chromosomes 3q, 7p, and 17q and 9p21 deletions (p16 locus) are of special note which give them potential diagnostic and prognostic significance [8] (see Urovysion below).

Mutations

Mutations in bladder cancer (BC) mainly involve the genes responsible for neoplastic transformation, signal transduction, cell cycle regulation, DNA damage repair, transcription, and chromatin remodeling. Overall mutation rates in muscle invasive bladder carcinoma (MIBC) are very high (mean 8.2 and median 5.8 per megabase in coding regions according to The Cancer Genome Atlas (TCGA) data, only slightly fewer than lung cancer and melanoma [9, 10]). Recurrent genetic alterations include mutations in the coding region of many genes such as *FGFR3*, *PIK3CA*, *KDM6A*, *STAG2*, and *TP53* [10, 11] as well as in numerous non-coding regions such as *TERT*, *PLEKHS1*, *WDR74*, *TBC1D1*, *LEPROTL1*, and *GPR126* [12, 13].

D. Ertoy Baydar (✉)
Department of Pathology, Koc University Hospital, Istanbul, Turkey
e-mail: dertoy@kuh.ku.edu.tr

H. Zhou et al. (eds.), *Urinary Bladder Pathology*, https://doi.org/10.1007/978-3-030-71509-0_14

High mutation load in invasive UC is mainly thought to be driven by the APOBEC (apolipoprotein B mRNA editing enzyme catalytic polypeptide-like) mutagenesis. APOBEC is a member of the evolutionary conserved family of cytidine deaminases that are involved in the intrinsic response to infection, modification, and clearance of viral DNA. TCGA Bladder Cancer Group has shown that the somatic mutations in UC are dominated by a C:G → T:A [9]. This is characteristic of mutations caused by the APOBEC family [14]. APOBEC-a and APOBEC-b mutation signatures account for 67% of all single nucleotide variants (SNVs) within MIBC. A second frequent mutational signature is associated with ERCC2 mutations and thought to be responsible for ~20% of all SNVs. ERCC2 encodes a DNA helicase that has a central role in the nucleotide excision DNA repair pathway. A third signature in the TCGA analysis is likely related to 5-methylcytosine deamination and has been associated with 8% of SNVs.

The most frequently mutated gene in the bladder cancer is the *TERT* (telomerase reverse transcriptase) promoter [13, 15, 16]. *TERT* encodes the catalytic subunit of the telomerase complex which is upregulated in the majority of cancers and is essential for vanquishing senescence and apoptosis by maintaining the 3′ telomere length at the ends of chromosomes [17]. Somatic *TERT* promoter mutations occur early in the process of bladder carcinogenesis [16, 18, 19]. Mutations generate consensus binding motifs for ETS transcription factors, increasing TERT expression and activity. Given that telomere shortening acts as a mitotic clock, the activation of telomerase elongates telomeres at the ends of chromosomes, which is essential for the continued growth of cancer cells [20].

Activating mutations of *FGFR3*, a gene located at chromosome 4p16.3, are common in bladder UC, particularly in the subset of low-grade and low-stage tumors, where their frequency reaches up to 70–80% [18]. They map to three mutation hotspots in exons 7 (codons 248 and 249), 10 (codons 372, 373, 375, 382, and 393), and 15 (codon 653) [21].

One of the most frequently mutated gene is *TP53* in muscle-invasive UCs and has been detected in nearly 50% of the cases [9]. Mouse double minute 2 homolog (*MDM2*) is another gene functioning in cell cycle regulation. *MDM2* amplification and overexpression are seen in 7% of UCs and mutually exclusive with *TP53* mutation. *RB1* mutation is a frequent accompaniment of *TP53* mutation, is observed in 17% of cases, and is mutually exclusive with *CDKN2A* deletion.

Mixed-lineage leukemia 2 (*MLL2*) gene belongs to the group of chromatin remodeling genes involved in epigenetic regulation. It is another frequently mutated gene and found in around 28% of UCs. Other frequently mutated genes include lysine (K)-specific methyltransferase 2C (*KMT2C*), ataxia telangiectasia mutation (*ATM*), FAT atypical cadherin 1 (*FAT1*), CREB-binding protein (*CREBBP*), *ERBB2*, spectrin alpha non-erythrocytic 1 (*SPTAN1*), and lysine (K)-specific methyltransferase 2A (*KMT2A*).

The recurrent gene fusions are rarely observed in UC [10]. Less than 5% of bladder cancers harbor *FGFR3-TACC3* (transforming acidic coiled-coil containing protein 3) fusions and even less frequently *TSEN2* (tRNA splicing endonuclease subunit 2)-*PPARG* (peroxisome proliferator-activated receptor gamma) and *MKRN2* (makorin ring finger protein 2)-*PPARG* translocations [22].

Epigenetic Alterations

Aberrant DNA methylation and histone modification play a role in regulating gene expression and may contribute to carcinogenesis. Several groups have documented that hypermethylation of *RARB*, *RASSF1*, and *DAPK* is linked to aggressiveness in UC [23].

Chromatin-modifying genes (CMGs) are the regulators of gene expression and commonly mutated in the malignancies [10, 24]. It was found that the two most commonly mutated CMGs in NMIBC were *KDM6A* (38%) and *ARID1A* (28%) [25]. *KDM6A* mutation frequency is 52% in low grade (LG) Ta, 38% in high grade (HG) Ta, 32% in HGT1, and 24% in

MIBC, whereas *ARID1A* mutation frequency is 9% in LGTa, 28% in HGTa, 18% in HGT1, and 24% in MIBC cases. Frequency of *KDM6A* mutations was found elevated in the female patients with Ta tumors (72%) compared to men (42%). *ARID1A* has been associated with increased risk of recurrence, which may be linked to increased aggressiveness or BCG resistance [25].

Molecular Pathways

Bladder UC is believed to develop via a field effect that involves multiple sites in the mucosa, leading to multifocal and metachronous tumorigenesis [18, 26]. Urothelial cells in the affected field gain additional genetic alterations and become malignant by clonal evolution.

UC develops along two oncogenic tracks: papillary (~80% of bladder cancers) and nonpapillary (~20% of bladder cancers), with some overlapping molecular profile (Fig. 14.1). Low-grade (LG) papillary tumors are superficial, and they arise from premalignant lesions referred to as urothelial dysplasia (low-grade intraurothelial neoplasia), whereas nonpapillary lesions are generally high grade (HG) and develop from urothelial dysplasia that progresses to carcinoma in situ (high-grade intraurothelial neoplasia). Low-grade papillary UCs have high propensity for recurrence after transurethral resections, but they usually do not penetrate the basement membrane of surface epithelium to invade the bladder wall. On the other hand, urothelial CIS is notorious for frequent transformation to invasive and metastatic cancer. It is also known that some of the low-grade papillary tumors (~10 to 15%) may progress to the noninvasive high-grade papillary UC and subsequently invasive UC. The MIBC cohort in The Cancer Genome Atlas (TCGA) study has demonstrated the mutual exclusiveness of alterations between *CDKN2A* and *TP53*, *CDKN2A* and *RB1*, *TP53* and *MDM2*, and *FGFR3* and *RB1* gene pairs. Similar analyses showed the co-occurrence of mutations in the *TP53* and *RB1* genes and in the *FGFR3* and *CDKN2A* genes [10]. It has now been widely accepted that the Ras pathway is a major driver of the papillary track, whereas the p53/RB1 and PTEN-related pathways contribute to the aggressive and invasive phenotype [2, 18, 27, 28]. Most CIS lesions gain TP53 mutations early in evolution and do not acquire FGFR3 mutations [29]. On the other hand, some low-grade papillary

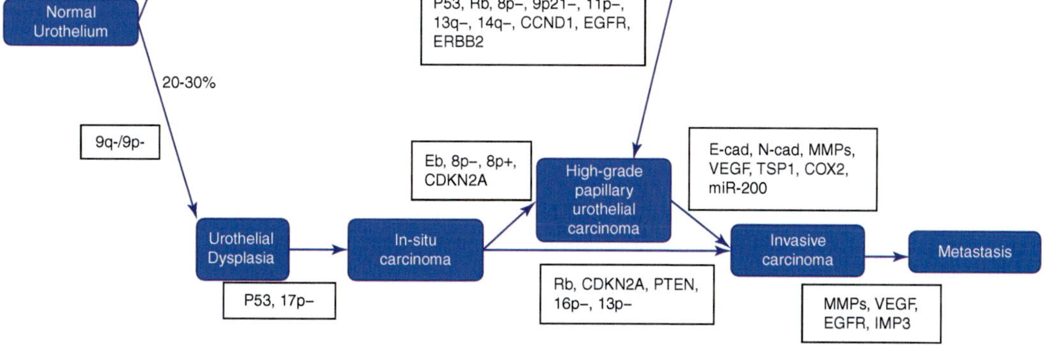

Fig. 14.1 Molecular pathways of urothelial carcinoma

tumors with *FGFR3* mutation may acquire additional mutations of the *TP53* gene and chromosomal losses of 9p21 (the locus that includes *CDKN2A*) and may progress to high-grade and invasive carcinoma [29–31].

Low-Grade Tumors

FGFR3/RAS Pathway: The FGFR3/RAS pathway is active mainly in low-grade noninvasive papillary UC. FGFR3 signals through Ras (RAS-MAPK-ERK pathway) and regulates cell cycle entry and proliferation. The most common *FGFR3* mutations facilitate ligand-independent receptor dimerization, leading to transphosphorylation and downstream signaling. Activating point mutation in *FGFR3* is most common in Ta tumors (~80%), with decreased frequency in high-grade Ta (59%), T1 (10–34%), and MIBC (10–20%) [25, 32, 33]. *FGFR3* mutations have been associated with a higher risk of recurrence in noninvasive papillary bladder cancer and favorable clinical outcomes in pT1 tumors [18, 27, 34, 35]. Approximately 10% of low-grade bladder carcinomas harbor mutations in *RAS* genes (*HRAS*, *KRAS*, or *NRAS)* [36] which do not co-occur with *FGFR3* mutations [37]. *FGFR3* fusion proteins are also implicated in bladder cancer pathogenesis, with in-frame *FGFR3-TACC3* fusions being the most common [10]. TACC3 is upstream of FGFR3 signaling, and fusion protein causes constitutive activation of the MAPK-ERK pathway [38]. *FGFR3-TACC3* fusions appear more commonly associated with MIBC.

High-Grade Tumors

TP53/RB1 Pathway: The TP53/RB1 pathway is an important regulator of cell cycle progression and plays an important role in the development of aggressive UCs [18, 39]. The mutation or deletion of *TP53* has been observed predominantly in CIS and MIBC. According to TCGA cohort data [10], 89% of MIBCs have an inactivated TP53 cell cycle pathway, with *TP53* mutations in 48%, *MDM2* amplification in 6%, and *MDM2* overexpression in 19% of cases. Seventeen percent of MIBCs harbor *RB1* mutations often with concurrent *TP53* mutations [40]. *CDKN2A* (*p16*), which functions as a negative regulator of the RB1 pathway, is found to be mutated (7%) or deleted (22%).

Evidence suggests LG noninvasive papillary UC, which classically has a high frequency of *FGFR3* mutation, progresses to high-grade and invasive carcinoma through mutations in *TP53* and chromosomal losses of 9p21, the locus that includes *CDKN2A* [30, 31]. In contrast, most CIS lesions develop *TP53* mutations early and do not acquire *FGFR3* mutations [29].

PIK3/AKT/MTOR Pathway: In vitro studies show that the ablation of p53 in a background of mutant Ras induces superficial papillary tumors but is insufficient to trigger cancer invasion, suggesting that additional complex genetic events are needed to induce a thoroughly aggressive and invasive phenotype [41]. Up to 40% of bladder UCs show the activation of the phosphoinositide 3-kinase/protein kinase B (or AKT)/mechanistic target of rapamycin (PI3K/AKT/mTOR) pathway. The PIK3/AKT/MTOR pathway regulates important steps in tumorigenesis and tumor progression. This pathway is activated by receptor tyrosine kinases including ERBB2, ERBB3, and FGFR3. The upstream pathway activator *ERBB2* encodes human epidermal growth factor receptor 2 (Her2), which is mitogenic for cell growth. It is amplified, mutated, or overexpressed in 12% of MIBCs or a subset of high-grade NMIBC cases [9, 25, 28]. When present in NMIBC, *ERBB2* amplification is associated with high risk of progression and concomitant CIS [42–44]. *ERBB2* mutations are commonly found in the extracellular domain and are likely reflect APOBEC mutational signature [10]. *PIK3CA* (cancer-associated phosphatidylinositol 3-kinase) encodes the catalytic subunit of PI3K, and its mutations are seen more frequently in NMIBC than in MIBC (Ta, 40–50%; T1, 6–20%; MIBC, 22%) [10, 13, 45]. They are more commonly located in the helical domain than in the kinase domain, likely due to the mutagenic activity of APOBEC. *PIK3CA* mutations appear to be associated with a favorable outcome in patients who undergo radical cystectomy [46]. The reduced expression of phosphatase and tensin homolog (PTEN) is a negative regulator of the PIK3/AKT/MTOR pathway. Inactivating deletions or mutations of the *PTEN* gene has been observed in many MIBC cases. Loss of PTEN was significantly associated with non-papillary, high-grade and invasive tumors, supporting that the involvement of the PI3K/AKT/mTOR pathway might be a potential driver of an invasive phenotype. *AKT1* and *TSC1* are other tumor suppressor genes and negative regulators of this pathway. However, they are not as frequently mutated [18].

Urothelial Proliferation of Unknown Malignant Potential (Urothelial Hyperplasia) and Dysplasia

The deletion of chromosome 9 is prevalent in urothelial hyperplasia and dysplasia [40, 47, 48], suggesting that this deletion occurs in the early stage of bladder cancer. In one study, chromosome 9 deletions were detected in 37% of cases of flat urothelial hyperplasia with or without associated papillary lesions, in addition to chromosome 8 deletions in 10% and *FGFR3* mutations in 23% of the cases [49]. The *FGFR3/HRAS* mutations are frequently found during the development of urothelial hyperplasia [2, 27, 28, 50, 51]. FGFR3/RAS pathway enables tumors to progress from urothelial hyperplasia to noninvasive papillary tumors with high recurrence rates. Expression of ectopic mutant FGFR3 in normal urothelial cells has been shown to induce aberrant activation of the MAPK and PLCg1 signaling pathways and increase cell proliferation [21]. In animal models the activating mutations of the Ras gene caused the development of urothelial dysplasia and low-grade superficial papillary UC [50, 52]. The dose of activated Ras was related to phenotypic change. A low copy number of mutant Ras induced urothelial dysplasia, whereas a high copy number led to the development of low-grade superficial papillary tumors.

Tumor Progression

Approximately, 15–20% of patients with NMIBC progress to muscle invasive disease [53] which is referred to as secondary MIBC. Two of the candidate genes proposed in tumor progression are E2F1 and CDKN2A. E2F1 is a regulator of cellular apoptosis that has been linked to tumor invasion and metastasis in various cancer types [53, 54]. Upregulation of E2F1 and its downstream targets, EZH2 and SUZ12, have been shown in patients with NMIBC progressing to muscle-invasive disease [55]. CDK2NA is a cell cycle regulator involved in G1-S arrest. CDKN2A is lost in the invasive portion of NMIBCs, and only tumors with progression lose both TP53 and CDK2NA [56].

Urothelial Papilloma (UP)

Results of molecular studies in UPs are variable. Rates of reported TERT promoter mutations vary from 46% to 0% [57, 58]. Similarly range of FGFR3 mutations varies from 75% [59] to 0% [58]. In a recent study, 10 of 11 UPs had oncogenic mutations in the RAS/ERK signaling pathway (seven *KRAS*, one *HRAS*, one *KRAS* plus *HRAS* and one *BRAF* mutations) [58]. Only one case harbored oncogenic *FGFR3* or *TERT* promoter mutations. This lesion was likely a recurrent carcinoma despite papilloma histology as the tumor also had oncogenic *PIK3CA*, *KMT2D*, and *CDKN1A* mutations and arose in a patient who had history of several low-grade noninvasive papillary urothelial carcinomas, prior and subsequent to UP.

Inverted Urothelial Papilloma (IUP)

There is variability in the reported results of molecular studies in inverted papillomas. Some groups report *FGFR3* mutations in 9.8–45% (a mean of 18%) of inverted papillomas [60, 61], but others have found no change in *FGFR3* gene [62]. Similarly, some tumors have been reported to harbor 9p deletions (in 3.9% of cases), 9q deletions (in 13.2%), and 17p deletions (in 51%) [60]. The most common molecular alterations in IUP appear in the MAP kinase/ERK pathway, *HRAS* and *KRAS* mutations being predominant. Recurrent *HRAS* mutations (Q61R) have been reported in 60% to over 90% of cases [57, 62].

TERT promoter mutations are rare in inverted urothelial papilloma, with most studies showing inverted papillomas lack these mutations [57, 60–63]. This information and the benign behavior and frequent mutations in the MAP kinase/ERK pathway in these lesions have been taken as evidence that IUPs are a distinct type of indolent low-grade urothelial neoplasia that does not progress to carcinoma [64].

Urothelial Carcinoma with Variant Histology

Urothelial Carcinoma with Divergent Differentiation

The literature on the molecular characteristics of divergent (glandular and/or squamous) differentiation in UC is scant, but it is very likely that there is overlap with those of UC, particularly in the presence of high rates of TERT promoter mutations [65, 66].

Plasmacytoid Urothelial Carcinoma (PUC)

PUCs are characterized by loss of E-cadherin expression similar to lobular or diffuse carcinomas of the breast and stomach. Somatic *CDH1* truncating mutations are mostly responsible from E-cadherin loss as they have been identified in 84% of PUC; *CDH1* promoter hypermethylation occurs less frequently [67]. Aside from *CDH1* alterations, the genomic landscape of PUC is generally similar to that of coexistent conventional UC, suggesting that both histologic subtypes potentially evolve from a common cell of origin [67, 68]. No germline *CDH1* mutations have been reported in PUC.

Micropapillary Urothelial Carcinoma (MPUC)

Genomic expression profile of micropapillary cancer reveals that more than 6000 genes are aberrantly expressed when compared to conventional UC [69]. The micropapillary expression signature is also present in conventional UC component accompanying MPUC, suggesting that micropapillary variant arises from a unique subset of conventional UCs.

Consistently higher rates of *ERBB2* amplification have been reported in MPUC than in conventional UC [70]. *ERBB2* amplification is associated with a worse outcome following radical cystectomy in some series [71]. A study has shown that *ERBB2* amplification is more commonly identified in the micropapillary variant than conventional UC when both components are present [72] although the rate of *ERBB2* amplification in the conventional urothelial component in these mixed (micropapillary + conventional urothelial) tumors is much higher than the reported rates in UC not containing micropapillary component [10, 73, 74].

It has been reported that in MPUC there is common downregulation of miR-296 and activation of chromatin-remodeling complex RUVBL1, with overexpression of its downstream target genes such as lysine-specific demethylase 4B (*KDM4B*), insulin-like growth factor-binding protein 3 (*IGFBP3*), and disintegrin and metalloproteinase domain-containing protein 15 (*ADAM15*) [75, 76]. These are known to be involved in cell growth, DNA damage repair, and metastasis.

Sarcomatoid Urothelial Carcinoma

The sarcomatous and urothelial components within the same tumor share common clonal origin. More recently, it has been shown that sarcomatoid UC is enriched with mutations *in TP53*, *RB1*, and *PIK3CA* and is associated with overexpression of epithelial-mesenchymal transition markers [77–80].

Nested Variant of Urothelial Carcinoma

Up to now, only a few molecular findings have been reported related to this tumor type, the most common being the high rate of *TERT* promoter mutations as well as occasional mutations in *TP53*, *JAK3*, and *CTNNB1*. These findings suggest that this UC subtype harbors molecular alterations similar to those of UC in general [81, 82]. Documentation of *TERT* promoter mutation can be beneficial in difficult cases such as small biopsies as it is not found in benign mimickers of nested UC.

Small Cell/Neuroendocrine Carcinoma of the Bladder (SmCC)

One of the most common findings in SmCC is the near ubiquitous presence of loss-of-function co-alterations of *TP53* and *RB1*. One study reported mutations of *TP53* and *RB1* in 90% and 87% of cases, respectively (80% of tumors displaying co-alterations of both) [83]. Even in tumors with no loss-of-function mutations in *RB1* gene, RB protein expression was lost immunohistochemically, suggesting an alternative mechanism for RB suppression, such as epigenetic silencing.

Small cell carcinoma has a high somatic mutational burden driven predominantly by an APOBEC-mediated mutational process [84]. Genes that are commonly mutated in UC are also found mutated in bladder SmCC, including *TERT* promoter mutations (95%) and truncating alterations in genes involved in chromatin modification such as *CREBBP*, *EP300*, *ARID1A*, and *KMT2D* in ~75% of cases [83, 84]. Unlike UC, there is near absence of *KDM6A* truncating mutations, *CDKN2A* deletion, and *CCND1* amplifications in SmCC [83]. SmCC is associated with a high level of chromosomal instability, and whole genome duplication is seen in 72% of tumors. RNA sequencing reveals novel fusion transcripts, including an in-frame Pvt1 oncogene (*PVT1*)-*ERBB2* fusion, which is associated with aberrant *ERBB2* expression.

Studies investigating the clonal connection between the small cell and urothelial components within the same tumor have shown that there are shared changes between the two components as well as different alterations in each component. These findings further support the common clonal origin for SmCC and coexisting conventional UC [83].

Micro-RNA (miRNA)

Over 200 miRNAs or miRNA families/clusters are aberrantly expressed in UC [85]. The downregulated miRNAs may serve as tumor suppressors. miR-145 appears to be the most frequently downregulated miRNA in bladder cancer. The upregulated miRNAs may contribute to tumor progression. miR-21 has been shown to be upregulated in the tissues, plasma, and urinary exosomes of patients with bladder carcinoma, but its role in UC still needs further investigation. Circulating miRNAs in body fluids, especially in urine, constitute an important cancer signature and carry the potential to be the useful molecular markers for diagnosis, prognosis, classification, and recurrence of UC. miR-146a-5p is frequently overexpressed in the urine of UC patients, which indicates its potential as a novel biomarker for the rapid and early diagnosis.

Inheritance

Upper tract UC is a characteristic tumor of Lynch syndrome (an autosomal dominant disorder caused by a defect in a DNA mismatch repair (MMR) gene). Invasive upper tract UCs are MSI-high/MMR-deficient in ~20% of cases [86]. Emerging evidence suggests an increased (but smaller) risk of urothelial neoplasia in the bladder as well [87]. The 10-year risk for urothelial cancer in patients already diagnosed with Lynch syndrome is 2%. The patients with Lynch syndrome seem to develop urothelial tumors mainly when MSH2 is affected by a germline mutation [88].

Bladder cancer has been reported in patients with hereditary retinoblastoma, possibly related to radiation and/or cyclophosphamide therapy. Bladder cancer can be a component of Costello syndrome. Patients with this syndrome have been reported to develop papillary UC during childhood [87].

Molecular Biomarkers for Tumor Detection and Surveillance

Analysis of desquamated urothelial cells in urine is a valuable source for noninvasive detection of bladder cancer. Urine cytology is an important tool in this respect for both diagnosis and follow-up of UC. However, its overall low sensitivity, especially in low-grade tumors, limits its utility. By the help of accumulating data about pathogenesis and molecular background of urothelial neoplasia, several urine-based noninvasive assays have now become available for early detection and surveillance of the disease with higher sensitivity and specificity.

- The Urovysion assay: This test is multitarget, multicolor fluorescence in situ hybridization (FISH) assay and explores four common chromosomal alterations (aneuploidy of chromosomes 3, 7, and 17 and losses in 9p21) in high-grade UC cells shed to the urine [89]. It was reported that almost all invasive tumors including pT1 as well as a large fraction of the noninvasive bladder tumors were identified by this assay. Most studies also claim that adding this test to standard urine cytology increases sensitivity for detecting recurrence [90].

- Mutation detection assays: Urine-based mutational tests performed on cellular DNA have higher sensitivity than urine cytology and can detect low-grade tumor, an advantage over FISH. They mainly evaluate the genes altered in bladder cancer, such as *TERT* promoter and *FGFR3*, with focus on mutational hotspots [91, 92]. The noninvasive test may be useful for monitoring patients and triage cystoscopy. A positive result may serve as a warning of future recurrence if the subsequent cystoscopy is unable to show a tumor. Mutations in the *TERT* promoter occur early and are very common in UC regardless of grade, stage, and morphologic variants including papillary urothelial neoplasm of low malignant potential [93, 94]. *TERT* promotor mutations do not occur in reactive urothelial proliferations. Thus, they also have great diagnostic utility in distinguishing UC from its benign mimics. *FGFR3* mutations in the cell-free DNA obtained from blood were identified in 68% of patients with advanced or metastatic UC in one study [95].

- UroSEEK: This is a urine-based molecular assay recently developed for the detection and surveillance of urothelial neoplasms [96]. It is designed to detect alterations in 11 genes (*TERT*, *FGFR3*, *PIK3CA*, *TP53*, *HRAS*, *KRAS*, *ERBB2*, *CDKN2A*, *MET*, *MLL*, and *VHL*) commonly mutated in bladder cancer and copy number changes on 39 chromosome arms. Combined with cytology, the test detects 95% of bladder UC, 75% of upper tract UC, and 68% of recurrent bladder carcinoma. The advantage of the assay over cytology is more evident in low-grade tumors as UroSEEK detects 67% of these cases whereas cytology does none.

Molecular Markers for Treatment

The potential therapeutic molecular targets have been identified overall in 70% of the bladder cancers; however, none of them has been integrated into clinical practice, waiting for the results of ongoing studies and clinical trials.

***FGFR Inhibitors*:** A very high proportion of bladder tumors are characterized by *FGFR3* dysregulation. Activating point mutations of *FGFR3* are found in up to 80% of low-grade and low-stage UC of the bladder. Upregulated expression of FGFR3 protein is also found in a significant number of tumors which lack point mutations and are predominantly muscle invasive [21]. Thus, *FGFR3* may be an important therapeutic target in both noninvasive and invasive UC. Several studies have shown in preclinical models that silencing or inhibition of *FGFR3* has a profound inhibitory effect on some UC cells leading to decreased proliferation, reduced anchorage-independent growth, and enhanced apoptosis [97–99]. Therefore, FGFR inhibitors have been proposed as novel therapeutic agents in the treatment of bladder tumors [100], and clinical trials of such agents have been initiated. In a phase II trial of erdafitinib (an FGFR inhibitor) for metastatic UC with *FGFR3* alterations, the overall response rate was 40% [101]. The study of BGJ398 and erdafitinib showed significant clinical activity in patients with refractory metastatic cancers whose tumors contained activating *FGFR3* mutations or fusions, which led to the recent US Food and Drug Administration (FDA) approval of erdafitinib. The US FDA also approved a companion diagnostic test for FGFR3 mutations and fusions. Given the high frequency of *FGFR3* mutation in NMIBC, *FGFR3* may be a rational target in NMIBC as well.

DNA Damage Response (DDR) Gene Alterations and Treatment: *ERCC2* is among the DDR-related genes, and its alterations are detected in 10–15% of MIBCs. Mutations in *ERCC2* and other genes involved in DNA damage response and repair have recently been shown to be associated with improved response not only to cisplatin-based chemotherapy but also to immune checkpoint blockade and radiation therapy for advanced UC [102–104]. Forty percent of responders to neoadjuvant chemotherapy (NAC) have been seen to have nonsynonymous *ERCC2* gene alteration versus 7% in non-responders [105]. Other DDR genes such as *ATM*, *RB1*, and *FANCC* appear as potential biomarkers for response to NAC as well [106, 107].

Mammalian Target of Rapamycin (mTOR) Inhibitors: The potential therapeutic vulnerabilities also include the targets in the PI-3 kinase/AKT/mTOR and in the receptor tyrosine kinase (RTK)/mitogen-activated protein kinase (MAPK) pathways. Patients with mutations that activate mTOR pathway may benefit from mTOR inhibitors. *TSC1* is the negative regulator of mTOR, and its loss may be associated with increased cell growth and survival in high-risk NMIBC [4]. mTOR inhibitors may be an effective therapy to prevent recurrence of tumors with *TSC1* loss.

Other Potential Targets: Urothelial carcinoma with carcinogenesis by *EGFR*, *ERBB2*, *ERBB3*, *PIK3CA*, or *RAS* alterations may benefit from targeted therapy. Chromatin regulatory genes have been found more frequently mutated in UC than other common cancers, further supporting additional therapeutic options [10]. Long non-coding RNAs (lncRNAs) are long RNA transcripts greater than 200 nucleotides in length that do not code for any proteins. The lncRNA urothelial cancer-associated 1 (UCA1) has been associated with cisplatin chemotherapy resistance through activation of Wnt signaling [108].

Bacillus Calmette-Guérin (BCG) Responsiveness

Certain glutathione pathway genomic variations and immune system gene single nucleotide polymorphisms reveal potential to predict recurrence and progression-free survival after BCG therapy [109–111]. *IL-8* (−251 T > A) polymorphism has been associated with an increased recurrence-free survival (RFS) in BCG-treated patients [112]. Gene polymorphisms in *XPA*, *XPC*, *XPD*, *XPG*, *XPF*, *ERCC1*, *ERCC2*, *XRCC1*, *XRCC4*, *APEX1*, *GSTM1*, *CCNB1*, *PON1*, and *SLCO1B* have been linked to reduced RFS or increased recurrence risk after BCG treatment. High tumor mutation burden and loss of *CDK2NA* may predict progression to MIBC in high-risk NMIBC treated with BCG [56]. *ARID1A* mutation has been associated with increasing stage and aggressiveness and may serve as a predictive biomarker of resistance in patients undergoing BCG therapy or a potential therapeutic target to enhance BCG response [25].

Conclusions

The discovery of the molecular changes and pathways involved in bladder cancer is fundamental to understand its biological heterogeneity. Analysis of specific alterations can be used to plan targeted therapies, and predict clinical outcomes and responsiveness to personalized therapies.

References

1. Sandberg AA. Cytogenetics and molecular genetics of bladder cancer: a personal view. Am J Med Genet. 2002;115(3):173–82. https://doi.org/10.1002/ajmg.10693.
2. Wu XR. Urothelial tumorigenesis: a tale of divergent pathways. Nat Rev Cancer. 2005;5(9):713–25. https://doi.org/10.1038/nrc1697.
3. Matsuyama H, Ikemoto K, Eguchi S, et al. Copy number aberrations using multicolour fluorescence in situ hybridization (FISH) for prognostication in non-muscle-invasive bladder cancer (NIMBC). BJU Int. 2014;113(4):662–7. https://doi.org/10.1111/bju.12232.
4. Hurst CD, Alder O, Platt FM, et al. Genomic subtypes of non-invasive bladder cancer with distinct metabolic profile and female gender bias in KDM6A mutation frequency. Cancer Cell. 2017;32(5):701–715.e7. https://doi.org/10.1016/j.ccell.2017.08.005.
5. Granberg-Ohman I, Tribukait B, Wijkström H. Cytogenetic analysis of 62 transitional cell bladder carcinomas. Cancer Genet Cytogenet. 1984;11(1):69–85. https://doi.org/10.1016/0165-4608(84)90100-6.
6. Richter J, Jiang F, Görög JP, et al. Marked genetic differences between stage pTa and stage pT1 papillary bladder cancer detected by comparative genomic hybridization. Cancer Res. 1997;57(14):2860–4.
7. Hurst CD, Knowles MA. Mutational landscape of non-muscle-invasive bladder cancer [published online ahead of print, 2018 Nov 13]. Urol Oncol. 2018;S1078-1439(18)30398-3.; https://doi.org/10.1016/j.urolonc.2018.10.015.
8. Kawauchi S, Sakai H, Ikemoto K, et al. 9p21 index as estimated by dual-color fluorescence in situ hybridization is useful to predict urothelial carcinoma recurrence in bladder washing cytology. Hum Pathol. 2009;40(12):1783–9. https://doi.org/10.1016/j.humpath.2009.06.011.
9. Cancer Genome Atlas Research Network. Comprehensive molecular characterization of urothelial bladder carcinoma. Nature. 2014;507(7492):315–22. https://doi.org/10.1038/nature12965.
10. Robertson AG, Kim J, Al-Ahmadie H, et al. Comprehensive molecular characterization of muscle-invasive bladder cancer [published correction appears in Cell. 2018 Aug 9;174(4):1033]. Cell. 2017;171(3):540–556.e25. https://doi.org/10.1016/j.cell.2017.09.007.
11. Ward DG, Gordon NS, Boucher RH, et al. Targeted deep sequencing of urothelial bladder cancers and associated urinary DNA: a 23-gene panel with utility for non-invasive diagnosis and risk stratification. BJU Int. 2019;124(3):532–44. https://doi.org/10.1111/bju.14808.
12. Jeeta RR, Gordon N, Baxter L, Goel A, Noyvert B, Ott S, Boucher R, Humayun-Zakaria N, Arnold R, James N, Zeegers M, Cheng K, Bryan R, Ward D. Non-coding mutations in urothelial bladder cancer: biological and clinical relevance and potential utility as biomarkers. Bladder Cancer. 2019;5:263–72. https://doi.org/10.3233/BLC-190251.
13. Hurst CD, Knowles MA. Mutational landscape of non-muscle-invasive bladder cancer [published online ahead of print, 2018 Nov 13]. Urol Oncol. 2018;S1078-1439(18)30398-3; https://doi.org/10.1016/j.urolonc.2018.10.015.
14. Lawrence MS, Stojanov P, Polak P, et al. Mutational heterogeneity in cancer and the search for new cancer-associated genes. Nature. 2013;499(7457):214–8. https://doi.org/10.1038/nature12213.
15. Liu X, Wu G, Shan Y, Hartmann C, von Deimling A, Xing M. Highly prevalent TERT promoter mutations in bladder cancer and glioblastoma. Cell Cycle. 2013;12(10):1637–8. https://doi.org/10.4161/cc.24662.
16. Allory Y, Beukers W, Sagrera A, et al. Telomerase reverse transcriptase promoter mutations in bladder cancer: high frequency across stages, detection in urine, and lack of association with outcome. Eur Urol. 2014;65(2):360–6. https://doi.org/10.1016/j.eururo.2013.08.052.
17. Colebatch AJ, Dobrovic A, Cooper WA. *TERT* gene: its function and dysregulation in cancer. J Clin Pathol. 2019;72(4):281–4. https://doi.org/10.1136/jclinpath-2018-205653.
18. Moch H, Humphrey PA, Ulbright TM, Reuter VE. WHO classification of tumours of the urinary system and male genital organs. 4th ed. Lyon: IARC Press; 2016.
19. Wang CC, Huang CY, Jhuang YL, Chen CC, Jeng YM. Biological significance of TERT promoter mutation in papillary urothelial neoplasm of low malignant potential. Histopathology. 2018;72(5):795–803. https://doi.org/10.1111/his.13441.
20. Günes C, Rudolph KL. The role of telomeres in stem cells and cancer. Cell. 2013;152(3):390–3. https://doi.org/10.1016/j.cell.2013.01.010.
21. di Martino E, Tomlinson DC, Knowles MAA. Decade of FGF receptor research in bladder cancer: past, present, and future challenges. Adv Urol. 2012;2012:429213. https://doi.org/10.1155/2012/429213.
22. Guo CC, Czerniak B. Bladder cancer in the genomic era. Arch Pathol Lab Med. 2019;143(6):695–704. https://doi.org/10.5858/arpa.2018-0329-RA.
23. Netto GJ, Cheng L. Emerging critical role of molecular testing in diagnostic genitourinary pathology. Arch Pathol Lab Med. 2012;136(4):372–90. https://doi.org/10.5858/arpa.2011-0471-RA.
24. Guo G, Sun X, Chen C, et al. Whole-genome and whole-exome sequencing of bladder cancer identifies frequent alterations in genes involved in sister chromatid cohesion and segregation. Nat Genet. 2013;45(12):1459–63. https://doi.org/10.1038/ng.2798.
25. Pietzak EJ, Bagrodia A, Cha EK, et al. Next-generation sequencing of nonmuscle invasive blad-

der cancer reveals potential biomarkers and rational therapeutic targets. Eur Urol. 2017;72(6):952–9. https://doi.org/10.1016/j.eururo.2017.05.032.
26. Jones TD, Wang M, Eble JN, et al. Molecular evidence supporting field effect in urothelial carcinogenesis. Clin Cancer Res. 2005;11(18):6512–9. https://doi.org/10.1158/1078-0432.CCR-05-0891.
27. Knowles MA, Hurst CD. Molecular biology of bladder cancer: new insights into pathogenesis and clinical diversity. Nat Rev Cancer. 2015;15(1):25–41. https://doi.org/10.1038/nrc3817.
28. Sanli O, Dobruch J, Knowles MA, et al. Bladder cancer. Nat Rev Dis Primers. 2017;3:17022. Published 2017 Apr 13. https://doi.org/10.1038/nrdp.2017.22.
29. Amin MB, Eble JN. Urological pathology. Philadelphia: Wolters Kluwer Health/Lippincott Williams & Wilkins; 2014.
30. Rebouissou S, Hérault A, Letouzé E, et al. CDKN2A homozygous deletion is associated with muscle invasion in FGFR3-mutated urothelial bladder carcinoma. J Pathol. 2012;227(3):315–24. https://doi.org/10.1002/path.4017.
31. Downes MR, Weening B, van Rhijn BW, Have CL, Treurniet KM, van der Kwast TH. Analysis of papillary urothelial carcinomas of the bladder with grade heterogeneity: supportive evidence for an early role of CDKN2A deletions in the FGFR3 pathway. Histopathology. 2017;70(2):281–9. https://doi.org/10.1111/his.13063.
32. Billerey C, Chopin D, Aubriot-Lorton MH, et al. Frequent FGFR3 mutations in papillary non-invasive bladder (pTa) tumors. Am J Pathol. 2001;158(6):1955–9. https://doi.org/10.1016/S0002-9440(10)64665-2.
33. Kimura T, Suzuki H, Ohashi T, Asano K, Kiyota H, Eto Y. The incidence of thanatophoric dysplasia mutations in FGFR3 gene is higher in low-grade or superficial bladder carcinomas [published correction appears in Cancer 2002 Apr 1;94(7):2117]. Cancer. 2001;92(10):2555–61. https://doi.org/10.1002/1097-0142(20011115)92:10<2555::aid-cncr1607>3.0.co;2-m.
34. Hernández S, López-Knowles E, Lloreta J, et al. Prospective study of FGFR3 mutations as a prognostic factor in nonmuscle invasive urothelial bladder carcinomas. J Clin Oncol. 2006;24(22):3664–71. https://doi.org/10.1200/JCO.2005.05.1771.
35. van Rhijn BW, van der Kwast TH, Liu L, et al. The FGFR3 mutation is related to favorable pT1 bladder cancer. J Urol. 2012;187(1):310–4. https://doi.org/10.1016/j.juro.2011.09.008.
36. Kompier LC, Lurkin I, van der Aa MN, van Rhijn BW, van der Kwast TH, Zwarthoff EC. FGFR3, HRAS, KRAS, NRAS and PIK3CA mutations in bladder cancer and their potential as biomarkers for surveillance and therapy. PLoS One. 2010;5(11):e13821. Published 2010 Nov 3. https://doi.org/10.1371/journal.pone.0013821.
37. Jebar AH, Hurst CD, Tomlinson DC, Johnston C, Taylor CF, Knowles MA. FGFR3 and Ras gene mutations are mutually exclusive genetic events in urothelial cell carcinoma. Oncogene. 2005;24(33):5218–25. https://doi.org/10.1038/sj.onc.1208705.
38. Glaser AP, Fantini D, Shilatifard A, Schaeffer EM, Meeks JJ. The evolving genomic landscape of urothelial carcinoma [published online ahead of print, 2017 Feb 7]. Nat Rev Urol. 2017;14(4):215–29. https://doi.org/10.1038/nrurol.2017.11.
39. Hartmann A, Schlake G, Zaak D, et al. Occurrence of chromosome 9 and p53 alterations in multifocal dysplasia and carcinoma in situ of human urinary bladder. Cancer Res. 2002;62(3):809–18.
40. Kim J, Akbani R, Creighton CJ, et al. Invasive bladder cancer: genomic insights and therapeutic promise. Clin Cancer Res. 2015;21(20):4514–24. https://doi.org/10.1158/1078-0432.CCR-14-1215.
41. Hedegaard J, Lamy P, Nordentoft I, et al. Comprehensive transcriptional analysis of early-stage urothelial carcinoma. Cancer Cell. 2016;30(1):27–42. https://doi.org/10.1016/j.ccell.2016.05.004.
42. Kiss B, Wyatt AW, Douglas J, et al. Her2 alterations in muscle-invasive bladder cancer: Patient selection beyond protein expression for targeted therapy. Sci Rep. 2017;7:42713. Published 2017 Feb 16. https://doi.org/10.1038/srep42713.
43. Chen PC, Yu HJ, Chang YH, Pan CC. Her2 amplification distinguishes a subset of non-muscle-invasive bladder cancers with a high risk of progression. J Clin Pathol. 2013;66(2):113–9. https://doi.org/10.1136/jclinpath-2012-200944.
44. Breyer J, Otto W, Wirtz RM, et al. ERBB2 expression as potential risk-stratification for early cystectomy in patients with pT1 bladder cancer and concomitant carcinoma in situ. Urol Int. 2017;98(3):282–9. https://doi.org/10.1159/000453670.
45. López-Knowles E, Hernández S, Malats N, et al. PIK3CA mutations are an early genetic alteration associated with FGFR3 mutations in superficial papillary bladder tumors. Cancer Res. 2006;66(15):7401–4. https://doi.org/10.1158/0008-5472.CAN-06-1182.
46. Kim PH, Cha EK, Sfakianos JP, et al. Genomic predictors of survival in patients with high-grade urothelial carcinoma of the bladder. Eur Urol. 2015;67(2):198–201. https://doi.org/10.1016/j.eururo.2014.06.050.
47. Obermann EC, Junker K, Stoehr R, et al. Frequent genetic alterations in flat urothelial hyperplasias and concomitant papillary bladder cancer as detected by CGH, LOH, and FISH analyses. J Pathol. 2003;199(1):50–7. https://doi.org/10.1002/path.1259.
48. Chow NH, Cairns P, Eisenberger CF, et al. Papillary urothelial hyperplasia is a clonal precursor to papillary transitional cell bladder cancer. Int J Cancer. 2000;89(6):514–8.
49. Adar R, Monsonego-Ornan E, David P, Yayon A. Differential activation of cysteine-substitution

mutants of fibroblast growth factor receptor 3 is determined by cysteine localization. J Bone Miner Res. 2002;17(5):860–8. https://doi.org/10.1359/jbmr.2002.17.5.860.
50. Mo L, Zheng X, Huang HY, et al. Hyperactivation of Ha-ras oncogene, but not Ink4a/Arf deficiency, triggers bladder tumorigenesis. J Clin Invest. 2007;117(2):314–25. https://doi.org/10.1172/JCI30062.
51. van Oers JM, Adam C, Denzinger S, et al. Chromosome 9 deletions are more frequent than FGFR3 mutations in flat urothelial hyperplasias of the bladder. Int J Cancer. 2006;119(5):1212–5. https://doi.org/10.1002/ijc.21958.
52. Zhang ZT, Pak J, Huang HY, et al. Role of Ha-ras activation in superficial papillary pathway of urothelial tumor formation. Oncogene. 2001;20(16):1973–80. https://doi.org/10.1038/sj.onc.1204315.
53. Chamie K, Litwin MS, Bassett JC, et al. Recurrence of high-risk bladder cancer: a population-based analysis. Cancer. 2013;119(17):3219–27. https://doi.org/10.1002/cncr.28147.
54. Pützer BM, Engelmann D. E2F1 apoptosis counterattacked: evil strikes back. Trends Mol Med. 2013;19(2):89–98. https://doi.org/10.1016/j.molmed.2012.10.009.
55. Lee SR, Roh YG, Kim SK, et al. Activation of EZH2 and SUZ12 regulated by E2F1 predicts the disease progression and aggressive characteristics of bladder cancer. Clin Cancer Res. 2015;21(23):5391–403. https://doi.org/10.1158/1078-0432.CCR-14-2680.
56. Meeks JJ, Carneiro BA, Pai SG, et al. Genomic characterization of high-risk non-muscle invasive bladder cancer. Oncotarget. 2016;7(46):75176–84. https://doi.org/10.18632/oncotarget.12661.
57. Isharwal S, Hu W, Sarungbam J, et al. Genomic landscape of inverted urothelial papilloma and urothelial papilloma of the bladder. J Pathol. 2019;248(3):260–5. https://doi.org/10.1002/path.5261.
58. Wang X, Lopez-Beltran A, Osunkoya AO, et al. TERT promoter mutation status in sarcomatoid urothelial carcinomas of the upper urinary tract. Future Oncol. 2017;13(8):705–14. https://doi.org/10.2217/fon-2016-0414.
59. van Rhijn BW, Montironi R, Zwarthoff EC, Jöbsis AC, van der Kwast TH. Frequent FGFR3 mutations in urothelial papilloma. J Pathol. 2002;198(2):245–51. https://doi.org/10.1002/path.1202.
60. Collomp K, Ahmaidi S, Audran M, Chanal JL, Préfaut C. Effects of caffeine ingestion on performance and anaerobic metabolism during the Wingate Test. Int J Sports Med. 1991;12(5):439–43. https://doi.org/10.1055/s-2007-1024710.
61. Lott S, Wang M, Zhang S, et al. FGFR3 and TP53 mutation analysis in inverted urothelial papilloma: incidence and etiological considerations. Mod Pathol. 2009;22(5):627–32. https://doi.org/10.1038/modpathol.2009.28.
62. McDaniel AS, Zhai Y, Cho KR, et al. HRAS mutations are frequent in inverted urothelial neoplasms. Hum Pathol. 2014;45(9):1957–65. https://doi.org/10.1016/j.humpath.2014.06.003.
63. Cheng L, Davidson DD, Wang M, et al. Telomerase reverse transcriptase (TERT) promoter mutation analysis of benign, malignant and reactive urothelial lesions reveals a subpopulation of inverted papilloma with immortalizing genetic change. Histopathology. 2016;69(1):107–13. https://doi.org/10.1111/his.12920.
64. Akgul M, MacLennan GT, Cheng L. Distinct mutational landscape of inverted urothelial papilloma. J Pathol. 2019;249(1):3–5. https://doi.org/10.1002/path.5307.
65. Brown NA, Lew M, Weigelin HC, et al. Comparative study of TERT promoter mutation status within spatially, temporally and morphologically distinct components of urothelial carcinoma. Histopathology. 2018;72(2):354–6. https://doi.org/10.1111/his.13318.
66. Vail E, Zheng X, Zhou M, et al. Telomerase reverse transcriptase promoter mutations in glandular lesions of the urinary bladder. Ann Diagn Pathol. 2015;19(5):301–5. https://doi.org/10.1016/j.anndiagpath.2015.06.007.
67. Al-Ahmadie HA, Iyer G, Lee BH, et al. Frequent somatic CDH1 loss-of-function mutations in plasmacytoid variant bladder cancer. Nat Genet. 2016;48(4):356–8. https://doi.org/10.1038/ng.3503.
68. Palsgrove DN, Taheri D, Springer SU, et al. Targeted sequencing of plasmacytoid urothelial carcinoma reveals frequent TERT promoter mutations. Hum Pathol. 2019;85:1–9. https://doi.org/10.1016/j.humpath.2018.10.033.
69. Guo CC, Dadhania V, Zhang L, et al. Gene expression profile of the clinically aggressive micropapillary variant of bladder cancer. Eur Urol. 2016;70(4):611–20. https://doi.org/10.1016/j.eururo.2016.02.056.
70. Tschui J, Vassella E, Bandi N, et al. Morphological and molecular characteristics of HER2 amplified urothelial bladder cancer. Virchows Arch. 2015;466(6):703–10. https://doi.org/10.1007/s00428-015-1729-4.
71. Schneider SA, Sukov WR, Frank I, et al. Outcome of patients with micropapillary urothelial carcinoma following radical cystectomy: ERBB2 (HER2) amplification identifies patients with poor outcome. Mod Pathol. 2014;27(5):758–64. https://doi.org/10.1038/modpathol.2013.201.
72. Isharwal S, Huang H, Nanjangud G, et al. Intratumoral heterogeneity of ERBB2 amplification and HER2 expression in micropapillary urothelial carcinoma. Hum Pathol. 2018;77:63–9. https://doi.org/10.1016/j.humpath.2018.03.015.
73. Iyer G, Al-Ahmadie H, Schultz N, et al. Prevalence and co-occurrence of actionable genomic alterations in high-grade bladder cancer. J Clin Oncol. 2013;31(25):3133–40. https://doi.org/10.1200/JCO.2012.46.5740.
74. Fleischmann A, Rotzer D, Seiler R, Studer UE, Thalmann GN. Her2 amplification is signifi-

cantly more frequent in lymph node metastases from urothelial bladder cancer than in the primary tumours. Eur Urol. 2011;60(2):350–7. https://doi.org/10.1016/j.eururo.2011.05.035.
75. Vaira V, Faversani A, Dohi T, et al. miR-296 regulation of a cell polarity-cell plasticity module controls tumor progression. Oncogene. 2012;31(1):27–38. https://doi.org/10.1038/onc.2011.209.
76. Gentili C, Castor D, Kaden S, et al. Chromosome missegregation associated with RUVBL1 deficiency. PLoS One. 2015;10(7):e0133576. Published 2015 Jul 22. https://doi.org/10.1371/journal.pone.0133576.
77. Sanfrancesco J, McKenney JK, Leivo MZ, Gupta S, Elson P, Hansel DE. Sarcomatoid Urothelial carcinoma of the bladder: analysis of 28 cases with emphasis on clinicopathologic features and markers of epithelial-to-mesenchymal transition. Arch Pathol Lab Med. 2016;140(6):543–51. https://doi.org/10.5858/arpa.2015-0085-OA.
78. Sung MT, Wang M, MacLennan GT, et al. Histogenesis of sarcomatoid urothelial carcinoma of the urinary bladder: evidence for a common clonal origin with divergent differentiation. J Pathol. 2007;211(4):420–30. https://doi.org/10.1002/path.2129.
79. Guo CC, Majewski T, Zhang L, et al. Dysregulation of EMT drives the progression to clinically aggressive sarcomatoid bladder cancer. Cell Rep. 2019;27(6):1781–1793.e4. https://doi.org/10.1016/j.celrep.2019.04.048.
80. Genitsch V, Kollár A, Vandekerkhove G, et al. Morphologic and genomic characterization of urothelial to sarcomatoid transition in muscle-invasive bladder cancer. Urol Oncol. 2019;37(11):826–36. https://doi.org/10.1016/j.urolonc.2019.09.025.
81. Weyerer V, Weisser R, Moskalev EA, et al. Distinct genetic alterations and luminal molecular subtype in nested variant of urothelial carcinoma. Histopathology. 2019;75(6):865–75. https://doi.org/10.1111/his.13958.
82. Zhong M, Tian W, Zhuge J, et al. Distinguishing nested variants of urothelial carcinoma from benign mimickers by TERT promoter mutation. Am J Surg Pathol. 2015;39(1):127–31. https://doi.org/10.1097/PAS.0000000000000305.
83. Chang MT, Penson A, Desai NB, et al. Small-cell carcinomas of the bladder and lung are characterized by a convergent but distinct pathogenesis. Clin Cancer Res. 2018;24(8):1965–73. https://doi.org/10.1158/1078-0432.CCR-17-2655.
84. Shen P, Jing Y, Zhang R, et al. Comprehensive genomic profiling of neuroendocrine bladder cancer pinpoints molecular origin and potential therapeutics. Oncogene. 2018;37(22):3039–44. https://doi.org/10.1038/s41388-018-0192-5.
85. Li Q, Wang H, Peng H, et al. MicroRNAs: key players in bladder Cancer. Mol Diagn Ther. 2019;23(5):579–601. https://doi.org/10.1007/s40291-019-00410-4.
86. Rouprêt M, Fromont G, Azzouzi AR, et al. Microsatellite instability as predictor of survival in patients with invasive upper urinary tract transitional cell carcinoma. Urology. 2005;65(6):1233–7. https://doi.org/10.1016/j.urology.2005.01.019.
87. Mueller CM, Caporaso N, Greene MH. Familial and genetic risk of transitional cell carcinoma of the urinary tract. Urol Oncol. 2008;26(5):451–64. https://doi.org/10.1016/j.urolonc.2008.02.016.
88. Engel C, Loeffler M, Steinke V, et al. Risks of less common cancers in proven mutation carriers with lynch syndrome. J Clin Oncol. 2012;30(35):4409–15. https://doi.org/10.1200/JCO.2012.43.2278.
89. Bubendorf L, Grilli B, Sauter G, Mihatsch MJ, Gasser TC, Dalquen P. Multiprobe FISH for enhanced detection of bladder cancer in voided urine specimens and bladder washings. Am J Clin Pathol. 2001;116(1):79–86. https://doi.org/10.1309/K5P2-4Y8B-7L5A-FAA9.
90. Hajdinjak T. UroVysion FISH test for detecting urothelial cancers: meta-analysis of diagnostic accuracy and comparison with urinary cytology testing. Urol Oncol. 2008;26(6):646–51. https://doi.org/10.1016/j.urolonc.2007.06.002.
91. Kandimalla R, Masius R, Beukers W, et al. A 3-plex methylation assay combined with the FGFR3 mutation assay sensitively detects recurrent bladder cancer in voided urine. Clin Cancer Res. 2013;19(17):4760–9. https://doi.org/10.1158/1078-0432.CCR-12-3276.
92. Beukers W, van der Keur KA, Kandimalla R, et al. FGFR3, TERT and OTX1 as a urinary biomarker combination for surveillance of patients with bladder cancer in a large prospective multicenter study. J Urol. 2017;197(6):1410–8. https://doi.org/10.1016/j.juro.2016.12.096.
93. Rodriguez Pena MDC, Tregnago AC, Eich ML, et al. Spectrum of genetic mutations in de novo PUNLMP of the urinary bladder. Virchows Arch. 2017;471(6):761–7. https://doi.org/10.1007/s00428-017-2164-5.
94. Wang CC, Huang CY, Jhuang YL, Chen CC, Jeng YM. Biological significance of TERT promoter mutation in papillary urothelial neoplasm of low malignant potential. Histopathology. 2018;72(5):795–803. https://doi.org/10.1111/his.13441.
95. Pal SK, Rosenberg JE, Hoffman-Censits JH, et al. Efficacy of BGJ398, a fibroblast growth factor receptor 1-3 inhibitor, in patients with previously treated advanced urothelial carcinoma with *FGFR3* alterations. Cancer Discov. 2018;8(7):812–21. https://doi.org/10.1158/2159-8290.CD-18-0229.
96. Springer SU, Chen CH, Rodriguez Pena MDC, et al. Non-invasive detection of urothelial cancer through the analysis of driver gene mutations and aneuploidy [published correction appears in Elife. 2018 Nov 12;7:]. Elife. 2018;7:e32143. Published 2018 Mar 20. https://doi.org/10.7554/eLife.32143
97. Bernard-Pierrot I, Brams A, Dunois-Lardé C, et al. Oncogenic properties of the mutated forms of fibro-

blast growth factor receptor 3b. Carcinogenesis. 2006;27(4):740–7. https://doi.org/10.1093/carcin/bgi290.
98. Tomlinson DC, Hurst CD, Knowles MA. Knockdown by shRNA identifies S249C mutant FGFR3 as a potential therapeutic target in bladder cancer. Oncogene. 2007;26(40):5889–99. https://doi.org/10.1038/sj.onc.1210399.
99. Lamont FR, Tomlinson DC, Cooper PA, Shnyder SD, Chester JD, Knowles MA. Small molecule FGF receptor inhibitors block FGFR-dependent urothelial carcinoma growth in vitro and in vivo. Br J Cancer. 2011;104(1):75–82. https://doi.org/10.1038/sj.bjc.6606016.
100. Knowles MA. Novel therapeutic targets in bladder cancer: mutation and expression of FGF receptors. Future Oncol. 2008;4(1):71–83. https://doi.org/10.2217/14796694.4.1.71.
101. Loriot Y, Necchi A, Park SH, et al. Erdafitinib in locally advanced or metastatic urothelial carcinoma. N Engl J Med. 2019;381(4):338–48. https://doi.org/10.1056/NEJMoa1817323.
102. Teo MY, Bambury RM, Zabor EC, et al. DNA damage response and repair gene alterations are associated with improved survival in patients with platinum-treated advanced urothelial carcinoma. Clin Cancer Res. 2017;23(14):3610–8. https://doi.org/10.1158/1078-0432.CCR-16-2520.
103. Teo MY, Seier K, Ostrovnaya I, et al. Alterations in DNA damage response and repair genes as potential marker of clinical benefit from PD-1/PD-L1 blockade in advanced urothelial cancers. J Clin Oncol. 2018;36(17):1685–94. https://doi.org/10.1200/JCO.2017.75.7740.
104. Desai NB, Scott SN, Zabor EC, et al. Genomic characterization of response to chemoradiation in urothelial bladder cancer. Cancer. 2016;122(23):3715–23. https://doi.org/10.1002/cncr.30219.
105. Liu D, Plimack ER, Hoffman-Censits J, et al. Clinical validation of chemotherapy response biomarker ERCC2 in muscle-invasive urothelial bladder carcinoma. JAMA Oncol. 2016;2(8):1094–6. https://doi.org/10.1001/jamaoncol.2016.1056.
106. Plimack ER, Dunbrack RL, Brennan TA, et al. Defects in DNA repair genes predict response to neoadjuvant cisplatin-based chemotherapy in muscle-invasive bladder cancer. Eur Urol. 2015;68(6):959–67. https://doi.org/10.1016/j.eururo.2015.07.009.
107. Lotan Y, Woldu SL, Sanli O, Black P, Milowsky MI. Modelling cost-effectiveness of a biomarker-based approach to neoadjuvant chemotherapy for muscle-invasive bladder cancer. BJU Int. 2018;122(3):434–40. https://doi.org/10.1111/bju.14220.
108. Fan Y, Shen B, Tan M, et al. Long non-coding RNA UCA1 increases chemoresistance of bladder cancer cells by regulating Wnt signaling. FEBS J. 2014;281(7):1750–8. https://doi.org/10.1111/febs.12737.
109. Ke HL, Lin J, Ye Y, et al. Genetic variations in glutathione pathway genes predict cancer recurrence in patients treated with transurethral resection and Bacillus Calmette-Guerin instillation for non-muscle invasive bladder cancer. Ann Surg Oncol. 2015;22(12):4104–10. https://doi.org/10.1245/s10434-015-4431-5.
110. Kim YJ, Ha YS, Kim SK, et al. Gene signatures for the prediction of response to Bacillus Calmette-Guerin immunotherapy in primary pT1 bladder cancers. Clin Cancer Res. 2010;16(7):2131–7. https://doi.org/10.1158/1078-0432.CCR-09-3323.
111. Kiselyov A, Bunimovich-Mendrazitsky S, Startsev V. Treatment of non-muscle invasive bladder cancer with Bacillus Calmette-Guerin (BCG): Biological markers and simulation studies. BBA Clin. 2015;(4):27–34. Published 2015 Jun 10. https://doi.org/10.1016/j.bbacli.2015.06.002.
112. Ahirwar DK, Mandhani A, Mittal RD. IL-8 -251 T > A polymorphism is associated with bladder cancer susceptibility and outcome after BCG immunotherapy in a northern Indian cohort. Arch Med Res. 2010;41(2):97–103. https://doi.org/10.1016/j.arcmed.2010.03.005.

15 Surgical Treatment in Urinary Bladder Cancer

Dalsan You, Bumjin Lim, and Choung-Soo Kim

Introduction

Bladder cancer (BC) accounts for approximately 3% of all the human malignancies. In 2018, there were approximately 550,000 new cases of BC and 200,000 deaths from BC worldwide. BC was ranked as the tenth most common cancer and the 14th leading cause of cancer deaths in the world [1]. In 2020, an estimated 81,300 new cases (62,100 for men and 19,200 for women) and 17,980 deaths (13,050 for men and 4,930 for women) occurred in the United States [2]. Approximately 70% of BC cases present as non-muscle-invasive tumors (NMIBC) [3].

Despite recent advances in chemotherapy and radiation therapy, surgery continues to be the mainstay of the management of BC. The initial assessment, diagnosis, and staging of BC are determined with transurethral resection of bladder tumor (TURBT). TURBT serves to establish the pathologic diagnosis and the local extent of the disease. Especially in the setting of NMIBC, TURBT with intravesical cytotoxic chemotherapy and immunotherapy is the main treatment procedure.

D. You · B. Lim · C.-S. Kim (✉)
Department of Urology, Asan Medical Center, University of Ulsan College of Medicine, Seoul, South Korea
e-mail: dalsanyou@amc.seoul.kr; cskim@amc.seoul.kr

However, regarding muscle-invasive tumors, TURBT does not provide adequate local control. To maximize the chance for cure, radical cystectomy with regional lymph node dissection is necessary for muscle-invasive bladder cancer (MIBC). In this chapter, we summarize the contemporary surgical management of bladder cancer.

Transurethral Resection of Bladder Tumor (TURBT)

TURBT is the first-line surgical treatment for any bladder tumor. The first description of endoscopic fulguration of papillary bladder tumors was reported in 1910 [4]. It is very important to identify histological diagnosis, staging, and other prognostic factors [tumor grade, multifocality, size, and presence of carcinoma in situ (CIS)]. TURBT is performed in the following way. General anesthesia or spinal anesthesia is used. After positioning the patient in the lithotomy position, physical examination is performed. Physical examination should include the palpation of the abdomen and suprapubic region for any palpable mass. In men, digital rectal examination (DRE) can be used to assess prostatic involvement, and in women, bimanual examination can be used to evaluate anterior vaginal involvement. A thorough visual inspection is then performed using the 30/70 degree lens to examine the urethra in its entirety and then to perform

H. Zhou et al. (eds.), *Urinary Bladder Pathology*, https://doi.org/10.1007/978-3-030-71509-0_15

a preliminary evaluation of the bladder mucosa and ureteral orifices. It is important to record the tumor size (by comparing with the diameter of the loop), anatomic location (lateral walls, fundus, bladder neck, and ureteric orifices), and any mucosal abnormalities suggestive of CIS. If necessary, a more accurate lens, such as a 120° lens, can be used. After tumor mapping, resection can be performed with either monopolar or bipolar electrocautery. The goal of any resection should be the visual eradication of any tumor burden with an adequate depth of resection.

Important basic surgical skills required for complete TURBTs are:

(i) Resection of all visible tumors.
(ii) Resection of histologically normal mucosa on the border of the tumor. Bladder tumors frequently exhibit growth beyond the visible edge; resection should include an approximate 1 cm margin of normal-appearing tissue.
(iii) Resection of the muscle layer at the base of the tumor until normal muscle fibers are visible. Utilizing a cutting current, a loop electrode is used to resect the tumor with muscularis propria (Fig. 15.1).

Depending on the location of the tumor, sometimes it is difficult to resect the tumor, especially those at the lateral and ureteral orifice areas. The obturator nerve passes near the inferolateral bladder wall, bladder neck, and lateral prostatic urethra. When tumors are encountered on the lateral wall, there is a risk of an obturator reflex whereby the electric current stimulates the obturator nerve, causing the ipsilateral leg to adduct. This can lead to inadvertent lateral deflection of the instrument. It can cause bladder perforation. The reflex can be blocked by obturator nerve block or by muscle paralysis during general anesthesia [5]. To lessen this risk, we recommend the following techniques. First, it is important to avoid overfilling of the bladder. A distended bladder brings the lateral bladder wall closer to the obturator nerve. Second, using bipolar diathermy current is widely accepted to lower the risk of obturator reflex [6, 7]. Third, the use of a neuromuscular blockade agent can reduce the reflex of the obturator nerve if the patient is under a general anesthetic. Lastly, obturator nerve block can be performed to avoid unwanted stimulation of the obturator nerve and subsequent adductor contraction. In 1922, obturator nerve block was first described by Labat [8]. Since then, several researchers have suggested an effective obturator nerve block method using nerve stimulator and ultrasound, which has proven that complications are reduced [9–11]. Tumors overlying a ureteral orifice pose another

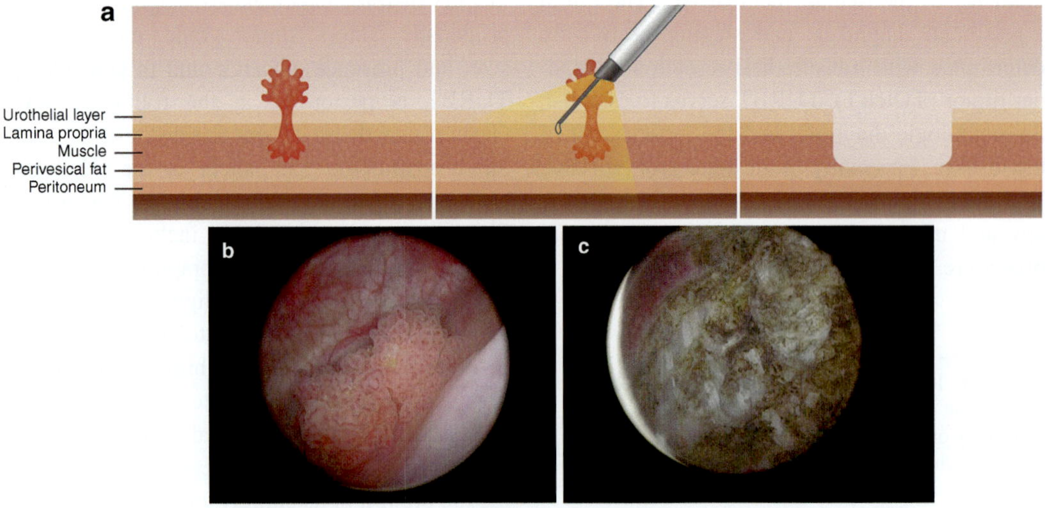

Fig. 15.1 (**a**) A loop electrode is used to resect the tumor with the muscularis propria. (**b**) Preoperative finding before TURBT. (**c**) Postoperative finding after TURBT

challenge. Although this complication is rare, the surgeon should be concerned about ureteral stenosis. In order to avoid the risk of stricture, only the cutting current should be used, and resection strokes should be as quick as possible. When resecting around the ureteral orifice area, ureteral stenting is sometimes used to prevent ureteral stenosis.

What do we need from pathology report?

1. Good gross description.
2. Tumor: papillary vs. flat; low grade vs. high grade, invasion, suburothelial connective tissue invasion (lamina propria, submucosa invasion) vs. proper muscle invasion, lymphovascular invasion.
3. Proper muscle (PM) present, no PM present, uncertain for PM.
4. Adjacent urothelial mucosa, normal, low-grade dysplasia, high grade/cis.

Re-staging Transurethral Resection

Re-staging transurethral resection, the so-called repeat TUR (re-TUR), is mandatory in patients who have an incomplete resection of a NMIBC or evidence of T1or high-grade Ta disease. Residual tumors are common after initial TUR for high-risk NMIBC. According to a recent meta-analysis of 2262 cases, tumor persistence rate is 19.4% to 56% and 15.2% to 55% in Ta and T1 diseases, respectively, and upstaging occurred in 0% to 14.3% of Ta and 0% to 24.4% of T1 at re-TUR, respectively [12]. Therefore, the guidelines recommended re-TUR for patients with high grade, T1 stage, or multifocal NMIBC. When re-TUR is performed, the remaining tumor is resected totally, and previously operated areas are cautiously resected to include the muscle layer but to avoid perforation.

What do we need from pathology report?

1. Residual tumor
2. PM present, no PM present, uncertain for PM
3. Urothelial mucosa, normal, low-grade dysplasia vs. high-grade dysplasia/cis

Partial Cystectomy

Partial cystectomy is a rarely performed procedure in MIBC. It is used as bladder-sparing surgery in the setting of primary adenocarcinoma arising from the urachus. It may provide oncological results similar to radical cystectomy in highly selected patients with invasive bladder cancer [13]. The advantage of this surgery is that the patient can preserve their bladder and doesn't need reconstructive surgery. Typically suitable candidates have a solitary tumor without CIS. Before partial cystectomy, systematic bladder biopsies are needed to confirm the absence of CIS and multiple lesions. In addition, it is necessary to predict postoperative urination status by evaluating preoperative bladder capacity.

Partial cystectomy should be performed with pelvic lymph node dissection (PLND). The first step of partial cystectomy is bladder mobilization. The tumor is then excised with a mucosal margin of 1 ~ 2 cm. If necessary, frozen section analysis is used to confirm the free resection margins. After excision of the tumor, the cystotomy is closed in two or three layers, and an instillation of fluid via a Foley catheter is performed to ensure a watertight closure. Normal saline or distilled water is usually used to irrigate the operation field. A closed drain should be placed. The cystotomy closure is confirmed with a cystogram on postoperative day 7, after which the catheter is removed (Fig. 15.2).

What do we need from pathology report?

1. Good gross description
2. Tumor: size, location, depth of invasion, grade, presence of necrosis, lymphovascular invasion
3. Uninvolved mucosa, normal, low-grade dysplasia, high-grade dysplasia/CIS
4. Margins

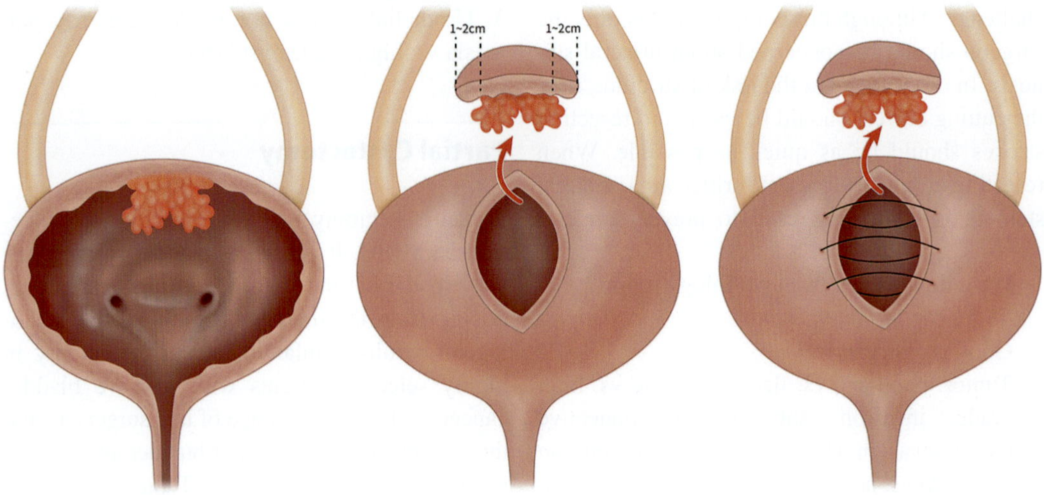

Fig. 15.2 Partial cystectomy. The tumor is excised with a mucosal margin of 1–2 cm, and the cystotomy in closed in two or three layers

Radical Cystectomy

Radical cystectomy has been considered the standard of therapy for MIBC. Recently, many patients are receiving neoadjuvant chemotherapy, which must be considered during preoperative planning [14, 15]. Traditionally in men, radical cystectomy typically includes removal of the prostate and seminal vesicles. In women, radical cystectomy also involves removal of the uterus, ovaries, and part of the vagina. All patients receive a mechanical and antibacterial bowel preparation. Mechanical and antibacterial bowel preparation have been thought to reduce postoperative complications such as anastomotic leak, intra-abdominal infection, and surgical wound infection. However, these practices were questioned based on the results of large randomized trials in colon and rectal surgery. Ren et al. and Zmora et al. revealed that mechanical bowel preparation had no significant effect on postoperative complications [16, 17]. The efforts to reduce mechanical preparation have been tried in radical cystectomy, but these have not been enough evidence. For this reason, some urologists do not advise bowel preparation for patients undergoing radical cystectomy, especially if only ileal segments are to be used. But we recommend bowel preparation.

Prophylactic antibiotics are administered within 1 h of surgical incision, and a broad-spectrum cephalosporin is usually used. Stockings or pneumatic compression can be used to prevent thromboembolism. The male patient is placed in the hyperextended supine position with the flexion point of the table at the level of the anterior superior iliac spine. In female patients, the vagina must be fully prepared and accessible. Therefore, the modified "frog-leg" or lithotomy position is used. A nasogastric tube is placed, and the patient is prepared from xiphoid to the upper portion of the thighs. After the patient is draped, a Foley catheter is placed in the bladder. A vertical midline incision is made extending from the pubic symphysis to the umbilicus superiorly. The incision should be directed 2–3 cm lateral to the umbilicus on the contralateral side of the marked stoma site (Fig. 15.3). After the midline is identified, the anterior rectus fascia is incised.

The rectus muscles are retracted laterally and the space of Retzius is entered. The posterior rectus sheath and peritoneum are entered inferiorly to the level of the umbilicus. The median umbilical ligament is identified; blunt dissection is performed releasing the bladder from both pelvic side wall attachments. This can be achieved at the vas deferens levels in men and round ligament levels in women (Fig. 15.4). Then the root of the

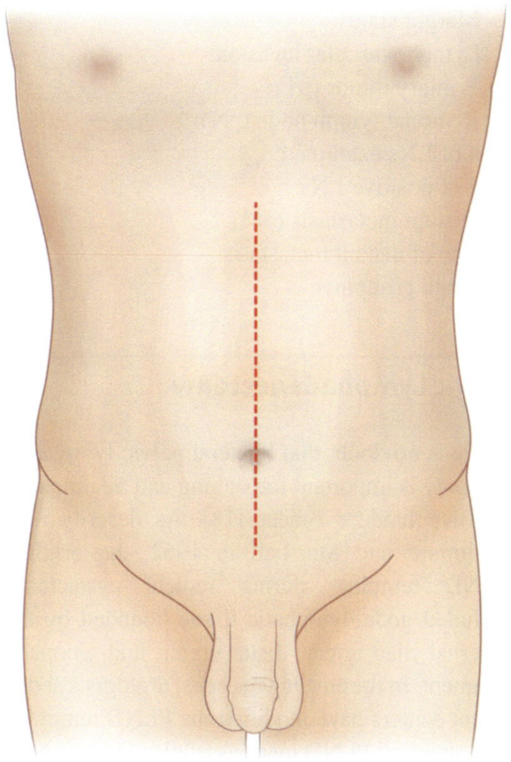

Fig. 15.3 The vertical midline incision which extends from the pubic symphysis to the umbilicus superiorly

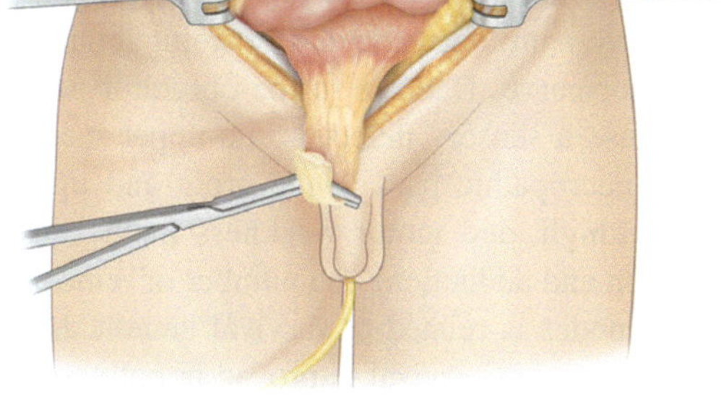

Fig. 15.4 The rectus muscles are retracted laterally to enter the space of Retzius. The median umbilical ligament is identified, and blunt dissection is performed to release the bladder from both pelvic side wall attachments

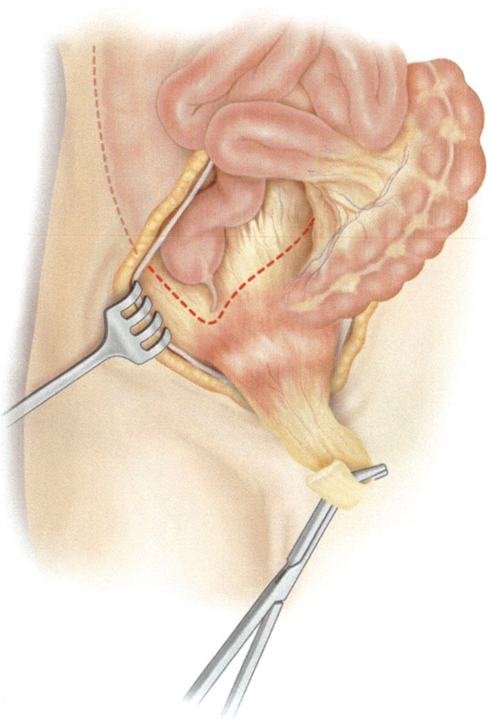

Fig. 15.5 The white line of Toldt is incised and carried around the cecum and ascending colon

small bowel mesentery and the left colon are mobilized to achieve proper exposure of large blood vessels and the ureter. On the right side, the white line of Toldt is incised, and it is carried around the cecum and ascending colon (Fig. 15.5). The mesentery to the small bowel is then mobilized off its retroperitoneal attachments. This dissection facilitates a tension-free urethro-enteric anastomosis. On the left side, the white line of Toldt is incised, and a window is created below the sigmoid colon mesentery. This window is used to allow the left ureter to pass through the uretero-enteric anastomosis. The ureters are easily visible around common iliac vessels. They are carefully dissected up to the bladder. The ureter separated from the bladder and suture ligature (Fig. 15.6). To ensure the absence of carcinoma, distal ureter margins are sent for frozen section analysis. The ureter is then slightly mobilized in a cephalad direction and

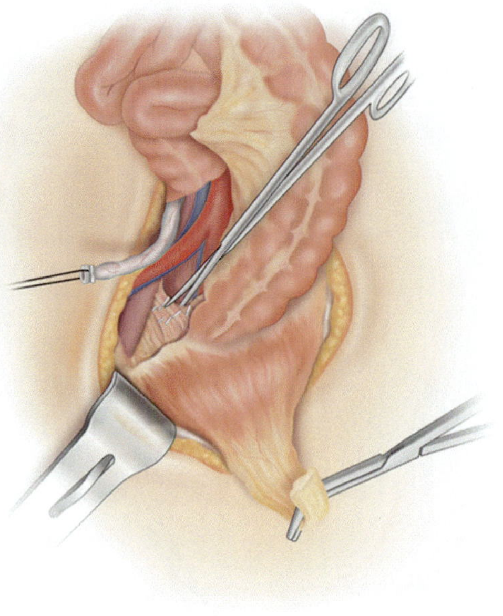

Fig. 15.6 The ureter is separated from the bladder and ligated using suture

tucked under the rolled towel to prevent inadvertent injury. The ureter is then moved toward the abdomen to prevent unexpected damage. Control of the main pedicle to the bladder, including the superior, middle, and inferior vesical arteries, can be achieved with a vascular stapler, surgical clips, or vascular sealing instruments.

What do we need from pathology report?

1. Good gross description
2. Tumor: size, location, depth of invasion, grade, presence of necrosis, lymphovascular invasion
3. Margins: ureters, urethra, perivesical soft tissue margin
4. Tumor synoptic report
   Procedure type:
   Tumor site:
   Tumor size:
   Histologic type:
   Histologic grade (low or high):
   Tumor extension:
   Margin status:
   Lymphovascular invasion:
   Primary tumor (pT):
   Regional lymph node (pN):
   # of LNs examined:
   # of positive LNs:
   Distant metastasis (pM):
   Site of distant metastasis:
   Stage grouping:

Pelvic Lymphadenectomy

There is no doubt that bilateral pelvic lymphadenectomy is important for staging and treatment of invasive bladder cancer [18]. As described by Whitmore and Marshall in 1962, the original PLND template during radical cystectomy included nodal/lymphatic tissue bounded by the external iliac artery, distal ureter, and Cooper's ligament. In the ensuing decades, urologists at different centers have modified the PLND template. The standard PLND margins of dissection consist of the genitofemoral nerves laterally, the internal iliac artery medially, Cooper ligament inferiorly, and the point at which the ureter crosses the common iliac artery superiorly. In case of advance disease, an extended dissection including the entire common iliac lymph node and presacral lymph node can be obtained.

Pelvic lymphadenectomy may be performed before removal of the bladder specimen depending on the surgeon. Completion of pelvic lymphadenectomy helps to identify the vascular pedicles of the bladder. During pelvic lymphadenectomy, a urologist should be careful about the obturator nerve. Damage to the obturator nerve can cause a sensory defect in the upper medial thigh, neuropathic pain in the groin and upper medial thigh, and motor weakness in the high flexation and adduction. The number of removed lymph nodes is related to survival benefit. Herr et al. found that survival improved in both node-positive and node-negative patients as the number of nodes removed increased when at least ten lymph nodes were removed [19].

What do we need from pathology report?

1. How many lymph nodes isolated and how many lymph node-positive
2. Size of largest metastatic lymph node (metastatic tumor size, not lymph node size)
3. Presence or absence of extranodal extension

Radical Cystectomy: Male

The lateral vascular pedicles are isolated, ligated, and divided. The rectovesical junction, or rectal cul-de-sac (pouch of Douglas), is identified, and an incision is made where the peritoneum covers the seminal vesicles (Fig. 15.7). The rectum is dissected with either blunt dissection or sharp dissection in the midline, and it is carried to the level of the prostate. An understanding of the fascia layer is important for proper dissection of this plane (Fig. 15.8). This is because Denonvilliers' fascia did not develop between the prostate and the seminal vesicles but between the prostate and the rectum. This allows proper and safe entry into and development of Denonvilliers' space between the anterior rectal wall and the posterior sheath of Denonvilliers' fascia. Once the posterior pedicles have been defined, the urethra should be palpable, and at this point the anterior dissection is initiated like a radical prostatectomy. The endopelvic fascia is incised sharply, allowing for identification of the urethra and the dorsal venous complex. Ligation and division of the dorsal venous complex allows for visualization of the anterior urethra, which is then incised, and a frozen section analysis of the urethral margin is performed to ensure a negative resection margin. For men with good erectile function who are not suspected to have extravesical tumor spread in the area of the neurovascular bundle, nerve fibers in the dorsomedial pedicles lateral to seminal vesicles and the periprostatic neurovascular bundle should be spared. Avoid any trauma to the pelvic plexus, including clamping or pinching of the tissue with forceps. However, the role of preservation of the neurovascular bundles, unlike in radical prostatectomy, remains controversial in radical cystectomy.

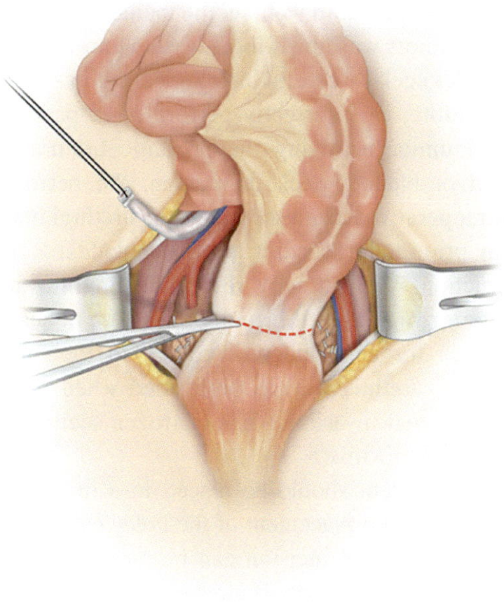

Fig. 15.7 The rectovesical junction and rectal cul-de-sac (pouch of Douglas) are identified, and an incision is made where the peritoneum covers the seminal vesicles

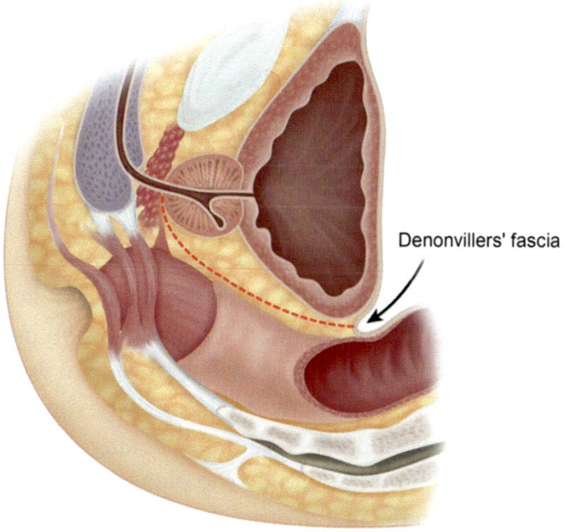

Fig. 15.8 Denonvilliers' fascia in the male pelvis

What do we need from pathology report?

1. Tumor involvement in prostatic urethra: in situ vs. invasion into stroma
2. Prostate parenchyma involvement: confined within ducts or acini vs. stromal invasion
3. Mention prostate cancer, if present

Radical Cystectomy: Female

In women, radical cystectomy also involves removal of the uterus, ovaries, and part of the vagina. When developing the posterior pedicles, the posterior vagina is incised at the cervical fornix (Fig. 15.9). This incision is carried anteriorly along the lateral and anterior vaginal wall forming a circumferential incision. The anterior lateral vaginal wall is then grasped. Applying countertraction to the anterior lateral vaginal wall facilitates dissection between the anterior vaginal wall and the bladder. A vaginal packing during this step can aid in defining the plane of separation between the bladder and the anterior vaginal wall in the midline.

In women, unlike men, dissection should not be done anterior to the urethra along the pelvic floor. The endopelvic fascia should remain undisturbed and unopened in women considering orthotopic diversion. This prevents damage to the rhabdosphincter region and corresponding nervous system, which is important in maintaining continuous mechanisms. Anatomical studies show that the innervation to this rhabdosphincter region in women arises from branches of the pudendal nerve that course along the pelvic floor posterior to the levator muscles. Any dissection anteriorly may injure these nerves and compromise the continence status [20]. This dissection is carried to the level of the bladder neck, which can easily be identified by use of the Foley catheter balloon as a guide. The specimen is removed, and a frozen section analysis of the urethral margin is performed. If the urethral margin is negative for malignancy, orthotopic diversion can be performed. The vaginal stump is closed with a 2-0 polyglactin suture.

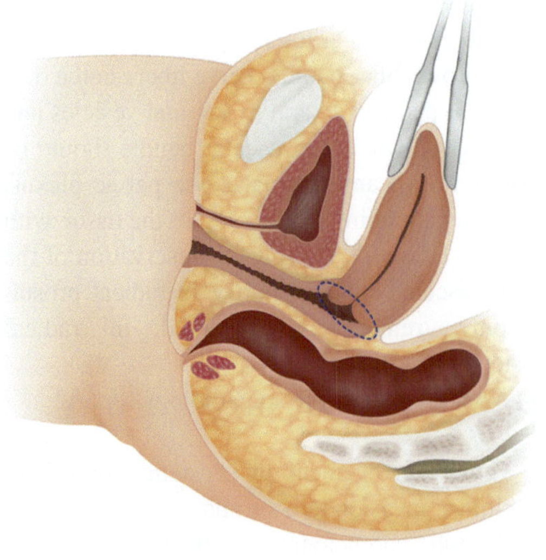

Fig. 15.9 During development of the posterior pedicles, the posterior vagina is incised at the cervical fornix

What do we need from pathology report?

1. Tumor involvement: vagina, uterine cervix, uterine corpus, fallopian tubes, and ovaries
2. Margins

Urethrectomy

Over the past 10 years, the indications for total urethrectomy at the time of cystectomy have undergone substantial modification. Historically urethrectomy was performed in patents with multifocal tumors, diffuse carcinoma in situ, and prostatic urethral involvement. In men, several studies have identified prostatic stromal invasion or diffuse CIS of the prostatic urethra as the primary risk factor. In women, the incidence of urethral tumors was low if there was no tumor in the bladder neck by careful histological studies [21]. Therefore, it is currently performed in patients with tumor involving the prostatic urethra in men or bladder neck in women. We perform intraoperative frozen section of the urethral margin prior to proceeding with neobladder construction. We routinely resect the urethra and anterior vaginal wall in women who are not candidates for neobladder diversion. In the male patient, urethrectomy is performed when prostate stromal invasion exists or frozen section of urethra is positive.

The patient should be placed in a lithotomy position. After placement of the Foley catheter, a vertical perineal incision can be made over the palpable urethral bulb. If greater exposure is necessary, an inverted U incision or a midline incision with lateral extension can be performed. The subcutaneous tissue and the bulbospongiosus muscle are divided along in the midline until the central perineal tendon and corpus spongiosum are encountered. Dissection should be done laterally around the corpus spongiosum. The corpus spongiosum should be completely isolated until the end of urethra is identified proximally. The distal urethra should be separated for the corpora cavernosa. The dissection should be carried up to the base of the glans. When this step is completed, we proceed to excise the distal urethra to remove the entire urethra en bloc. Then the distal urethra is excised, including the fossa navicularis, by wedge resection.

What do we need from pathology report?

1. Low-grade dysplasia vs. high-grade dysplasia/CIS vs. carcinoma with stromal invasion
2. Margins

Urinary Diversion

Once the bladder is removed, the urologist is confronted with a challenge in selecting the appropriate urinary diversion. These procedures can be divided into incontinent (ileal conduit and cutaneous urostomy) and continent procedures. The continent procedures can be further subdivided into cutaneous reservoirs (in which the reservoir is connected to the abdominal skin requiring intermittent catheterization) and orthotopic neobladder (in which the reservoir is connected to the urethra). Ileal conduits were the gold standard for urinary reconstruction before the advent of continent diversions, but continuously draining stoma can affect the quality of life of some patients. The urologist must analyze a variety of elements before selecting the optimal procedure for individual patient.

Incontinent Diversion (Ileal Conduit)

Incontinent urine diversion simply directs urine from the ureters through a segment of isolated bowel to the surface of the abdominal wall via a cutaneous stoma. There, urine drains continuously and is collected by an external appliance attached to the skin surface. The most common type of incontinent urinary diversion is an ileal conduit. A segment of ileum is selected; the terminal 15 to 20 cm of ileum at the ileocecal junction is typically preserved to maintain adequate absorption of nutrients. The 15–20-cm-long ileal segment is isolated, and the proximal end is closed with seromuscular running suture. The left ureter is passed over the aorta to the right paracaval area. The right ureter is dissected upward. The ileal segment is anastomosed with both ureters. The distal part of ileal segment is brought to the skin. It is sutured with the skin at eight sites.

Continent Diversion

All continent cutaneous reservoirs are made of a low-pressure pouch constructed of various detubularized bowel segments and use a functional mechanism that connects the reservoir to the skin designed to prevent involuntary urine flow. One of the continent cutaneous reservoirs is continent ileal reservoir (ileal W-reservoir and Mitrofanoff continent mechanism), and the most obvious advantage of this type of diversion is the ability to avoid continuous urine drainage with the need for an external appliance. This continent cutaneous diversion requires life-long intermittent clean self-catheterization through the stoma both to empty the reservoir and to remove mucus.

In patients with renal insufficiency (estimated glomerular filtration rate < 35 ml/min/1.73 m^2, serum creatinine levels >2.0 mg/L), orthotopic urinary diversion should be avoided. Ileal reservoirs (Hautmann W-neobladder, Studer, and Ghoneim) are the most common procedure. Koch ileocecal reservoirs, Indiana pouch, and Mainz pouch also can be used.

References

1. Bray F, Ferlay J, Soerjomataram I, Siegel RL, Torre LA, Jemal A. Global cancer statistics 2018: GLOBOCAN estimates of incidence and mortality worldwide for 36 cancers in 185 countries. CA Cancer J Clin. 2018;68(6):394–424.

2. Siegel RL, Miller KD, Jemal A. Cancer statistics, 2019. CA Cancer J Clin. 2020;70(1):7–29.
3. Shen PL, Lin ME, Hong YK, He XJ. Bladder preservation approach versus radical cystectomy for high-grade non-muscle-invasive bladder cancer: a meta-analysis of cohort studies. World J Surg Oncol. 2018;16(1):197.
4. Beer E. Landmark article May 28, 1910: removal of neoplasms of the urinary bladder. By Edwin Beer. JAMA. 1983;250(10):1324–5.
5. Khorrami MH, Javid A, Saryazdi H, Javid M. Transvesical blockade of the obturator nerve to prevent adductor contraction in transurethral bladder surgery. J Endourol. 2010;24(10):1651–4.
6. Venkatramani V, Panda A, Manojkumar R, Kekre NS. Monopolar versus bipolar transurethral resection of bladder tumors: a single center, parallel arm, randomized, controlled trial. J Urol. 2014;191(6):1703–7.
7. Xishuang S, Deyong Y, Xiangyu C, Tao J, Quanlin L, Hongwei G, et al. Comparing the safety and efficiency of conventional monopolar, plasmakinetic, and holmium laser transurethral resection of primary non-muscle invasive bladder cancer. J Endourol. 2010;24(1):69–73.
8. Labat G. Regional anesthesia; its technic and clinical application. Philadelphia/London: W. B. Saunders Company; 1922. xv, 496 p.
9. Bolat D, Aydogdu O, Tekgul ZT, Polat S, Yonguc T, Bozkurt IH, et al. Impact of nerve stimulator-guided obturator nerve block on the short-term outcomes and complications of transurethral resection of bladder tumour: a prospective randomized controlled study. Can Urol Assoc J. 2015;9(11–12):E780–4.
10. Shah NF, Sofi KP, Nengroo SH. Obturator nerve block in transurethral resection of bladder tumor: a comparison of ultrasound-guided technique versus ultrasound with nerve stimulation technique. Anesth Essays Res. 2017;11(2):411–5.
11. Wassef MR. Interadductor approach to obturator nerve blockade for spastic conditions of adductor thigh muscles. Reg Anesth. 1993;18(1):13–7.
12. Vianello A, Costantini E, Del Zingaro M, Bini V, Herr HW, Porena M. Repeated white light transurethral resection of the bladder in nonmuscle-invasive urothelial bladder cancers: systematic review and meta-analysis. J Endourol. 2011;25(11):1703–12.
13. Leveridge MJ, Siemens DR, Izard JP, Wei X, Booth CM. Partial cystectomy for urothelial carcinoma of the bladder: practice patterns and outcomes in the general population. Can Urol Assoc J. 2017;11(12):412–8.
14. Advanced Bladder Cancer Meta-analysis C. Neoadjuvant chemotherapy in invasive bladder cancer: update of a systematic review and meta-analysis of individual patient data advanced bladder cancer (ABC) meta-analysis collaboration. Eur Urol. 2005;48(2):202–205; discussion 5–6.
15. Grossman HB, Natale RB, Tangen CM, Speights VO, Vogelzang NJ, Trump DL, et al. Neoadjuvant chemotherapy plus cystectomy compared with cystectomy alone for locally advanced bladder cancer. N Engl J Med. 2003;349(9):859–66.
16. Ren L, Zhu D, Wei Y, Pan X, Liang L, Xu J, et al. Enhanced Recovery After Surgery (ERAS) program attenuates stress and accelerates recovery in patients after radical resection for colorectal cancer: a prospective randomized controlled trial. World J Surg. 2012;36(2):407–14.
17. Zmora O, Mahajna A, Bar-Zakai B, Rosin D, Hershko D, Shabtai M, et al. Colon and rectal surgery without mechanical bowel preparation: a randomized prospective trial. Ann Surg. 2003;237(3):363–7.
18. Brunocilla E, Pernetti R, Martorana G. The role of pelvic lymph node dissection during radical cystectomy for bladder cancer. Anticancer Res. 2011;31(1):271–5.
19. Herr HW, Bochner BH, Dalbagni G, Donat SM, Reuter VE, Bajorin DF. Impact of the number of lymph nodes retrieved on outcome in patients with muscle invasive bladder cancer. J Urol. 2002;167(3):1295–8.
20. Grossfeld GD, Stein JP, Bennett CJ, Ginsberg DA, Boyd SD, Lieskovsky G, et al. Lower urinary tract reconstruction in the female using the Kock ileal reservoir with bilateral ureteroileal urethrostomy: update of continence results and fluorourodynamic findings. Urology. 1996;48(3):383–8.
21. Kanaroglou A, Shayegan B. Management of the urethra in urothelial bladder cancer. Can Urol Assoc J. 2009;3(6 Suppl 4):S211–4.

Medical Treatment with Targeted Therapy for Metastatic Urothelial Bladder Carcinoma

16

Omar Alhalabi and Jianjun Gao

Introduction

Bladder cancer is the fourth most common cancer occurring in men and the 12th in women, with 81,400 new cases in 2020 in the USA and estimated 17,980 deaths [1]. While 75% of new urothelial carcinoma (UC) cases are non-muscle invasive, 25% of cases are muscle invasive or metastatic at presentation [2]. Traditionally, the 5-year survival for localized disease has been 68% compared to 5% in metastatic disease [3]. Muscle-invasiveness, multifocality, grade, and other risk factors help determine the further steps of management after endoscopic removal of localized tumors [4], which could include cystectomy. Cisplatin-based neoadjuvant chemotherapy has been shown to provide long-term survival benefit in patients with muscle invasive UC [5–10]. Similarly, platinum-based regimens remain the standard-of-care first-line therapy for platinum-eligible patients with metastatic UC [11], but they offer only a modest median overall survival (OS) of approximately 15 months [2, 12] and a very low 5-year survival of 4.8% [3]. Immune checkpoint therapy (ICT) finally shifted the paradigm with a better duration of response in platinum-refractory and platinum-ineligible frontline patients [13–20], although the majority of patients (about 75–80%) derive no benefit. In addition, antibody-drug conjugates (ADCs) targeting tumor-associated antigens (TAAs) in UC have shown promising results in patients failing platinum-based therapy and ICT [21]. Furthermore, genetic alterations involving the fibroblast growth factor receptor (FGFR) have been identified in about 15–20% of patients with advanced bladder UC and in close to 35% with upper tract UC [22–24]. There are several ongoing efforts to target these genetic alterations and better characterize distinct molecular subtypes of UC [25–28]. Here, we summarize the prominent strategies in targeted therapy for advanced-stage UC.

Discussion

Targeting Tumor-Associated Antigens (TAAs) Using Antibody-Drug Conjugates (ADCs)

ADCs are compounds that conjugate a monoclonal antibody targeting a specific TAA with a cytotoxic payload by a cleavable linker [29].

O. Alhalabi
Department of Genitourinary Medical Oncology, University of Texas MD Anderson Cancer Center, Houston, TX, USA
e-mail: oalhalabi@mdanderson.org

J. Gao (✉)
Department of Genitourinary Medical Oncology, The University of Texas MD Anderson Cancer Center, Houston, TX, USA
e-mail: JGao1@mdanderson.org

H. Zhou et al. (eds.), *Urinary Bladder Pathology*, https://doi.org/10.1007/978-3-030-71509-0_16

Following the binding of the antibody to the TAA on the surface of cancer cells, internalization of the conjugate occurs by way of endocytosis. Then the cytotoxic payload is released after lysosomal degradation [21]. The greatest challenge in using ADCs in solid tumors is the identification of specific antigen targets. Many TAAs are also expressed at a low level in healthy tissue, so internalization of the ADC could have serious toxicities. In UC, several TAAs have been studied as potentially attractive targets for ADC development (Fig. 16.1a), either as monotherapy or in combination with other therapeutic agents including ICT [21, 30].

Targeting Nectin-4 with Enfortumab Vedotin

Nectins [1 through 4] act as Ca2 + −independent cellular adhesion molecules [31]. In addition, nectin-4 is the epithelial receptor for the measles virus and has been investigated as serum tumor marker for several epithelial carcinomas, including ovarian, lung, and breast [32–35]. In particular, high nectin-4 mRNA expression levels were identified in bladder cancer [36]. The differential overexpression of nectin-4 in UC led to the development of enfortumab vedotin (EV). EV is a fully human antibody against nectin-4 linked via a cleavable drug linker to a microtubule-disrupting chemotherapy agent: monomethyl auristatin E (MMAE) (Fig. 16.1a, Table 16.1) [36]. In the phase I EV-101 dose-escalation trial (NCT02091999), 112 patients with metastatic UC were treated with 1.25 mg/kg of EV on days 1, 8, and 15 of a 28-day cycle [37]. Of the enrolled patients, 81% had received prior platinum therapy, and 75% had received prior ICT. In the most mature data report in 2019, confirmed overall response rate (RR) was 42%, median duration of response was 7.7 months, and median overall survival (OS) was 12.5 months [38]. The encouraging results from EV-101 were recaptured in the phase II trial EV-201 (NCT03219333), which showed a confirmed RR of 42% as a third-line therapy [39]. Treatment-related grade 3 or higher ($G \geq 3$) adverse events (AEs) included rash in 11% and peripheral neuropathy in 3%. On December 18, 2019, the US Food and Drug

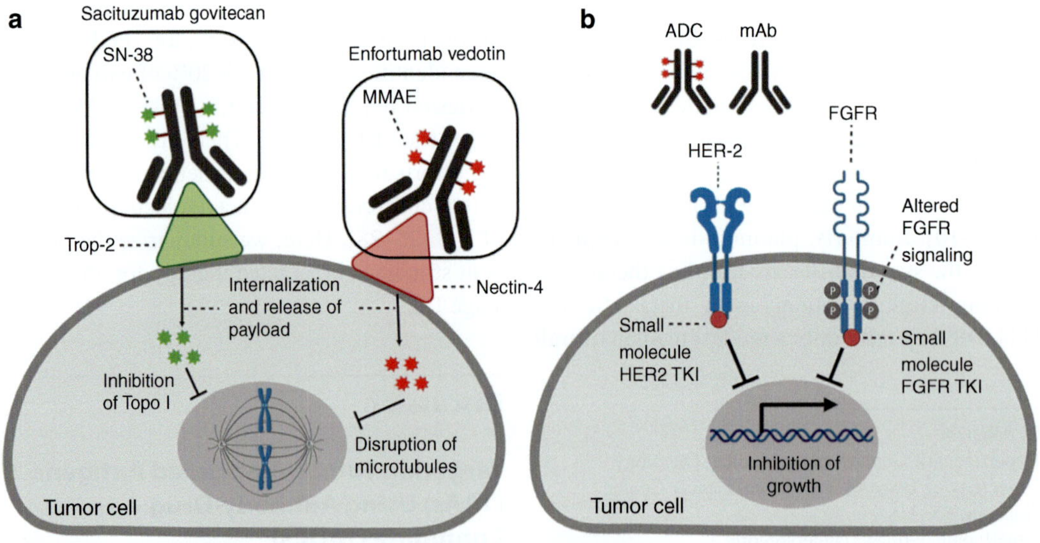

Fig. 16.1 Distinct strategies for targeting urothelial carcinoma. (**a**) Antibody drug conjugates (ADCs). Sacituzumab govitecan and enfortumab vedotin target trop-2 to deliver SN-38 and nectin-4 to deliver MMAE, respectively. SN-38 and MMAE have distinct mechanisms in inhibiting cellular growth and inducing apoptosis. (**b**) Mechanisms of targeting growth factor receptors in urothelial carcinoma. SN-38, active metabolite of irinotecan; Topo I, topoisomerase I; MMAE, monomethyl auristatin E; ADC, antibody drug conjugate; mAb, monoclonal antibody; HER-2, human epidermal growth factor receptor 2; FGFR, fibroblast growth factor receptor; TKI, tyrosine kinase inhibitor. (This figure was created using biorender.com)

Table 16.1 Characteristics of ADCs at or beyond phase I drug development in UC

ADC (alternative name)	Developer	Target TAA	Linker	Payload	Payload's mechanism of cytotoxicity
Enfortumab Vedotin	Seattle genetics and Astellas	Nectin-4	Protease-cleavable	Monomethyl auristatin E (MMAE)	Microtubule-disrupting agent
Sacituzumab Govitecan (IMMU-132)	Immunomedics	Trop-2	Protease-cleavable	Active metabolite of irinotecan (SN-38)	Topoisomerase I inhibitor leading to DNA damage
Sirtratumab vedotin (ASG-15ME)	Seattle genetics and Astellas	SLITRK6	Protease-cleavable	Monomethyl auristatin E (MMAE)	Microtubule-disrupting agent

Adapted from Alhalabi et al. (2019)

Administration (FDA) granted accelerated approval to EV in the third-line setting for patients with advanced UC who previously received anti-PD(L)-1 and a platinum-containing chemotherapy. A global, randomized, controlled, phase III trial EV-301 (NCT03474107) is ongoing to compare EV against standard single-agent chemotherapy in patients with locally advanced or metastatic UC previously treated with platinum chemotherapy and anti-PD-1/PD-L1. Furthermore, EV combined with pembrolizumab is being tested as a "chemotherapy-free" regimen in the frontline setting for cisplatin-ineligible patients with locally advanced or metastatic UC in the EV-103 trial (NCT03288545). Preliminary data presented at the American Society of Clinical Oncology (ASCO) Genitourinary Cancers Symposium 2020 (San Francisco, CA) showed an overall RR of 73.3% including 15.6% complete response. The overall RR in patients with liver metastasis was 53.3% (8/15) [40].

Targeting trop-2 with Sacituzumab Govitecan

Trophoblast cell-surface antigen 2 (Trop-2) is overexpressed in several carcinomas, including breast carcinoma and UC [41–43]. In UC, expression of trop-2 correlates with invasiveness of tumors, advanced clinical stage [44], and worse prognosis [45]. Sacituzumab govitecan (SG) is a humanized antibody against Trop-2 linked to the cytotoxic payload SN-38 (active metabolite of irinotecan), which inhibits topoisomerase I, leading to DNA damage and cellular death (Fig. 16.1a, Table 16.1) [46, 47]. In a phase I/II study (NCT03547973), 45 patients with metastatic UC who progressed after ≥1 prior systemic therapy were treated with SG 10 mg/kg on days 1 and 8 of a 21-day cycle. Overall RR was 31%, duration of response was 12.9 months, and OS was 18.9 months [48]. Grade ≥ 3 AEs were neutropenia (38%), anemia (11%), hypophosphatemia (11%), diarrhea (9%), fatigue (9%), and febrile neutropenia (7%). Along with grade 4 neutropenia or febrile neutropenia, 65% had a polymorphism in UGT1A1, which is higher than expected for an unselected patient population and could explain the relatively high rate of neutropenia [49].

Targeting SLITRK6 with Sirtratumab Vedotin (ASG-15ME)

SLIT and NTRK expression, like that of family member 6 (SLITRK6), was seen in 88% of bladder cancer specimens based on a tissue microarray that involved more than 500 samples [50]. Sirtratumab vedotin (SV) is composed of a SLITRK6-specific human antibody conjugated to MMAE via a protease-cleavable linker [50]. NCT01963052 was a phase I dose-escalation trial that had 42 evaluable patients treated at doses considered active (≥0.5 mg/kg) for SV; overall RR was 33%, including 4/11 patients (36%) with liver metastases and 5/12 patients (42%) who failed prior ICT [51].

Targeting Growth Factor Receptors

Targeting the Fibroblast Growth Factor Receptor (FGFR) with Tyrosine Kinase Inhibitors (TKIs)

In bladder cancer, aberrations in the FGFR signaling pathway, particularly *FGFR1* and *FGFR3* genetic aberrations, have been linked to oncogenesis and tumor angiogenesis [52, 53]. The expression of a constitutively activated FGFR3 in UC and its oncogenic role was first established 20 years ago [54]. According to The Cancer Genome Atlas (TCGA) data, which includes 412 muscle-invasive UC primary tumors, *FGFR3* alterations have a 14% frequency and cluster in the luminal I subtype [23]. Multiple mechanisms, such as mutations and fusions, are involved in FGFR3 pathway dysregulation and lead to constitutive activation of the kinase domain of FGFR3 [55]. Here, we summarize the data on small-molecule FGFR TKIs that are FDA approved or in an advanced phase of investigation in UC (Fig. 16.1b, Table 16.2).

Table 16.2 Examples of fibroblast growth factor receptor (FGFR) tyrosine kinase inhibitors (TKIs) that are being tested in UC

Compound (alternative name)	Spectrum of FGFR inhibition	Recombinant FGFR3 IC_{50} (nmol/L, in vitro)	Developer
AZD4547 [56]	1,2,3	1.8	AstraZeneca
Dovitinib (CHIR258, TKI258) [72]	1,3	500	Novartis
Erdafitinib (JNJ-42756493) [73]	1,2,3,4	3.1	Janssen
BAY1163877 (rogaratinib) [74]	1,2,3	19	Bayer
BGJ398 (infigratinib) [75]	1,2,3	1	Novartis
INCB054828 (pemigatinib) [76]	1,2,3	1	Incyte

AZD4547

AZD4547 is an FGFR1–3 inhibitor [56] studied in the BISCAY trial (NCT02546661), which enrolled patients with UC who progressed on prior platinum therapy. Patients who had activating *FGFR1–3* mutations or fusions received AZD4547 with or without durvalumab. Patients with mutations in homologous recombination repair genes were assigned to receive olaparib with durvalumab. Patients with RICTOR amplification or deleterious mutations in *TSC1* or *TSC2* were assigned to vistusertib with durvalumab. Finally, an unselected arm was assigned to durvalumab monotherapy alone to serve as a control arm to interpret RRs in the other arms [57]. AZD4547 had activity in the *FGFR* mutants with RR of 20% [57]; however, it was not statistically different from durvalumab plus AZD4547 with RR of 28.6%.

Dovitinib

Dovitinib (TKI258) is a broad-targeted inhibitor of tyrosine kinases, including FGFR3, which was evaluated in patients with previously treated advanced FGFR3-mutated or FGFR3 – wild-type UC [58]. The study was terminated as dovitinib had very limited single-agent activity (RR 0% in FGFR3-mutated and 3.2% in FGFR3 – wild type) among patients with previously treated advanced UC. Agents that are more specific have been prioritized over dovitinib in UC.

Erdafitinib

Erdafitinib (JNJ-42756493) is a pan-FGFR [1 through 4] inhibitor approved by the FDA on April 12, 2019, for the treatment of metastatic UC with susceptible *FGFR2* or *FGFR3* genetic alterations after platinum failure. The FDA also approved the therascreen® FGFR RGQ RT-PCR Kit, developed by QIAGEN, for use as a companion diagnostic for this therapeutic indication [59]. In a phase I study using intermittent dosing of erdafitinib, 21% of UC patients responded, and dose-dependent elevations in serum phosphate were found to represent a pharmacodynamic effect of the medication [60]. The FDA approval was based on the results of the BLC2001 phase II trial of erdafitinib in advanced UC [24]. In this trial, erdafitinib was given at 8 mg per day in a continuous regimen, and dose was escalated to 9 mg if the serum phosphate level had not reached the target of 5.5 mg per deciliter (1.8 mmol/L), a level that had been associated with an improved RR in the phase I study. The rate of confirmed overall RR was 40%, and disease control rate (DCR) was 79% [24]. Median time to response was around 6 weeks, indicating quick responses. Among patients with prior ICT, RR was 59%. The median PFS was 5.5 months, and the median OS was 13.8 months. AEs were manageable: 13% of patients discontinued therapy due to treatment-related adverse events (TRAEs), and there were no treatment-related deaths [24]. Common G $\geq$ 3 AEs were hyponatremia (11%), stomatitis (10%), and asthenia (7%). To clarify the ideal sequence of erdafitinib and ICT in the second-line setting, the phase 3 THOR trial (NCT03390504) is comparing erdafitinib to chemotherapy or pembrolizumab for patients with platinum-refractory advanced UC with selected *FGFR* gene alterations. Furthermore, NCT03473743 is a phase Ib/II trial assessing the combination of erdafitinib plus cetrelimab (JNJ-63723283; anti-PD-1) in cisplatin-ineligible patients with metastatic UC harboring selected *FGFR* gene alterations.

Rogaratinib

Rogaratinib (BAY1163877) is an oral pan-FGFR inhibitor that was studied in patients with UC and high FGFR1–3 mRNA expression levels, with particular attention to activity in patients with evidence of activating mutations in potential resistance genes, including *PIK3CA* and *RAS*. NCT01976741 showed an overall RR of 24%, and DCR was 73% [61]. FORT-2 (NCT03473756) is a phase Ib/II trial of rogaratinib plus atezolizumab in the frontline setting for cisplatin-ineligible, untreated, FGFR-positive metastatic UC.

Infigratinib

Infigratinib (BGJ398) is a potent, FGFR1–3 inhibitor that initially demonstrated antitumor activity in four of five patients with *FGFR3-mutated* advanced UC when it was in phase I testing [62]. Sixty-seven patients who were platinum-ineligible were subsequently enrolled in the expansion cohort. The majority (70.1%) had received two or more prior treatments. Overall RR was 25.4% and DCR was 64.2%. The most common treatment-emergent toxicities were hyperphosphatemia, elevated creatinine, fatigue, constipation, and decreased appetite [63].

Pemigatinib

Pemigatinib (NCT02872714) is a potent, selective, oral inhibitor of FGFR1–3. FIGHT-201 was a phase II, open-label, multicenter study of pemigatinib in patients with metastatic or unresectable UC harboring *FGFR3* genetic alterations (cohort A) or other *FGFR* alterations (cohort B). Overall RR was 25% in cohort A and 3% in cohort B [64].

Targeting the Human Epidermal Growth Factor Receptor 2 (HER2)

Molecular alterations involving the human epidermal growth factor receptor (including amplification, mutation, and overexpression) occur in up to 20–30% of UC patients [23]. HER2 alterations have gained significant interest in the past few years with agents specifically targeting this receptor in UC. HER2-targeted agents investigated in clinical trials of UC have various mechanisms of action, including (Fig. 16.1b) (a) monoclonal antibodies such as trastuzumab [65, 66]; (b) HER2 TKIs such as lapatinib [67], afatinib [68], and neratinib [69]; and (c) an ADC targeted against HER2 such as T-DM1 [70], as well as other investigational agents. A limitation to the clinical translation of HER2 as a predictive biomarker has been the discordance between HER2 immunohistochemistry (IHC) score, fluorescence in situ hybridization (FISH), and genomic-level molecular characterization [71]. However, with proper biomarkers and well-designed clinical trials, HER2-targeted agents could be an important part of the management of early or advanced UC, either as monotherapy or in combination with other agents.

Summary

With the FDA approval of an FGFR inhibitor and an ADC in 2019, targeted therapy strategies finally became a reality for patients with metastatic UC. Research efforts continue to identify new therapeutic targets, biomarkers of response, and mechanisms of resistance, thus leading to continued accumulation of our armamentarium against UC at the frontline and subsequent lines of therapy.

References

1. Siegel RL, Miller KD, Jemal A. Cancer statistics, 2020. CA Cancer J Clin. 2020;70(1):7–30. Epub 2020/01/09. https://doi.org/10.3322/caac.21590.
2. Kamat AM, Hahn NM, Efstathiou JA, Lerner SP, Malmström P-U, Choi W, Guo CC, Lotan Y, Kassouf W. Bladder cancer. Lancet. 2016;388(10061):2796–810. https://doi.org/10.1016/s0140-6736(16)30512-8.
3. NCI. Surveillance, epidemiology, and end results program. Cancer stat facts: bladder cancer 2018, cited 4 July 2018. Available from: https://seer.cancer.gov/statfacts/html/urinb.html
4. Herr HW, Sogani PC. Does early cystectomy improve the survival of patients with high risk superficial bladder tumors? J Urol. 2001;166(4):1296–9. Epub 2001/09/08
5. Plimack ER, Hoffman-Censits JH, Viterbo R, Trabulsi EJ, Ross EA, Greenberg RE, Chen DY, Lallas CD, Wong YN, Lin J, Kutikov A, Dotan E, Brennan TA, Palma N, Dulaimi E, Mehrazin R, Boorjian SA, Kelly WK, Uzzo RG, Hudes GR. Accelerated methotrexate, vinblastine, doxorubicin, and cisplatin is safe, effective, and efficient neoadjuvant treatment for muscle-invasive bladder cancer: results of a multicenter phase II study with molecular correlates of response and toxicity. J Clin Oncol Off J Am Soc Clin Oncol. 2014;32(18):1895–901. https://doi.org/10.1200/JCO.2013.53.2465. PubMed PMID: 24821881; PMCID: 4050203
6. Griffiths G, Hall R, Sylvester R, Raghavan D, Parmar MK. International phase III trial assessing neoadjuvant cisplatin, methotrexate, and vinblastine chemotherapy for muscle-invasive bladder cancer: long-term results of the BA06 30894 trial. J Clin Oncol Off J Am Soc Clin Oncol. 2011;29(16):2171–7. Epub 2011/04/20. 10.1200/jco.2010.32.3139. PubMed PMID: 21502557; PMCID: PMC3107740
7. Iyer G, Balar AV, Milowsky MI, Bochner BH, Dalbagni G, Donat SM, Herr HW, Huang WC, Taneja SS, Woods M, Ostrovnaya I, Al-Ahmadie H, Arcila ME, Riches JC, Meier A, Bourque C, Shady M, Won H, Rose TL, Kim WY, Kania BE, Boyd ME, Cipolla CK, Regazzi AM, Delbeau D, AS MC, Vargas HA, Berger MF, Solit DB, Rosenberg JE, Bajorin DF. Multicenter Prospective Phase II Trial of Neoadjuvant Dose-Dense Gemcitabine Plus Cisplatin in Patients With Muscle-Invasive Bladder Cancer. J Clin Oncol. 2018;36(19):1949–56. https://doi.org/10.1200/JCO.2017.75.0158.
8. Grossman HB, Natale RB, Tangen CM, Speights VO, Vogelzang NJ, Trump DL, deVere White RW, Sarosdy MF, Wood DP, Jr., Raghavan D, Crawford ED. Neoadjuvant chemotherapy plus cystectomy compared with cystectomy alone for locally advanced bladder cancer. N Engl J Med 2003;349(9):859–66. Epub 2003/08/29. https://doi.org/10.1056/NEJMoa022148349/9/859 [pii].
9. Sonpavde G, Goldman BH, Speights VO, Lerner SP, Wood DP, Vogelzang NJ, Trump DL, Natale RB, Grossman HB, Crawford ED. Quality of pathologic response and surgery correlate with survival for patients with completely resected bladder cancer after neoadjuvant chemotherapy. Cancer. 2009;115(18):4104–9. https://doi.org/10.1002/cncr.24466.
10. Rosenblatt R, Sherif A, Rintala E, Wahlqvist R, Ullen A, Nilsson S, Malmstrom PU. Pathologic downstaging is a surrogate marker for efficacy and increased survival following neoadjuvant chemotherapy and radical cystectomy for muscle-invasive urothelial bladder cancer. Eur Urol. 2012;61(6):1229–38. Epub 2011/12/23. https://doi.org/10.1016/j.eururo.2011.12.010.
11. Network NCC. Clinical practice guidelines in oncology: bladder cancer 2019, updated 7/10/19; cited 2019 8/1/19; Version 4.2019: NCCN clinical practice guidelines in oncology: bladder cancer, 2019. Available from: https://www.nccn.org/professionals/physician_gls/pdf/bladder.pdf
12. von der Maase H, Hansen SW, Roberts JT, Dogliotti L, Oliver T, Moore MJ, Bodrogi I, Albers P, Knuth A, Lippert CM, Kerbrat P, Rovira PS, Wersall P, Cleall SP, Roychowdhury DF, Tomlin I, Visseren-Grul CM, Conte PF. Gemcitabine and cisplatin versus methotrexate, vinblastine, doxorubicin, and cisplatin in advanced or metastatic bladder cancer: results of a large, randomized, multinational, multicenter, phase III study. J Clin Oncol. 2000; (0732-183X (Print))
13. Patel MR, Ellerton J, Infante JR, Agrawal M, Gordon M, Aljumaily R, Britten CD, Dirix L, Lee K-W, Taylor M, Schöffski P, Wang D, Ravaud A, Gelb AB, Xiong J, Rosen G, Gulley JL, Apolo AB. Avelumab in metastatic urothelial carcinoma after platinum failure (JAVELIN solid tumor): pooled results from two expansion cohorts of an open-label, phase 1 trial. Lancet Oncol. 2018;19(1):51–64. https://doi.org/10.1016/S1470-2045(17)30900-2.
14. Powles T, O'Donnell PH, Massard C, et al. Efficacy and safety of durvalumab in locally advanced or metastatic urothelial carcinoma: updated results from a phase 1/2 open-label study. JAMA Oncol. 2017;3(9):e172411. https://doi.org/10.1001/jamaoncol.2017.2411.

15. Rosenberg JE, Hoffman-Censits J, Powles T, van der Heijden MS, Balar AV, Necchi A, Dawson N, O'Donnell PH, Balmanoukian A, Loriot Y, Srinivas S, Retz MM, Grivas P, Joseph RW, Galsky MD, Fleming MT, Petrylak DP, Perez-Gracia JL, Burris HA, Castellano D, Canil C, Bellmunt J, Bajorin D, Nickles D, Bourgon R, Frampton GM, Cui N, Mariathasan S, Abidoye O, Fine GD, Dreicer R. Atezolizumab in patients with locally advanced and metastatic urothelial carcinoma who have progressed following treatment with platinum-based chemotherapy: a single-arm, multicentre, phase 2 trial. Lancet. 2016;387(10031):1909–20. https://doi.org/10.1016/S0140-6736(16)00561-4.
16. Sharma P, Callahan MK, Bono P, Kim J, Spiliopoulou P, Calvo E, Pillai RN, Ott PA, de Braud F, Morse M, Le DT, Jaeger D, Chan E, Harbison C, Lin CS, Tschaika M, Azrilevich A, Rosenberg JE. Nivolumab monotherapy in recurrent metastatic urothelial carcinoma (CheckMate 032): a multicentre, open-label, two-stage, multi-arm, phase 1/2 trial. Lancet Oncol. 2016;17(11):1590–8. Epub 2016/10/14. https://doi.org/10.1016/s1470-2045(16)30496-x. PubMed PMID: 27733243; PMCID: PMC5648054
17. Powles T, Eder JP, Fine GD, Braiteh FS, Loriot Y, Cruz C, Bellmunt J, Burris HA, Petrylak DP. Teng S-l, Shen X, Boyd Z, Hegde PS, Chen DS, Vogelzang NJ. MPDL3280A (anti-PD-L1) treatment leads to clinical activity in metastatic bladder cancer. Nature. 2014;515:558. https://doi.org/10.1038/nature13904.
18. Apolo AB, Infante JR, Balmanoukian A, Patel MR, Wang D, Kelly K, Mega AE, Britten CD, Ravaud A, Mita AC, Safran H, Stinchcombe TE, Srdanov M, Gelb AB, Schlichting M, Chin K, Gulley JL. Avelumab, an anti–programmed death-ligand 1 antibody, in patients with refractory metastatic urothelial carcinoma: results from a multicenter, phase Ib study. J Clin Oncol. 2017;35(19):2117–24. https://doi.org/10.1200/JCO.2016.71.6795.
19. Balar AV, Castellano D, O'Donnell PH, Grivas P, Vuky J, Powles T, Plimack ER, Hahn NM, de Wit R, Pang L, Savage MJ, Perini RF, Keefe SM, Bajorin D, Bellmunt J. First-line pembrolizumab in cisplatin-ineligible patients with locally advanced and unresectable or metastatic urothelial cancer (KEYNOTE-052): a multicentre, single-arm, phase 2 study. Lancet Oncol. 2017;18(11):1483–92. https://doi.org/10.1016/S1470-2045(17)30616-2.
20. Bellmunt J, de Wit R, Vaughn DJ, Fradet Y, Lee J-L, Fong L, Vogelzang NJ, Climent MA, Petrylak DP, Choueiri TK, Necchi A, Gerritsen W, Gurney H, Quinn DI, Culine S, Sternberg CN, Mai Y, Poehlein CH, Perini RF, Bajorin DF. Pembrolizumab as second-line therapy for advanced urothelial carcinoma. N Engl J Med. 2017;376(11):1015–26. https://doi.org/10.1056/NEJMoa1613683.
21. Nagayama A, Ellisen LW, Chabner B, Bardia A. Antibody-drug conjugates for the treatment of solid tumors: clinical experience and latest developments. Target Oncol. 2017;12(6):719–39. Epub 2017/11/09. https://doi.org/10.1007/s11523-017-0535-0.
22. Iyer G, Al-Ahmadie H, Schultz N, Hanrahan AJ, Ostrovnaya I, Balar AV, Kim PH, Lin O, Weinhold N, Sander C, Zabor EC, Janakiraman M, Garcia-Grossman IR, Heguy A, Viale A, Bochner BH, Reuter VE, Bajorin DF, Milowsky MI, Taylor BS, Solit DB. Prevalence and co-occurrence of actionable genomic alterations in high-grade bladder cancer. J Clin Oncol Off J Am Soc Clin Oncol. 2013;31(25):3133–40. Epub 2013/07/31. https://doi.org/10.1200/jco.2012.46.5740. PubMed PMID: 23897969; PMCID: PMC3753703.
23. Robertson AG, Kim J, Al-Ahmadie H, Bellmunt J, Guo G, Cherniack AD, Hinoue T, Laird PW, Hoadley KA, Akbani R, Castro MAA, Gibb EA, Kanchi RS, Gordenin DA, Shukla SA, Sanchez-Vega F, Hansel DE, Czerniak BA, Reuter VE, Su X, de Sa Carvalho B, Chagas VS, Mungall KL, Sadeghi S, Pedamallu CS, Lu Y, Klimczak LJ, Zhang J, Choo C, Ojesina AI, Bullman S, Leraas KM, Lichtenberg TM, Wu CJ, Schultz N, Getz G, Meyerson M, Mills GB, McConkey DJ, Weinstein JN, Kwiatkowski DJ, Lerner SP. Comprehensive molecular characterization of muscle-invasive bladder cancer. Cell. 2017;171(3):540–56.e25. Epub 2017/10/11. https://doi.org/10.1016/j.cell.2017.09.007. PubMed PMID: 28988769; PMCID: PMC5687509.
24. Loriot Y, Necchi A, Park SH, Garcia-Donas J, Huddart R, Burgess E, Fleming M, Rezazadeh A, Mellado B, Varlamov S, Joshi M, Duran I, Tagawa ST, Zakharia Y, Zhong B, Stuyckens K, Santiago-Walker A, De Porre P, O'Hagan A, Avadhani A, Siefker-Radtke AO. Erdafitinib in locally advanced or metastatic urothelial carcinoma. N Engl J Med. 2019;381(4):338–48. https://doi.org/10.1056/NEJMoa1817323.
25. Choi W, Czerniak B, Ochoa A, Su X, Siefker-Radtke A, Dinney C, McConkey DJ. Intrinsic basal and luminal subtypes of muscle-invasive bladder cancer. Nat Rev Urol. 2014;11(7):400–10. https://doi.org/10.1038/nrurol.2014.129.
26. McConkey DCW, Shen Y, Lee I, Porten S, Matin S, Kamat A, Corn P, Millikan R, Dinney C, Czerniak B, Siefker-Radtke A. A prognostic gene expression signature in the molecular classification of chemotherapy-naive urothelial Cancer is predictive of clinical outcomes from neoadjuvant chemotherapy: a phase 2 trial of dose-dense methotrexate, vinblastine, doxorubicin, and cisplatin with bevacizumab in urothelial cancer. Eur Urol. 2016;69:855–62.
27. McConkey DJ, Choi W, Ochoa A, Siefker-Radtke A, Czerniak B, Dinney CP. Therapeutic opportunities in the intrinsic subtypes of muscle-invasive bladder cancer. Hematol Oncol Clin North Am 2015;29(2):377–94, x–xi. Epub 2015/04/04. https://doi.org/10.1016/j.hoc.2014.11.003.
28. Choi W, Porten S, Kim S, Willis D, Plimack Elizabeth R, Hoffman-Censits J, Roth B, Cheng T, Tran M, Lee IL, Melquist J, Bondaruk J, Majewski T, Zhang S,

Pretzsch S, Baggerly K, Siefker-Radtke A, Czerniak B, Dinney Colin PN, McConkey DJ. Identification of distinct basal and luminal subtypes of muscle-invasive bladder cancer with different sensitivities to frontline chemotherapy. Cancer Cell. 2014;25(2):152–65. https://doi.org/10.1016/j.ccr.2014.01.009.
29. Vlachostergios PJ, Jakubowski CD, Niaz MJ, Lee A, Thomas C, Hackett AL, Patel P, Rashid N, Tagawa ST. Antibody-drug conjugates in bladder cancer. Bladder Cancer (Amsterdam, Netherlands). 2018;4(3):247–59. https://doi.org/10.3233/BLC-180169.
30. Alhalabi O, Rafei H, Shah A, Siefker-Radtke A, Campbell M, Gao J. Targeting advanced urothelial carcinoma-developing strategies Current opinion in oncology 2019. Epub 2019/03/08. https://doi.org/10.1097/cco.0000000000000532.
31. Samanta D, Almo SC. Nectin family of cell-adhesion molecules: structural and molecular aspects of function and specificity. Cell Mol Life Sci 2015;72(4):645–58. Epub 2014/10/20. https://doi.org/10.1007/s00018-014-1763-4.
32. Mühlebach MD, Mateo M, Sinn PL, Prüfer S, Uhlig KM, Leonard VHJ, Navaratnarajah CK, Frenzke M, Wong XX, Sawatsky B, Ramachandran S, McCray PB, Cichutek K, von Messling V, Lopez M, Cattaneo R. Adherens junction protein nectin-4 is the epithelial receptor for measles virus. Nature 2011;480:530. https://doi.org/10.1038/nature10639.; https://www.nature.com/articles/nature10639#supplementary-information.
33. Derycke MS, Pambuccian SE, Gilks CB, Kalloger SE, Ghidouche A, Lopez M, Bliss RL, Geller MA, Argenta PA, Harrington KM, Skubitz AP. Nectin 4 overexpression in ovarian cancer tissues and serum: potential role as a serum biomarker. Am J Clin Pathol. 2010;134(5):835–45. Epub 2010/10/21. https://doi.org/10.1309/ajcpgxk0fr4mhihb. PubMed PMID: 20959669; PMCID: PMC3042138.
34. Fabre-Lafay S, Garrido-Urbani S, Reymond N, Goncalves A, Dubreuil P, Lopez M. Nectin-4, a new serological breast cancer marker, is a substrate for tumor necrosis factor-alpha-converting enzyme (TACE)/ADAM-17. J Biol Chem. 2005;280(20):19543–50. Epub 2005/03/24. https://doi.org/10.1074/jbc.M410943200.
35. Takano A, Ishikawa N, Nishino R, Masuda K, Yasui W, Inai K, Nishimura H, Ito H, Nakayama H, Miyagi Y, Tsuchiya E, Kohno N, Nakamura Y, Daigo Y. Identification of nectin-4 oncoprotein as a diagnostic and therapeutic target for lung cancer. Cancer Res. 2009;69(16):6694–703. Epub 2009/08/15. https://doi.org/10.1158/0008-5472.Can-09-0016.
36. Challita-Eid PM, Satpayev D, Yang P, An Z, Morrison K, Shostak Y, Raitano A, Nadell R, Liu W, Lortie DR, Capo L, Verlinsky A, Leavitt M, Malik F, Avina H, Guevara CI, Dinh N, Karki S, Anand BS, Pereira DS, Joseph IB, Donate F, Morrison K, Stover DR. Enfortumab Vedotin antibody-drug conjugate targeting Nectin-4 is a highly potent therapeutic agent in multiple preclinical Cancer models. Cancer Res. 2016;76(10):3003–13. Epub 2016/03/26. https://doi.org/10.1158/0008-5472.Can-15-1313.
37. Rosenberg JE, Sridhar SS, Zhang J, Smith DC, Ruether JD, Flaig TW, Baranda JC, Lang JM, Plimack ER, Sangha RS, Heath EI, Merchan JR, Quinn DI, Srinivas S, Milowsky MI, Wu C, Gartner EM, Melhem-Bertrandt A, Petrylak DP. Updated results from the enfortumab vedotin phase 1 (EV-101) study in patients with metastatic urothelial cancer (mUC). J Clin Oncol. 2018;36(15_suppl) https://doi.org/10.1200/JCO.2018.36.15_suppl.4504.
38. Rosenberg JE, Sridhar SS, Zhang J, Smith DC, Ruether JD, Flaig TW, Baranda JC, Lang JM, Plimack ER, Sangha RS, Heath EI, Merchan JR, Quinn DI, Srinivas S, Milowsky MI, Wu C, Gartner EM, Melhem-Bertrandt A, Petrylak DP. Mature results from EV-101: a phase I study of enfortumab vedotin in patients with metastatic urothelial cancer (mUC). J Clin Oncol. 2019;37(7_suppl):377. https://doi.org/10.1200/JCO.2019.37.7_suppl.377.
39. Rosenberg JE, Heath EI, O'Donnell PH, Hahn NM, Balar AV, Gartner EM, Melhem-Bertrandt A, Petrylak DP. EV-201 study: a single-arm, open-label, multicenter study of enfortumab vedotin for treatment of patients with locally advanced or metastatic urothelial cancer who previously received immune checkpoint inhibitor therapy. J Clin Oncol. 2018;36(15_suppl):TPS4590-TPS. https://doi.org/10.1200/JCO.2018.36.15_suppl.TPS4590.
40. Rosenberg JE, Flaig TW, Friedlander TW, Milowsky MI, Srinivas S, Petrylak DP, Merchan JR, Bilen MA, Carret A-S, Yuan N, Sasse C, Hoimes CJ. Study EV-103: preliminary durability results of enfortumab vedotin plus pembrolizumab for locally advanced or metastatic urothelial carcinoma. J Clin Oncol. 2020;38(6_suppl):441. https://doi.org/10.1200/JCO.2020.38.6_suppl.441.
41. Shvartsur A, Bonavida B. Trop2 and its overexpression in cancers: regulation and clinical/therapeutic implications. Genes Cancer. 2015;6(3–4):84–105. https://doi.org/10.18632/genesandcancer.40.
42. Stepan LP, Trueblood ES, Hale K, Babcook J, Borges L, Sutherland CL. Expression of Trop2 cell surface glycoprotein in normal and tumor tissues: potential implications as a cancer therapeutic target. J Histochem Cytochem. 2011;59(7):701–10. Epub 2011/05/10. https://doi.org/10.1369/0022155411410430. PubMed PMID: 21551320; PMCID: PMC3201164.
43. Trerotola M, Cantanelli P, Guerra E, Tripaldi R, Aloisi AL, Bonasera V, Lattanzio R, de Lange R, Weidle UH, Piantelli M, Alberti S. Upregulation of Trop-2 quantitatively stimulates human cancer growth. Oncogene. 2013;32(2):222–33. Epub 2012/02/22. https://doi.org/10.1038/onc.2012.36.
44. Avellini C, Licini C, Lazzarini R, Gesuita R, Guerra E, Tossetta G, Castellucci C, Giannubilo SR, Procopio A, Alberti S, Mazzucchelli R, Olivieri F, Marzioni D. The trophoblast cell surface antigen 2 and miR-125b axis in urothelial bladder cancer. Oncotarget. 2017;8(35):58642–53. Epub 2017/09/25. https://doi.

org/10.18632/oncotarget.17407. PubMed PMID: 28938585; PMCID: PMC5601681.
45. Lin H, Huang JF, Qiu JR, Zhang HL, Tang XJ, Li H, Wang CJ, Wang ZC, Feng ZQ, Zhu J. Significantly upregulated TACSTD2 and cyclin D1 correlate with poor prognosis of invasive ductal breast cancer. Exp Mol Pathol. 2013;94(1):73–8. Epub 2012/10/04. https://doi.org/10.1016/j.yexmp.2012.08.004.
46. Starodub AN, Ocean AJ, Shah MA, Guarino MJ, Picozzi VJ, Vahdat LT, Thomas SS, Govindan SV, Maliakal PP, Wegener WA, Hamburger SA, Sharkey RM, Goldenberg DM. First-in-human trial of a novel anti-Trop-2 antibody-SN-38 conjugate, Sacituzumab Govitecan, for the treatment of diverse metastatic solid tumors. Clin Cancer Res. 2015;21(17):3870. https://doi.org/10.1158/1078-0432.CCR-14-3321.
47. Cardillo TM, Govindan SV, Sharkey RM, Trisal P, Goldenberg DM. Humanized anti-Trop-2 IgG-SN-38 conjugate for effective treatment of diverse epithelial cancers: preclinical studies in human Cancer xenograft models and monkeys. Clin Cancer Res. 2011;17(10):3157.
48. Tagawa ST, Faltas BM, Lam ET, Saylor PJ, Bardia A, Hajdenberg J, Morgans AK, Lim EA, Kalinsky K, Simpson PS, Galsky MD, Goswam T, Wegener WA, Petrylak DP. Sacituzumab govitecan (IMMU-132) in patients with previously treated metastatic urothelial cancer (mUC): results from a phase I/II study. J Clin Oncol. 2019;37(7_suppl):354. https://doi.org/10.1200/JCO.2019.37.7_suppl.354.
49. Ocean AJ, Starodub AN, Bardia A, Vahdat LT, Isakoff SJ, Guarino M, Messersmith WA, Picozzi VJ, Mayer IA, Wegener WA, Maliakal P, Govindan SV, Sharkey RM, Goldenberg DM. Sacituzumab govitecan (IMMU-132), an anti-Trop-2-SN-38 antibody-drug conjugate for the treatment of diverse epithelial cancers: safety and pharmacokinetics. Cancer. 2017;123(19):3843–54. https://doi.org/10.1002/cncr.30789.
50. Morrison K, Challita-Eid PM, Raitano A, An Z, Yang P, Abad JD, Liu W, Lortie DR, Snyder JT, Capo L, Verlinsky A, Aviña H, Doñate F, Joseph IBJ, Pereira DS, Morrison K, Stover DR. Development of ASG-15ME, a novel antibody–drug conjugate targeting *SLITRK6*, a new urothelial cancer biomarker. Mol Cancer Ther. 2016;15(6):1301.
51. Melhem-Bertrandt A, Morgans AK, Anand B, Eigl BJ, Petrylak D, Gartner E, Heath E, Yu EY, Sonpavde G, Picus J, Morrison K, Jackson L, Vincent M, Chu R, Cheng S, George S, Hotte SJ. Interim analysis of a phase I dose escalation trial of the antibody drug conjugate (ADC) AGS15E (ASG-15ME) in patients (Pts) with metastatic urothelial cancer (mUC). Ann Oncol. 2016;27(suppl_6). https://doi.org/10.1093/annonc/mdw373.08.
52. Dieci MV, Arnedos M, Andre F, Soria JC. Fibroblast growth factor receptor inhibitors as a cancer treatment: from a biologic rationale to medical perspectives. Cancer Discov. 2013;3(3):264–79. Epub 2013/02/19. https://doi.org/10.1158/2159-8290.Cd-12-0362.
53. di Martino E, Tomlinson DC, Knowles MA. A decade of FGF receptor research in bladder cancer: past, present, and future challenges. Adv Urol. 2012;2012:10. https://doi.org/10.1155/2012/429213.
54. Cappellen D, De Oliveira C, Ricol D, de Medina S, Bourdin J, Sastre-Garau X, Chopin D, Thiery JP, Radvanyi F. Frequent activating mutations of FGFR3 in human bladder and cervix carcinomas. Nat Genet. 1999;23:18. https://doi.org/10.1038/12615.
55. Williams SV, Hurst CD, Knowles MA. Oncogenic FGFR3 gene fusions in bladder cancer. Hum Mol Genet. 2013;22(4):795–803. Epub 2012/11/24. https://doi.org/10.1093/hmg/dds486. PubMed PMID: 23175443; PMCID: PMC3554204.
56. Gavine PR, Mooney L, Kilgour E, Thomas AP, Al-Kadhimi K, Beck S, Rooney C, Coleman T, Baker D, Mellor MJ, Brooks AN, Klinowska T. AZD4547: an orally bioavailable, potent, and selective inhibitor of the fibroblast growth factor receptor tyrosine kinase family. Cancer Res. 2012;72(8):2045–56. Epub 2012/03/01. https://doi.org/10.1158/0008-5472.Can-11-3034.
57. Powles T, Balar A, Gravis G, Jones R, Ravaud A, Florence J, Grivas P, Petrylak DP, Galsky M, Carles J, Sridhar S, Arkenau H-T, Carroll D, DeCesare J, Mercier F, Hodgson D, Stone J, Cosaert J, Landers D. 902O An adaptive, biomarker directed platform study in metastatic urothelial cancer (BISCAY) with durvalumab in combination with targeted therapies. Ann Oncol. 2019;30(Supplement_5). https://doi.org/10.1093/annonc/mdz249.001.
58. Milowsky MI, Dittrich C, Duran I, Jagdev S, Millard FE, Sweeney CJ, Bajorin D, Cerbone L, Quinn DI, Stadler WM, Rosenberg JE, Lochheed M, Sen P, Squires M, Shi M, Sternberg CN. Phase 2 trial of dovitinib in patients with progressive FGFR3-mutated or FGFR3 wild-type advanced urothelial carcinoma. Eur J Cancer (Oxford, England: 1990). 2014;50(18):3145–52. Epub 2014/12/03. https://doi.org/10.1016/j.ejca.2014.10.013.
59. FDA website [Internet]. TFaDA. FDA grants accelerated approval to erdafitinib for metastatic urothelial carcinoma. 2019. https://www.fda.gov/drugs/resources-information-approved-drugs/fda-grants-accelerated-approval-erdafitinib-metastatic-urothelial-carcinoma
60. Tabernero J, Bahleda R, Dienstmann R, Infante JR, Mita A, Italiano A, Calvo E, Moreno V, Adamo B, Gazzah A, Zhong B, Platero SJ, Smit JW, Stuyckens K, Chatterjee-Kishore M, Rodon J, Peddareddigari V, Luo FR, Soria JC. Phase I dose-escalation study of JNJ-42756493, an oral pan-fibroblast growth factor receptor inhibitor, in patients with advanced solid tumors. J Clin Oncol Off J Am Soc Clin Oncol. 2015;33(30):3401–8. Epub 2015/09/02. https://doi.org/10.1200/jco.2014.60.7341.

61. Joerger M, Cassier PA, Penel N, Cathomas R, Richly H, Schostak M, Janitzky A, Wermke M, Nogova L, Tai DW-M, Sayehli C, Grüllich C, Grande E, Navarro A, Park SH, Nogai H, Bender S, Ellinghaus P, Schuler MH. Rogaratinib in patients with advanced urothelial carcinomas prescreened for tumor FGFR mRNA expression and effects of mutations in the FGFR signaling pathway. J Clin Oncol. 2018;36(15_suppl):4513. https://doi.org/10.1200/JCO.2018.36.15_suppl.4513.
62. Sequist LV, Cassier P, Varga A, Tabernero J, Schellens JH, Delord J-P, LoRusso P, Camidge DR, Medina MH, Schuler M, Campone M, Tian GG, Wong S, Corral J, Isaacs R, Sen SK, Porta DG, Kulkarni SG, Lefebvre C, Wolf J. Abstract CT326: phase I study of BGJ398, a selective pan-FGFR inhibitor in genetically preselected advanced solid tumors. Cancer Res. 2014;74(19 Supplement):CT326-CT. https://doi.org/10.1158/1538-7445.Am2014-ct326.
63. Pal SK, Rosenberg JE, Hoffman-Censits JH, Berger R, Quinn DI, Galsky MD, Wolf J, Dittrich C, Keam B, Delord JP, Schellens JHM, Gravis G, Medioni J, Maroto P, Sriuranpong V, Charoentum C, Burris HA, Grunwald V, Petrylak D, Vaishampayan U, Gez E, De Giorgi U, Lee JL, Voortman J, Gupta S, Sharma S, Mortazavi A, Vaughn DJ, Isaacs R, Parker K, Chen X, Yu K, Porter D, Graus Porta D, Bajorin DF. Efficacy of BGJ398, a fibroblast growth factor receptor 1–3 Inhibitor, in patients with previously treated advanced urothelial carcinoma with FGFR3 alterations. Cancer Discov. 2018;8(7):812–21. Epub 2018/06/01. https://doi.org/10.1158/2159-8290.Cd-18-0229.
64. Necchi A, Pouessel D, Leibowitz-Amit R, Flechon A, Gupta S, Barthelemy P, Maio M, Zhu X, Asatiani E, Serbest G, Zhen H, Loriot Y. Interim results of fight-201, a phase II, open-label, multicenter study of INCB054828 in patients (pts) with metastatic or surgically unresectable urothelial carcinoma (UC) harboring fibroblast growth factor (FGF)/FGF receptor (FGFR) genetic alterations (GA). Ann Oncol. 2018;29:viii319–viii20. https://doi.org/10.1093/annonc/mdy283.109.
65. Hussain MH, MacVicar GR, Petrylak DP, Dunn RL, Vaishampayan U, Lara PN, Jr., Chatta GS, Nanus DM, Glode LM, Trump DL, Chen H, Smith DC. Trastuzumab, paclitaxel, carboplatin, and gemcitabine in advanced human epidermal growth factor receptor-2/neu-positive urothelial carcinoma: results of a multicenter phase II National Cancer Institute trial. J Clin Oncol Off J Am Soc Clin Oncol. 2007;25(16):2218–24. Epub 2007/06/01. https://doi.org/10.1200/jco.2006.08.0994.
66. Oudard S, Culine S, Vano Y, Goldwasser F, Theodore C, Nguyen T, Voog E, Banu E, Vieillefond A, Priou F, Deplanque G, Gravis G, Ravaud A, Vannetzel JM, Machiels JP, Muracciole X, Pichon MF, Bay JO, Elaidi R, Teghom C, Radvanyi F, Beuzeboc P. Multicentre randomised phase II trial of gemcitabine+platinum, with or without trastuzumab, in advanced or metastatic urothelial carcinoma overexpressing Her2. Eur J Cancer (Oxford, England: 1990). 2015;51(1):45–54. Epub 2014/12/03. https://doi.org/10.1016/j.ejca.2014.10.009.
67. Powles T, Huddart RA, Elliott T, Sarker SJ, Ackerman C, Jones R, Hussain S, Crabb S, Jagdev S, Chester J, Hilman S, Beresford M, Macdonald G, Santhanam S, Frew JA, Stockdale A, Hughes S, Berney D, Chowdhury S. Phase III, double-blind, randomized trial that compared maintenance lapatinib versus placebo after first-line chemotherapy in patients with human epidermal growth factor receptor 1/2-positive metastatic bladder cancer. J Clin Oncol Off J Am Soc Clin Oncol. 2017;35(1):48–55. Epub 2016/12/31. https://doi.org/10.1200/jco.2015.66.3468.
68. Choudhury NJ, Campanile A, Antic T, Yap KL, Fitzpatrick CA, Wade JL, 3rd, Karrison T, Stadler WM, Nakamura Y, O'Donnell PH. Afatinib activity in platinum-refractory metastatic urothelial carcinoma in patients with ERBB alterations. J Clin Oncol Off J Am Soc Clin Oncol. 2016;34(18):2165–71. Epub 2016/04/06. https://doi.org/10.1200/jco.2015.66.3047. PubMed PMID: 27044931; PMCID: PMC5569685.
69. Hyman DM, Piha-Paul SA, Won H, Rodon J, Saura C, Shapiro GI, Juric D, Quinn DI, Moreno V, Doger B, Mayer IA, Boni V, Calvo E, Loi S, Lockhart AC, Erinjeri JP, Scaltriti M, Ulaner GA, Patel J, Tang J, Beer H, Selcuklu SD, Hanrahan AJ, Bouvier N, Melcer M, Murali R, Schram AM, Smyth LM, Jhaveri K, Li BT, Drilon A, Harding JJ, Iyer G, Taylor BS, Berger MF, Cutler RE, Jr., Xu F, Butturini A, Eli LD, Mann G, Farrell C, Lalani AS, Bryce RP, Arteaga CL, Meric-Bernstam F, Baselga J, Solit DB. HER kinase inhibition in patients with HER2- and HER3-mutant cancers. Nature. 2018;554(7691):189–194. Epub 2018/02/09. https://doi.org/10.1038/nature25475. PubMed PMID: 29420467; PMCID: PMC5808581.
70. Li BT, Makker V, Buonocore DJ, Offin MD, Olah ZT, Panora E, Shen R, Ho AL, Yaeger R, Iyer G, Ginsberg MS, Ulaner G, Solit DB, Hyman DM, Rudin CM, Berger MF, Baselga J, Scaltriti M, Arcila ME, Kris MG. A multi-histology basket trial of ado-trastuzumab emtansine in patients with HER2 amplified cancers. J Clin Oncol. 2018;36(15_suppl):2502. https://doi.org/10.1200/JCO.2018.36.15_suppl.2502.
71. Kiss B, Wyatt AW, Douglas J, Skuginna V, Mo F, Anderson S, Rotzer D, Fleischmann A, Genitsch V, Hayashi T, Neuenschwander M, Buerki C, Davicioni E, Collins C, Thalmann GN, Black PC, Seiler R. Her2 alterations in muscle-invasive bladder cancer: patient selection beyond protein expression for targeted therapy. Sci Rep. 2017;7:42713. https://doi.org/10.1038/srep42713.
72. Lamont FR, Tomlinson DC, Cooper PA, Shnyder SD, Chester JD, Knowles MA. Small molecule FGF receptor inhibitors block FGFR-dependent urothelial carcinoma growth in vitro and in vivo. Br J Cancer. 2011;104(1):75–82. https://doi.org/10.1038/sj.bjc.6606016.
73. Perera TPS, Jovcheva E, Mevellec L, Vialard J, De Lange D, Verhulst T, Paulussen C, Van De Ven K,

King P, Freyne E, Rees DC, Squires M, Saxty G, Page M, Murray CW, Gilissen R, Ward G, Thompson NT, Newell DR, Cheng N, Xie L, Yang J, Platero SJ, Karkera JD, Moy C, Angibaud P, Laquerre S, Lorenzi MV. Discovery and pharmacological characterization of JNJ-42756493 (Erdafitinib), a functionally selective small-molecule FGFR family inhibitor. Mol Cancer Ther. 2017;16(6):1010–1020. Epub 2017/03/28. https://doi.org/10.1158/1535-7163.Mct-16-0589.

74. Collin M-P, Lobell M, Hübsch W, Brohm D, Schirok H, Jautelat R, Lustig K, Bömer U, Vöhringer V, Héroult M, Grünewald S, Hess-Stumpp H. Discovery of Rogaratinib (BAY 1163877): a pan-FGFR inhibitor. ChemMedChem. 2018;13(5):437–45. https://doi.org/10.1002/cmdc.201700718.
75. Guagnano V, Furet P, Spanka C, Bordas V, Le Douget M, Stamm C, Brueggen J, Jensen MR, Schnell C, Schmid H, Wartmann M, Berghausen J, Drueckes P, Zimmerlin A, Bussiere D, Murray J, Graus Porta D. Discovery of 3-(2,6-dichloro-3,5-dimethoxy-phenyl)-1-{6-[4-(4-ethyl-piperazin-1-yl)-phenylamino]-pyrimidin-4-yl}-1-methyl-urea (NVP-BGJ398), a potent and selective inhibitor of the fibroblast growth factor receptor family of receptor tyrosine kinase. J Med Chem. 2011;54(20):7066–7083. Epub 2011/09/23. https://doi.org/10.1021/jm2006222.
76. Liu PCC, Wu L, Koblish H, Bowman K, Zhang Y, Klabe R, Leffet L, DiMatteo D, Rupar M, Gallagher K, Hansbury M, Zhang C, He C, Collier P, Covington M, Wynn R, Yeleswaram S, Vaddi K, Burn T, Yao W, Huber R, Scherle P, Hollis G. Abstract 771: preclinical characterization of the selective FGFR inhibitor INCB054828. Cancer Res. 2015;75(15 Supplement):771. https://doi.org/10.1158/1538-7445.AM2015-771.

Bladder Cancer: Specimen Handling and Reporting

17

Yong Mee Cho and Jae Y. Ro

Introduction

The urinary tract is lined by the urothelium and runs from the renal calyces and pelvis to the ureter and urinary bladder and to the proximal two-thirds of the urethra. Most tumors of these organs are derived from the urothelial lining. The most common specimens from the urinary bladder are obtained by cystoscopic biopsies and transurethral resections of the bladder tumor (TURBT), both of which contain urothelium with subepithelial tissue and muscularis propria of varying depths [1]. Other specimens can be obtained from a partial cystectomy, radical cystectomy, cystoprostatectomy, pelvic exenteration, or resection of diverticula [1]. Surgical excision of an urachal carcinoma usually includes the bladder dome, urachal remnant, and umbilicus [1].

Pathology reports on cystoscopic biopsy and TURBT specimens provide the important information that determines subsequent patient management, while reports of curative resections (e.g., cystectomy) may help determine the need for further surgery, adjuvant chemo/radiotherapy, or appropriate surveillance [2].

Information for Bladder Cancer Diagnosis

Clinical History

The most common presenting symptom in bladder cancer patients is painless gross hematuria, which is observed in 85% of newly diagnosed bladder cancer patients [3]. The microscopic hematuria occurs in virtually all patients. Lower urinary tract symptoms, such as urgency, nocturia, and dysuria, may be signs of bladder cancer, especially in patients with concomitant urothelial carcinoma in situ [3]. However, these lower urinary tract symptoms are also classic signs of more common diseases, such as inflammatory cystitis and urethritis. Therefore, patients presenting with persistent lower urinary tract symptoms, especially older patients, should raise concern for bladder cancer.

A thorough clinical history should be obtained, as urinary tract stones, infection, instrumentation, radiation, or previous intravesical therapy may influence the interpretation of biopsy specimens. This is especially important for the differential diagnosis of flat urothelial lesions, such as reactive urothelial atypia versus urothelial carcinoma in situ.

Y. M. Cho (✉)
Department of Pathology, Asan Medical Center, University of Ulsan College of Medicine, Seoul, South Korea
e-mail: yongcho@amc.seoul.kr

J. Y. Ro
Department of Pathology and Genomic Medicine, Weill Medical College of Cornell University/Houston Methodist Hospital, Houston, TX, USA
e-mail: jaero@houstonmethodist.org

H. Zhou et al. (eds.), *Urinary Bladder Pathology*, https://doi.org/10.1007/978-3-030-71509-0_17

Pathological Examination History

Because urothelial tumors frequently recur with similar histologic features and grade, any previously diagnosed tumor should be noted and reviewed for their histologic type, primary site, and histologic grade. Previous pathology information is very helpful when a recurrent or metastatic tumors present with predominant divergent differentiation and variant histology. For example, when the previous urothelial tumor had areas of squamous differentiation, it is unlikely that the recurrent or metastatic tumor is of pure squamous cell carcinoma.

Clinical and pathological examination history can also help determine the clinical significance of denuded urothelium in bladder biopsy samples, as prior instrumentation and intravesical therapy are contributors to denudation. Urothelial carcinoma in situ is often associated with prominent cellular discohesion and exfoliation of neoplastic cells in the urine, mimicking denuding cystitis (Fig. 17.1a). In these cases, review of simultaneously tested urine cytology slides would help to ensure detection of the few residual discohesive cells of carcinoma in situ (Fig. 17.1b). In summary, extensive urothelial denudation in biopsy samples should be reported with caution [4].

Imaging

Computer tomography (CT) scan or magnetic resonance imaging (MRI) of the abdomen and pelvis is usually performed before biopsy and intervention, as post-procedural changes may cause inflammation and scarring, resulting in erroneous interpretation [5]. Imaging is used to localize the tumor within the urinary bladder and to estimate the depth of invasion. However, the final determination of tumor invasiveness and the depth of invasion should be assessed by pathologic examination of TURBT and/or subsequent cystectomy specimens. Additional workup, preferably with CT urography, is usually performed to check synchronous upper urinary tract lesions.

Cystoscopy Findings

Cystoscopic findings serve as an alternative to gross examination of urothelial tumors on biopsy and TURBT specimens. They are useful for the differential diagnosis between low-grade papillary urothelial tumors and non-neoplastic papillary urothelial lesions, such as redundant urothelial mucosa and papillary/polypoid cystitis (Fig. 17.2a and b). Papillary urothelial tumors present as an arborizing papillary mass, where the papillae are composed of a reddish blood-containing fibrovascular core lined by a whitish outer layer of urothelial tumor cells. In higher-grade tumors, irregularity in the thickness of the tumor cell layer is increased, and the fibrovascular cores are more often fused (Fig. 17.2b and c). The tumor could be a solid sessile mass in an infiltrating high-grade urothelial carcinoma, but

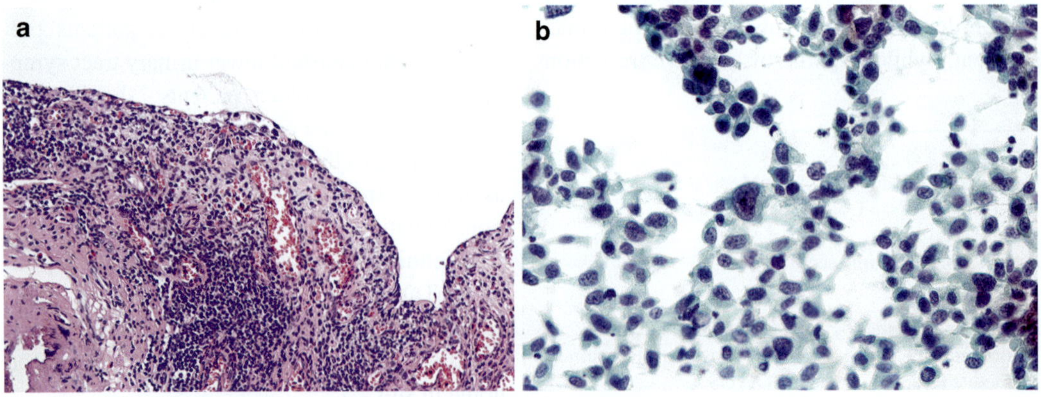

Fig. 17.1 Urothelial carcinoma in situ mimicking denuding cystitis. Extensive urothelial denudation in a biopsy sample (**a**) and abundant tumor cells in the simultaneously collected urine sample (**b**)

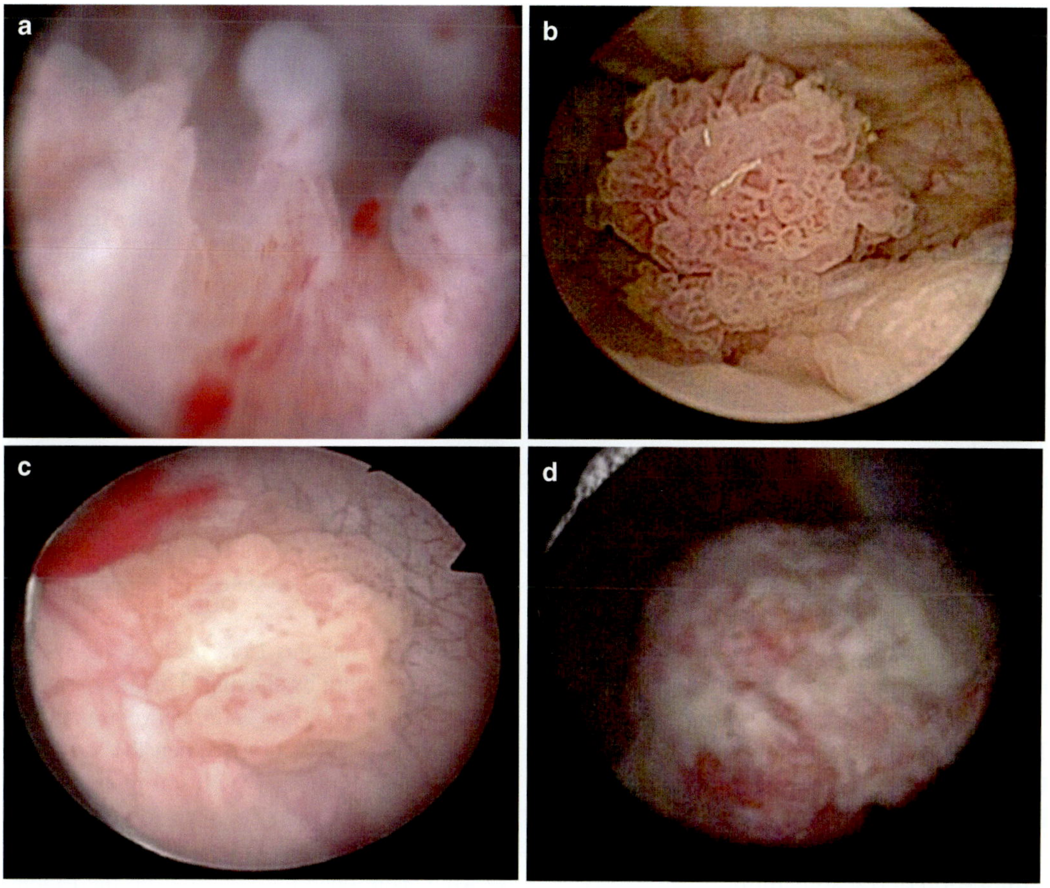

Fig. 17.2 Cystoscopic findings of papillary/polypoid cystitis (**a**), low-grade noninvasive papillary urothelial carcinoma (**b**), high-grade noninvasive papillary urothelial carcinoma (**c**), and invasive urothelial carcinoma (**d**)

in that case, its diagnosis is usually evident on histologic examination alone (Fig 17.2d).

Handling and Sampling of Bladder Cancer Specimens

Handling and reporting of bladder cancer specimens are described based on the current guidelines by the College of American Pathologists (CAP, Revised: February 2019) with modification [6, 7].

Biopsy and Transurethral Resection of Bladder Tumors

Small, noninvasive papillary neoplasms are often excised with cold-cup forceps, diathermy forceps, or small diathermy loops. These biopsy specimens should be entirely submitted for histopathologic examination and transferred in a fixative with minimal handling to avoid tissue distortion [1]. At least three levels of sectioning should be obtained on each small biopsy specimen [8].

Larger neoplasms are often sampled using TURBT with a diathermy loop that produces 6-mm-diameter tissue strips of variable lengths [1]. It has become a common practice to resect all visible tumors and take more deeply the underlying muscularis propria for evaluation of the depth of tumor invasion [7]. If the muscularis propria is not adequately sampled, repeat sampling is required to stage properly, especially in all invasive tumors [5]. Those specimens that need a separate diagnosis, such as deep biopsy for muscularis propria invasion and random biopsies for in situ carcinoma evaluation, should be submitted separately in a different container to ensure that they are not combined with TURBT specimens.

TURBT specimens should be weighted in aggregate [7]. It is important to avoid overfilling specimen cassettes with tissue fragments. According to the general rule of gross examination, one cassette per centimeter of tumor diameter may be prepared, up to ten cassettes. However, if the tumor appears noninvasive in initial sampling, or is invasive into the subepithelial connective tissue, additional sampling of tissue (possibly including all the tissue) is necessary for the evaluation of tumor invasiveness and muscularis propria invasion, respectively.

Thermocoagulation often produces severe artifact, such as detachment of epithelial cells from the basement membrane and spindling or palisading of the nuclei [9]. A comment on the thermocoagulation effect may be reported if it makes diagnostic evaluation difficult [1].

Total Cystectomy, Radical Cystoprostatectomy, and Pelvic Exenteration

Orientation of the Specimens

Anatomic landmarks of the urinary bladder and simultaneously resected pelvic organs can be used to orient specimens. In the male, the bladder adjoins the rectum and seminal vesicles posteriorly, the prostate inferiorly, and the pubis anteriorly, and peritoneum superiorly [8]. In the female, the vagina is located posteriorly, and the uterus is located superiorly [8]. The perivesical fat surrounding the bladder is lined by peritoneum along the superior surface and upper part of the bladder. In both males and females, the peritoneum descends further along the posterior wall of the bladder than it does along the anterior wall. Both ureters are located within the lateral perivesical fatty connective tissues.

Dissection of the Specimens

1. Once the specimen is opened anteriorly from the urethra to the bladder dome, examine the bladder mucosal surface for ulcerations, for exophytic or nodular tumors, or for more subtle mucosal alterations of in situ lesions, such as velvety erythematous mucosae. The number, size, gross appearance, and location of any lesion in the bladder should be documented.
2. The tumors may appear flat, papillary, nodular, or ulcerated. Examine whether the tumor infiltrates the muscularis propria or the perivesical fat of the bladder or other adjacent organs. Meticulous gross evaluation of the prostatic urethra is required to identify independent primary lesions involving the urethral lining [5]. Note any gross abnormality, such as tumor penetrating the serosa or at a surgical margin.
3. Take photographs of the opened specimen. Fresh tissue may be collected for special studies, and this must be stated in the pathological report.
4. Secure the margins from each of the ureters and the urethra by shaving. This is not necessary if the ureters and urethra have been evaluated by frozen sections. When the specimen includes the prostate, the distal prostatic urethral margin should be taken from the distal end of the prostate.
5. After then, open the ureters from the trigone orifices using a small pair of scissors. Look for ureteral strictures and dilatations, and examine the mucosa for ulcerations, diverticula, or exophytic lesions. Document these findings in the gross description. Submit transverse sections of the ureters.
6. Be sure to search for lymph nodes, which are sometimes present in the perivesical fat.

Sampling of the Specimens

Sections are taken in such a way as to show the relationship of the tumor to the adjacent urothelium, the tumor's maximal level of invasion, and external soft tissue margins with inking.

Sampling the Tumor If a tumor is identified in the bladder, make a full-thickness cut through the tumor and the bladder wall to demonstrate the tumor's maximal depth of invasion. For large exophytic tumors, take several sections from the tumor base to adequately assess the extent of invasion [8]. At least one section should be taken for each centimeter of the tumor's diameter.

Any previous TURBT scar and/or neoadjuvant chemotherapeutic effect may make it difficult to define the outline of the tumor. In such cases, generous sampling of the bladder, with particular attention to abnormal-appearing mucosa and to sites of previously documented tumor resection, is necessary for proper staging of the tumor. If no visible tumor is identified in the initial sections of the previous TURBT scar, the entire lesion should be prepared for histologic examination to document any residual tumor.

Sampling the Non-tumoral Mucosa Carefully inspect and generously sample the normal-appearing bladder mucosa and those of the ureter and prostatic urethra because many in situ lesions of the urinary tract present as flat or subtle red velvety flat mucosal lesions. Submit several sections of the mucosa away from the carcinoma, especially if abnormal-appearing mucosae are present, including the lateral wall(s), dome, and trigone.

Sampling the Prostate Gland If the tumor appears to invade the prostate parenchyma, sections that clearly demonstrate whether it invades from the prostatic urethra (pT2) or directly through the bladder wall (pT4) should be taken. Slice the prostate from apex to base perpendicular to the urethra at 5 mm intervals. It is important to take sections from the bladder neck, as this is an important route for urothelial carcinoma to invade the prostatic stroma. Representative sections of the peripheral zone, transition zone, central zone, and seminal vesicles should be included. Careful gross examination may help target sampling of selective abnormal-appearing areas.

If there are good reasons for additional sampling for prostatic adenocarcinoma (e.g., raised serum PSA levels, the presence of extensive prostatic carcinoma, Gleason patterns 4 or 5 on the initial sections), then consideration should be given to treating the organ as a radical prostatectomy with full staging and assessment of margins [2].

Sampling the Seminal Vesicle Inclusion of seminal vesicles is particularly important in tumors at the bladder neck, and these should be sampled in continuity with the tumor.

Sampling the Lymph Nodes
All nodal and perivesical fat samples should be thoroughly searched for lymph nodes. Submit one section from each grossly positive lymph node. All other grossly benign lymph nodes should be entirely submitted, as the presence of nodal disease may be used as an indication for adjuvant therapy.

Sampling the Margins Submit one section each of the ureteral margins and one section of the urethral margin, unless submitted separately as frozen section specimens. If a long segment of the ureter is present, then, after careful examination of the entire ureter, additional sections from the suspicious areas or a random section from the mid-portion of a grossly unremarkable ureter may be necessary, as urothelial cancer is often multifocal.

Sampling Other Organs If the submitted organs are grossly unremarkable, submit one or more sections of the uterus, vagina, and other organs. If the tumor grossly appears to invade the uterus or vagina, sections should be targeted, such that the relationship of the infiltrating tumor in the bladder wall and the adjacent viscus is clearly demonstrated.

Partial Cystectomy

Partial cystectomy specimens, including resections of diverticula, should be fixed and dissected according to the guidelines given for radical cystectomy specimens. However, unlike in a radical cystectomy specimen, in the partial cystectomy specimen the mucosal edges of the specimen represent the surgical margins of the bladder wall. Ink the edges and assess these margins for tumor involvement by taking perpendicular sections from all edges of the specimen at regular intervals.

The partial cystectomy specimen for urachal carcinoma consists of the dome of the urinary bladder in continuity with the urachal ligament and may include the umbilicus. Sections should be taken at right angles to the long axis of the urachal ligament and submitted for histologic examination. Remember to sample two additional margins in the partial cystectomy specimens: the soft tissue margin surrounding the urachal ligament and the skin margin around the umbilicus. The bladder portion of the specimen should be processed like other partial cystectomy specimens.

Evaluation of Diagnostic and Prognostic Information

The pathology report should provide clinically useful information derived from the macroscopic and microscopic pathologic evaluations.

Histologic Tumor Type

It is recommended to follow the current 2016 WHO classification of urinary tract tumors found in Table 17.1 [3]. More than 95% of carcinomas of the urinary bladder, ureter, and renal pelvis are of urothelial origin. The presence of histologic variants in urothelial carcinoma should be documented. Focal squamous, glandular, and/or Müllerian divergent differentiation may be present in the tumor and must be clearly reported with its relative proportion of the aberrant tumor histology. Occasionally, the divergent differentiation is extensive but should still be classified as urothelial, unless the cancer is composed purely of the alternative histology. In other words, bladder cancer with a recognizable papillary, invasive, or urothelial carcinoma in situ component should be classified as urothelial carcinoma with divergent differentiation. A key challenge is managing patients who present with squamous cell carcinoma or adenocarcinoma on initial biopsy or transurethral resection. Because of limited sampling at initial biopsy or resection, exclusion of a high-grade urothelial carcinoma with squamous or glandular differentiation is often difficult. This distinction typically can only be made after radical cystectomy when the entire lesion is available for histologic analysis [4].

The histologic subtype may reflect the risk of disease progression and different genetic etiology and, subsequently, determine whether a more aggressive treatment approach should be taken. Some variants, such as micropapillary, plasmacytoid, and sarcomatoid variants, are associated with reduced survival [5]. A malignant neoplasm with a small cell neuroendocrine carcinoma component arising in the urinary tract is designated as small cell carcinoma for treatment purposes.

Histologic Tumor Grade

There have been various grading systems for urothelial tumor. The International Society of Urological Pathology (ISUP) proposed a consensus classification in 1998 that was adopted by the WHO in 2004 and incorporated into the 2016 WHO classification system with minor modification (Table 17.1) [3]. The older WHO system (1973) may be concurrently used, according to institutional preference. Flat intraepithelial lesions and papillary and invasive lesions are graded separately.

The great majority of invasive urothelial carcinomas are high-grade. Since significant outcome differences have been reported between low- and high-grade invasive tumors, tumor grade should be reported [3]. Deceptively bland variants, such as nested or microcystic variants, that histologically appear low-grade tend to behave like invasive high-grade tumors of a similar stage [4].

Tumor Extent

Clinical stage classification (cTNM) is usually conducted by the referring physician before treatment during initial evaluation of the patient or when pathologic classification is not possible. Pathologic information obtained from cystoscopic biopsy or transurethral resection is used for clinical tumor staging (cT) along with the cystoscopic assessment, bimanual examination, and radiographic evaluation. Pathological staging (pT) of bladder cancer relies on pathologic information obtained from gross and microscopic assessment of partial or radical cystectomy specimens.

The latest TNM Staging System of the American Joint Committee on Cancer (AJCC)/

Table 17.1 Pathologic information to be included in the pathology report

Information	Comments
Procedure (R & B)	Biopsy, transurethral resection of bladder tumor (TURBT), partial cystectomy, radical cystectomy (total cystectomy), radical cystoprostatectomy, anterior exenteration, other (specify), not specified
Tumor site (R & B)	Trigone, right lateral wall, left lateral wall, anterior wall, posterior wall, dome, other (specify), not specified
Tumor number (R)	Single, multiple (specify)
Tumor size (R)	Greatest dimension
Histologic type (R & B)	**Urothelial tumors** Infiltrating urothelial carcinoma Infiltrating urothelial carcinoma with divergent differentiation: Squamous, glandular, trophoblastic, or Möllerian Specify the percentage of divergent differentiation Infiltrating urothelial carcinoma with variant histology: Nested (including large nested), microcystic, micropapillary, lymphoepithelioma-like, plasmacytoid/signet ring/diffuse, sarcomatoid, giant cell, poorly differentiated, lipid-rich, or clear cell Urothelial carcinoma in situ Noninvasive papillary urothelial carcinoma Papillary urothelial neoplasm of low malignant potential Urothelial papilloma Inverted urothelial papilloma Urothelial proliferation of uncertain malignant potential Urothelial dysplasia **Squamous cell neoplasms** Pure squamous cell carcinoma Verrucous carcinoma Squamous cell carcinoma in situ Squamous papilloma **Glandular neoplasms** Adenocarcinoma, NOS Adenocarcinoma, enteric, mucinous, mixed Adenocarcinoma in situ Villous adenoma **Urachal carcinoma** **Tumors of Möllerian type** Clear cell carcinoma Endometrioid carcinoma **Neuroendocrine tumors** Small cell neuroendocrine carcinoma Large cell neuroendocrine carcinoma Well-differentiated neuroendocrine carcinoma Paraganglioma **Melanocytic tumor** Malignant melanoma Nevus Melanosis **Mesenchymal tumors** Rhabdomyosarcoma Leiomyosarcoma Angiosarcoma Inflammatory myofibroblastic tumor Perivascular epithelioid cell tumor, benign, malignant Solitary fibrous tumor Leiomyoma Hemangioma Granular cell tumor Neurofibroma **Urothelial tract hematopoietic and lymphoid tumors** **Miscellaneous tumors** Carcinoma of Skene, Cowper, and Littre glands Metastatic tumors and tumors extending from other organs Epithelial tumors of the upper urinary tract Tumors arising in a bladder diverticulum Urothelial tumors of the urethra

Table 17.1 (continued)

Information	Comments
Histologic grade (R & B)	Urothelial: Low-grade, high-grade Squamous or adenocarcinoma: Well, moderately, poorly differentiated
Tumor extension (B)	Noninvasive papillary carcinoma Carcinoma in situ Tumor invades subepithelial connective tissue Tumor invades muscularis propria Urothelial carcinoma involving prostatic urethra, prostatic ducts, and acini
Tumor extension (R)	Noninvasive papillary carcinoma Carcinoma in situ Tumor invades lamina propria: Subepithelial connective tissue Tumor invades muscularis propria: Superficial, deep Tumor invades perivesical soft tissue: Microscopically, macroscopically tumor invades adjacent structures Male: Prostate (transmural invasion from the bladder tumor)[a], seminal vesicles Female: Uterus, vagina, adnexae Male/female: Pelvis wall, abdominal wall, rectum Other (specify)
Muscularis propria (B)	No muscularis propria (detrusor muscle) identified Muscularis propria (detrusor muscle) present Cannot be determined (explain)
Margin involvement (R)	Uninvolved by invasive carcinoma and carcinoma in situ/noninvasive urothelial carcinoma Involved by invasive carcinoma, carcinoma in situ/noninvasive high-grade urothelial carcinoma, noninvasive low-grade urothelial carcinoma/urothelial dysplasia
Positive margin site (R)	Right ureteral margin, left ureteral margin, urethral margin, soft tissue margin, other margin(s) (specify)
Lymphovascular invasion (R & B)	Not identified, present, cannot be determined
Regional lymph nodes (R)	No lymph nodes submitted or found Number of lymph nodes examined Number of lymph nodes involved Size of largest metastatic deposit and specify site Extranodal extension: Not identified, present, cannot be determined
Associated epithelial lesions (R & B)	Urothelial papilloma, inverted urothelial papilloma, urothelial proliferation of uncertain malignant potential, urothelial dysplasia
Additional pathologic findings (R & B)	Inflammation/regenerative changes, therapy-related changes, cautery artifact, cystitis cystica et glandularis, keratinizing squamous metaplasia, intestinal metaplasia, adenocarcinoma of prostate, other (specify)

R represents curative surgical resection specimens, such as partial and radical cystectomy. *B* represents cystoscopic biopsy and TURBT specimens

[a]Use the tumor staging system of urethral cancer for tumors that involve the urethral mucosa without invasion, tumors that involve the urethral mucosa with invasion of subepithelial connective tissue/prostate stroma, or tumors that involve prostatic ducts and acini with or without stromal invasion

International Union Against Cancer (UICC), revised in 2016, is recommended to be used for carcinomas of the urinary tract (Table 17.2) [5]. The tumor stage of bladder cancer is based on the level of invasion: noninvasive limited to urothelium (Ta or Tis); invasion into the subepithelial connective tissue also called lamina propria or submucosa (T1); invasion into the muscularis propria also called detrusor muscle (T2); and invasion into the perivesical fat or soft tissue (T3). Extravesical tumor invading adjacent organs is classified as T4 (Table 17.2). In the male, direct invasion into the prostate is included as part of the primary stage of the bladder tumor (pT4). However, initial spread along the prostatic urethral mucosa and prostate glands as in situ or noninvasive papillary urothelial carcinoma and then subsequent invasion to the prostatic stroma

Table 17.2 Pathologic stage classification of bladder cancer (pTNM, AJCC eighth Edition)

TNM			Definition
Primary tumor	pTX		Primary tumor cannot be assessed
	pT0		No evidence of primary tumor
	pTa		Noninvasive papillary carcinoma
	pTis		Urothelial carcinoma in situ: "Flat tumor"
	pT1		Tumor invades lamina propria (subepithelial connective tissue)
	pT2		Tumor invades muscularis propria
		pT2a	Tumor invades superficial muscularis propria (inner half)
		pT2b	Tumor invades deep muscularis propria (outer half)
	pT3		Tumor invades perivesical soft tissue
		pT3a	Microscopically
		pT3b	Macroscopically (extravesical mass)
	pT4		Extravesical tumor directly invades any of the following: Prostatic stroma, seminal vesicles, uterus, vagina, pelvic wall, abdominal wall
		pT4a	Extravesical tumor directly invades prostatic stroma, uterus, vagina
		pT4b	Extravesical tumor invades pelvic wall, abdominal wall
Regional lymph nodes	pNX		Lymph nodes cannot be assessed
	pN0		No lymph node metastasis
	pN1		Single regional lymph node metastasis in the true pelvis (perivesical, obturator, internal and external iliac, or sacral lymph node)
	pN2		Multiple regional lymph node metastasis in the true pelvis (perivesical, obturator, internal and external iliac, or sacral lymph node metastasis)
	pN3		Lymph node metastasis to the common iliac lymph nodes
Distant metastasis[a]	pM0		No distant metastasis
	pM1		Distant metastasis
		pM1a	Distant metastasis limited to lymph nodes beyond the common iliacs
		pM1b	Non-lymph node distant metastases

[a]pM is required only if confirmed pathologically

should be staged according to the staging system of the male urethra [5]. If a biopsied tumor is not resected for any reason (e.g., when technically unfeasible) and the highest T and N categories or the M1 category of the tumor can still be confirmed microscopically, the pathologic stage could be applied without total removal of the primary cancer.

Noninvasive Versus Invasive Bladder Cancer

The pathologist should pay careful attention to the diagnosis of tumors infiltrating the subepithelial connective tissue (T1). Recognition of subepithelial connective tissue invasion is challenging because of various diagnostic pitfalls, including tangential sectioning, poor specimen orientation, obscuring inflammation, thermal injury, deceptively bland cytology in some variants of urothelial carcinoma, and pseudoinvasive nests of benign proliferative urothelial cells [8]. In papillary tumors, invasion occurs most often at the base of the tumor and not infrequently in the stalk. Sometimes tentacular or finger-like extensions arise from the base of the papillary tumor (Fig. 17.3a) [8]. Invasive carcinoma cells often infiltrate the underlying stroma as single cells or irregularly shaped nests of tumor cells (Fig. 17.3b). The invading nests appear cytologically different from cells of the noninvasive component and often have more abundant cytoplasm and less nuclear pleomorphism, a feature known as paradoxical differentiation (Fig. 17.3c) [8]. The stromal reaction of subepithelial connective tissue to invasive tumor may be myxoid, fibrous, pseudosarcomatous, desmoplastic, or inflammatory [8].

Tumor cells may involve von Brunn's nests, either by pagetoid spread or by direct extension from adjacent tumors, and can be confused with subepithelial connective tissue invasion. When urothelial carcinoma involves von Brunn's nests as an in situ component, the basement membrane preserves a regular contour. A parallel array of thin-walled vessels often lines the basement membrane of noninvasive nests, whereas these vessels are usually absent next to invasive nests [8]. In some cases, retraction artifacts around microinvasive individual tumor cells, especially

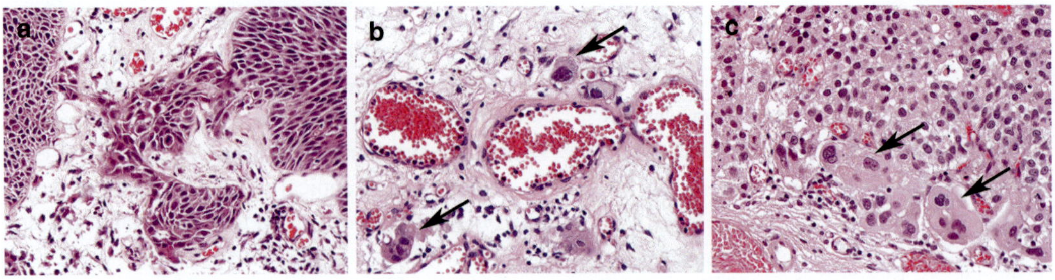

Fig. 17.3 Various patterns of early invasion in urothelial carcinoma. Tentacular extensions arising from the base of the noninvasive tumor (**a**), invasion as single cells or irregularly shaped nests of tumor cells (**b**), and paradoxical differentiation of infiltrating tumor cells (**c**) (arrows, infiltrating tumor cells)

in micropapillary variants, may mimic vascular invasion. This finding is often focal and may itself be an early sign of subepithelial connective tissue invasion. Immunohistochemistry may help distinguish tumor cells (pancytokeratin) and retraction artifacts from true vascular invasion (CD31, CD34, and ERG).

T1 Substaging

Although not formally endorsed in the AJCC cancer staging system, pT1 substaging appears to have prognostic value, with early invasion into the subepithelial connective tissue showing better outcomes than more advanced pT1 disease. The method of pT1 substaging has not been fully agreed upon, but pathologists are encouraged to provide an assessment of the extent of subepithelial connective tissue invasion: by the level of invasion (above, at, or below muscularis mucosae), by maximum dimension, or by depth of invasive focus in millimeters. Microinvasive urothelial carcinomas have been defined by different groups as invasive tumors of <1 high power field in content, greatest invasive tumor diameter of <1 mm, extending to a depth of 2 mm or less, or invasive tumor above the muscularis mucosae.

T1 Stage Versus T2 Stage

Pathologists play a critical role in patient management by distinguishing non-muscularis propria-invasive bladder cancers (Ta, Tis, and T1) from muscularis propria-invasive bladder cancers (T2 and higher). Generally, the former is managed by complete resection of the tumor through TURBT, followed by the initiation and maintenance of either immunotherapy with intravesical BCG instillation or intravesical chemotherapy [10]. For muscularis propria-invasive bladder cancer, multimodal treatment involving radical cystectomy with neoadjuvant chemotherapy offers the best chance for cure [10]. Therefore, in the biopsy and TURBT specimens, the presence or absence of muscularis propria, regardless of whether there is invasion or not, should be reported as an indication of resection adequacy. Designation of a tumor as merely muscle-invasive is inappropriate: the type of muscle invasion – i.e., muscularis mucosae invasion (T1 tumors) versus muscularis propria invasion (T2 tumors) – needs to be clearly stated. Descriptive terminology, such as "urothelial carcinoma with muscle invasion, indeterminate for the type of muscle invasion," may be used when it is not possible to assess the type of muscle invaded by the tumor. The muscle bundles of muscularis mucosae are typically thin, slender, and arranged in a single layer or a few layers of interrupted, dispersed, or continuous muscle frequently associated with large, thin-walled blood vessels [11]. On the other hand, muscles of the muscularis propria are usually thick, compact, and divided into distinct bundles.

Two patterns of hyperplastic muscularis mucosae have been described. One is aggregates of thin muscle fibers with haphazard orientation and irregular outlines morphologically distinct from that of the muscularis propria. The other is hyperplastic compact muscle bundles with small parallel muscle fibers and regular outlines arranged singly or in small groups, which may strongly resemble the muscularis propria. The most reliable feature to distinguish muscularis mucosae from the muscularis propria is its location in the subepithelial connective tissue; however, this is not always possible to determine when limited specimens are collected, such as with TURBT [4]. In the trigone, the subepithelial connective tissue is thin and merges imperceptibly into the muscularis propria. Furthermore, the muscle bundles in the trigone are smaller and thinner, especially in superficial muscularis propria compared to those from other regions of the urinary bladder (Fig. 17.4). Immunohistochemical staining with anti-smoothelin may help with this distinction [7]. However, in any situation, when the distinction between hyperplastic muscularis mucosae muscle versus proper muscle is difficult, discuss with an urologist for a clinical correlation, and if necessary, another deeper biopsy can be performed.

T2 Staging

In TURBT specimens, no attempt should be made to substage the depth of muscularis propria invasion because TURBT specimens lack orientation with respect to bladder anatomy. It is not uncommon for tumor cells to abut but not penetrate bundles of muscularis propria. The muscle-tumor interface may even have a smooth contour. Even without direct invasion into the muscularis propria wall, tumor cells immediately adjacent to broad smooth muscle fibers should be categorized as pT2 carcinoma [8]. When the proper muscle layer is extensively invaded and destructed by tumor cells, muscularis propria may also look like muscularis mucosae (Fig. 17.5). In such

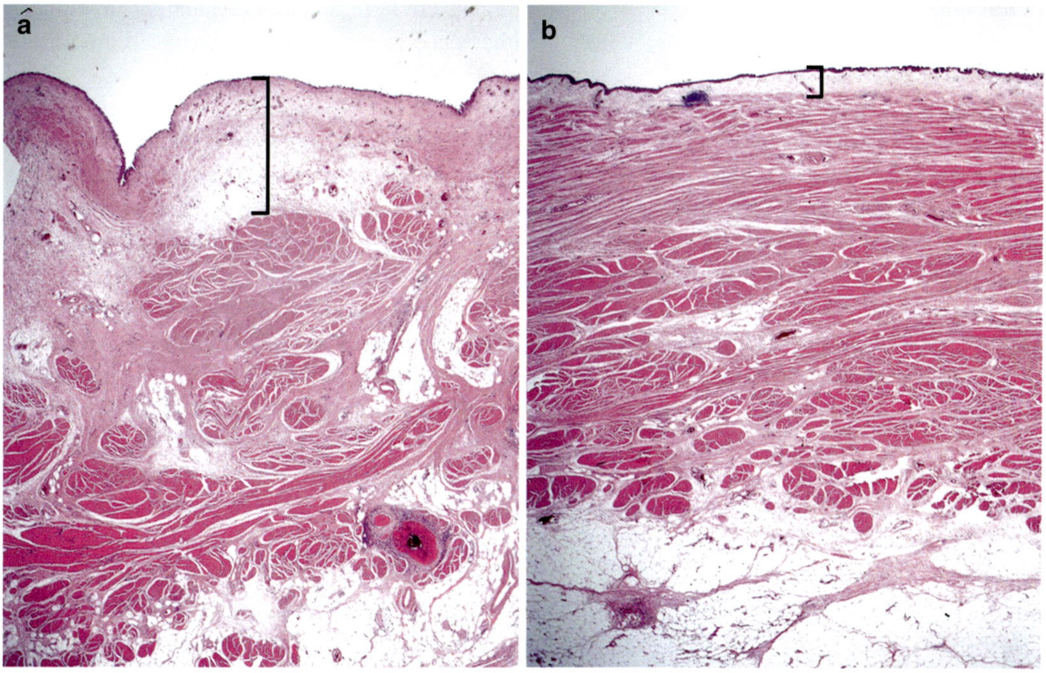

Fig. 17.4 Comparison of the histology of the trigone and other bladder walls. Compared to the lateral wall (**a**) of the urinary bladder, the trigone has thinner subepithelial connective tissue and smaller muscle bundles in the superficial muscularis propria (**b**). Both photographs are taken from the urinary bladder removed from one bladder cancer patient and are at the same magnification. The subepithelial connective tissue is marked with square brackets

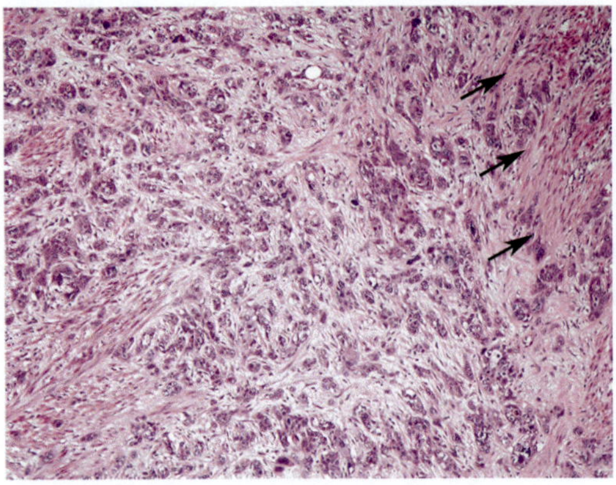

Fig. 17.5 Muscularis propria invasion mimicking muscularis mucosae invasion. The muscle bundles of the surrounding muscularis propria are indicated by arrows

cases, surrounding muscle bundles uninvolved by the tumor may help determine the type of invaded muscle.

T3 Staging

Besides the perivesical area, adipose tissue is frequently present in the subepithelial connective tissue and muscularis propria of the urinary bladder, usually scant in the former and abundant in the latter. Therefore, involvement of adipose tissue by the tumor in biopsy or TURBT specimens should not be interpreted as perivesical fat involvement or pT3 disease [12]. The determination of extravesical spread should be assessed on cystectomy specimens. Substaging of pT3 disease is not tenable in TURBT specimens [4].

Resection Margins

Tumor involving the resection margin on pathologic examination may be assumed to correspond to residual tumor in the patient and may be classified as microscopic (R1) or macroscopic (R2) according to the findings at the specimen margins. Statements about deep soft tissue margins should specify whether the peritoneal surface is involved by tumor. In cases of urachal adenocarcinoma, in which partial cystectomy with excision of the urachal ligament and umbilicus is performed, the margins of the urachal ligament (i.e., the soft tissue surrounding the urachus) and the skin around the umbilicus should be specified.

Venous/Lymphatic Vascular Invasion

Lymphovascular invasion (LVI) has been associated with poor clinical outcomes in invasive tumors; however, its overall value as an independent factor remains controversial. Assessment of LVI is performed using light microscopic analysis on invasive tumors of any stage [5]. Immunohistochemistry to identify vascular or lymphatic spaces is not currently recommended, but in suspicious cases, blood vessels can be highlighted by immunohistochemical staining for factor VIII-related antigen, ERG, CD31, or CD34 [5]. In general, we recommend an evaluation of LVI: [1] at the peritumoral area, at least one high power field distance from the tumor edge; [2] for plump endothelial lining cells; and [3] for attached space or association with organizing clots. In addition, evaluating invasion in the space associated with vascular route (artery and vein) is recommended.

Urothelial Carcinoma in Situ

The presence of urothelial carcinoma in situ has been associated with the presence of multifocal disease in the urinary tract, tumor recurrence, and increased risk of invasive disease [5]. Urothelial carcinoma in situ that occurs in association with high-grade papillary urothelial carcinoma should be reported [5]. In such cases, care must be taken to distinguish a separate focus of urothelial carcinoma in situ from the "shoulder," which refers to the lateral extension or base of a high-grade papillary carcinoma, because both lesions may appear flat [5, 13]. While no consensus guidelines for this situation exist, it is recommended that [1] the carcinoma in situ should be located away from the papillary tumor or present in an entirely different tissue fragment; [2] if present in the same tissue fragment, a strip of non-neoplastic urothelium is present between the in situ component and the papillary tumor; or [3] the in situ component looks histologically distinct from the papillary tumor [8].

Involvement of the Prostate

Invasion of the prostate may occur in three ways with different tumor staging. First, tumors can initially spread along the prostatic urethral mucosa and prostate glands as carcinoma in situ or noninvasive papillary urothelial carcinoma and then subsequently invade the prostatic stroma (transurethral mucosal route, pT2). Second, tumors may invade through the bladder wall and the base of the prostate directly into the prostate gland (pT4). Third, tumors can also invade into extravesical fat and then extend back into the prostate gland (pT4). The latter two routes are considered direct transmural invasion. In other circumstances in which involvement by urothelial carcinoma is seen in both sites, separate urinary bladder and prostatic urethral staging should be assigned.

Lymph Nodes and Distant Spread

Confirming the presence of nodal metastasis is a critical diagnostic role for pathologists, as the presence of nodal disease may indicate the need for adjuvant therapy. The primary regional lymph nodes of the urinary bladder are the perivesical, internal, and external iliac, obturator, and sacral nodes. The primary regional lymph nodes drain into the common iliac nodes, which constitute a secondary drainage region [5]. In contrast, the regional lymph nodes of the urethra and penis include the superficial and deep inguinal lymph nodes (Fig. 17.6). Therefore, when an inguinal lymph node is histologically indicative of urothelial or squamous cell carcinoma, the urethra and penis should be considered as primary sites for the metastatic tumor.

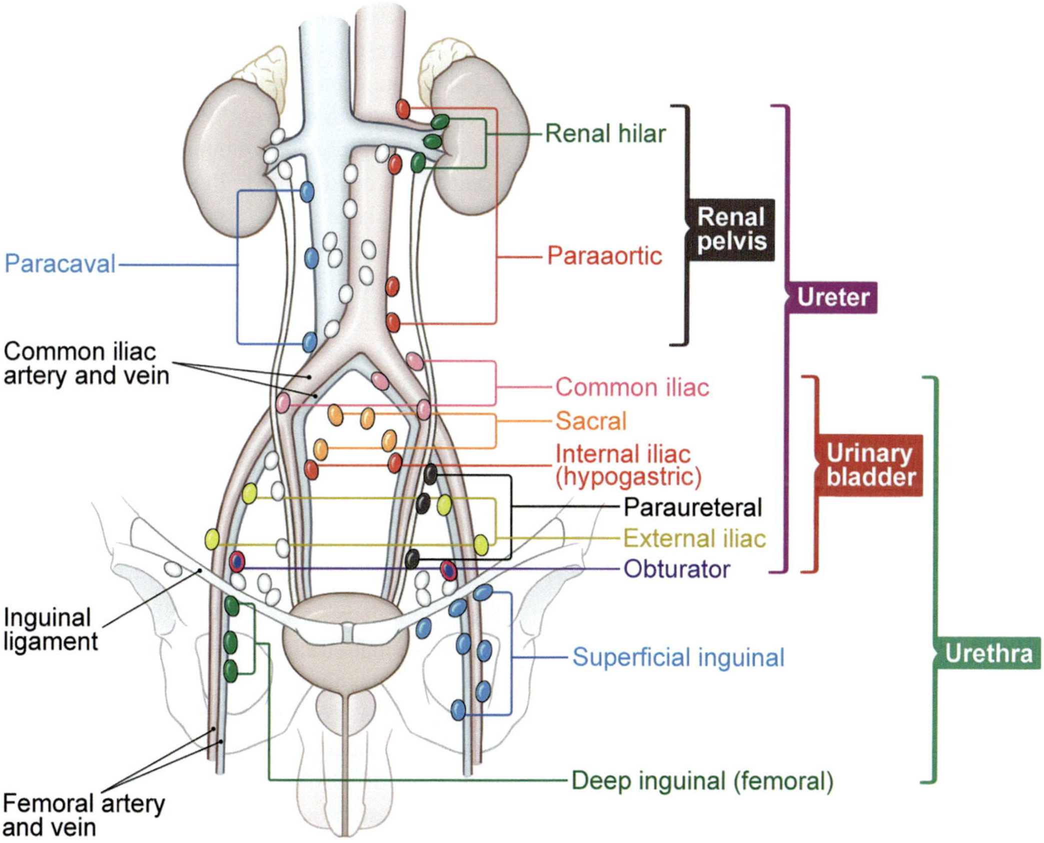

Fig. 17.6 Regional lymph nodes of the urinary tract

The total number of lymph nodes resected has been associated with improved outcomes in patients undergoing radical cystectomy. In addition, the number of resected lymph nodes involved by metastatic disease has been associated with diminished outcomes. However, neither factor has consistently been an independent factor. Nevertheless, it is recommended that both numbers are reported [5]. Pathology reports should include the number of lymph nodes submitted by the urologist, the number of lymph nodes involved by metastatic disease and, in cases of positive lymph nodes, the size of the largest lymph nodes for TNM staging, and the presence or absence of extranodal extension.

Distant spread is most common to the retroperitoneal lymph nodes, lung, bone, and liver. Lymph node involvement beyond the common iliac nodes (e.g., paracaval or intra-aortocaval) is considered metastatic (M1a).

Predictive Tissue Markers for Neoadjuvant Chemotherapy

The surgical treatment for bladder cancer is radical cystectomy and bilateral pelvic lymphadenectomy, which is often preceded by neoadjuvant cisplatin-based chemotherapy. Pathologic response is a surrogate marker to predict clinical efficacy of neoadjuvant chemotherapy and patient survival [10, 14]. Complete pathologic response is defined as pT0/pTis in surgical specimens and is observed in 26–38% of patients with neoadjuvant chemotherapy [10, 14]. There has been active research to determine the predictive biomarkers for successful neoadjuvant chemotherapy. Although none is currently widely accepted, mutations in *ERCC2* and in genes encoding proteins involved in repairing DNA damage (*ATM*, *FANCC*, *RB1*) have been proposed as predictive biomarkers for therapeutic response [15–18]. As such, molecular classification based on gene expression signature has been proposed as a potential predictive biomarker [19].

Predictive Tissue Markers for Immunotherapy

The current FDA-approved immunotherapies for advanced bladder cancers are the PD-L1 inhibitors atezolizumab (Tecentriq®), durvalumab (Imfinzi®), and avelumab (Bavencio®) and the PD-1 inhibitors nivolumab (Opdivo®) and pembrolizumab (Keytruda®). Immunostaining for PD-L1 and proteins involved in mismatch repair pathways are companion or complementary diagnostics that offer predictive value for immunotherapy efficacy [20–22]. PD-L1 immunostaining is required in the first-line setting for cisplatin-ineligible advanced bladder cancer patients to use atezolizumab and pembrolizumab. For second-line treatment, all above immunotherapeutic agents are approved without PD-L1 testing. Tumor mutation burden (TMB) and gene expression signatures have also been proposed as predictive markers for immunotherapy response in bladder cancer [20, 21].

PD-L1 Immunohistochemistry

PD-L1 immunohistochemistry is the most widely used predictive marker for the assessment of treatment response; however, given that the response rate even in PD-L1-positive patients is 20–40% and that even PD-L1-negative/low patients also respond to immunotherapy [22], this biomarker is not definitive. PD-L1 assays in clinical trials have used the Ventana SP142 (Atezolizumab), the 22C3 pharmDx (Pembrolizumab), the Ventana PD-L1 SP263 (Durvalumab), and the 28–8 pharmDx (Nivolumab) assays to quantify PD-L1 levels. The scoring algorithms and cutoff system used in clinical trials are summarized in Table 17.3 and Fig. 17.7 [23].

Mismatch Repair Deficient Tumors

All patients with tumors that are mismatch repair deficient (dMMR) or microsatellite instability (MSI)-high have been approved by FDA for pembrolizumab treatment regardless of tumor type [24], including bladder cancer. Mismatch repair (MMR) proteins repair DNA mismatches caused by misincorporation of bases during DNA replication. If DNA damage is not adequately repaired, these proteins induce apoptosis. When the MMR pathway does not function properly, mismatch errors increase and result in MSI. dMMR is diagnosed in the pathology laboratory

Table 17.3 Immunohistochemical PD-L1 assays for bladder cancer

Drug	Assay	Platform	Algorithm	Cutoffs	Comment
Atezolizumab (Tecentriq®)	Ventana SP142	Ventana	Ventana immune cell algorithm	5%	Plasma cells not included
Pembrolizumab (Keytruda®)	Dako 22c3	Dako link 48[a]	Combined positive score	10	Neutrophils and plasma cells not included
Durvalumab (Imfinzi®)	Ventana SP263	Ventana	Ventana immune cell and/or tumor cell algorithm[b]	25%	Plasma cells not included
Nivolumab (Opdivo®)	Dako 28–8	Dako link 48[a]	Tumor cell algorithm[b]	1%, 5%	

[a]Currently exclusively approved for the Dako Link 48 platform, approval process for Omnis platform is ongoing
[b]This algorithm is currently not prescribed and only explored in clinical trials

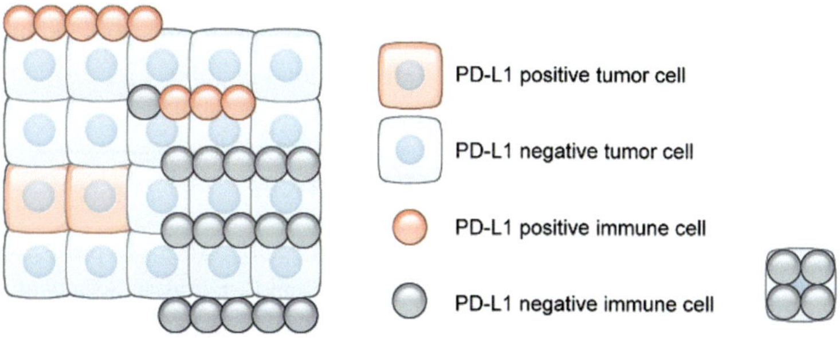

Drug	Scoring Algorithm		Example
Atezolizumab	IC score (%)	$\frac{\text{Area of PD-L1 positive immune cells}}{\text{Area of tumor cells}} \times 100$	$\frac{2}{20} \times 100 = 10\%$
Pembrolizumab	CPS score	$\frac{\text{Total number of PD-L1 positive tumor cells and immune cells}}{\text{Total number of tumor cells}} \times 100$	$\frac{10}{20} \times 100 = 10$
Durvalumab Avelumab Nivolumab	TC score (%)*	$\frac{\text{Total number (area) of PD-L1 positive tumor cells}}{\text{Total number (area) of tumor cells}} \times 100$	$\frac{2}{20} \times 100 = 10\%$
Durvalumab	IC score (%)*	$\frac{\text{Total number (area) of PD-L1positive immune cells}}{\text{Total number (area) of immune cells}} \times 100$	$\frac{8}{24} \times 100 = 33\%$

Fig. 17.7 PD-L1 scoring algorithms applied in clinical trials of urothelial carcinoma. Those algorithms that are currently not prescribed are indicated by asterisks (*)

by determining MSI through immunohistochemistry or polymerase chain reaction (PCR) tests. The immunohistochemistry-based test detects MSI by demonstrating negative staining of one or more of the four MMR proteins: MLH1, MSH2, MSH6, and PMS2 [20]. The PCR-based test measures the length of repetitive DNA sequences, known as microsatellites, in normal and tumoral tissue using five markers: BAT25, BAT26, D2S123, D5S346, and D17S250. Based on this, tumors are classified as MSI-high, MSI-low, or MSI-stable (MSS) [20]. MSI is common in colorectal cancer, occurring in 15% of patients, whereas MSI-high is reported in only 3% of urothelial carcinoma patients [20].

Tumor Mutation Burden

Mutations in tumor cells often modify the expression and function of proteins, resulting in neoantigen formation. T cells recognize these neoantigens, triggering an anti-tumor immune response [20]. Therefore, it is not surprising that cancers with high mutation rates – such as melanoma, non-small cell lung cancer, and bladder cancer – are highly responsive to immunotherapy, which boosts T cells' ability to recognize and target mutated tumor cells. Tumor mutation burden (TMB) is an estimate of somatic mutations and a good surrogate measurement of neoantigens, as it is easy to measure and use clinically. TMB can be assessed by whole exome sequencing or next-generation sequencing of selected gene panels comprised of hundreds of genes [20]. TMB cutoffs are currently in the range of 10–12 mutations per megabase, but this threshold needs to be standardized with a consistent cutoff [20].

Gene Expression Signature

There has been active research on gene expression patterns in bladder cancer, and various molecular classification systems have been proposed. Recently, a consensus classification was determined [19]. According to the consensus classification, muscle-invasive bladder cancer is classified into six subtypes: luminal papillary (24%), luminal nonspecified (LumNS, 8%), luminal unstable (LumU, 15%), stroma-rich (15%), basal/squamous (Ba/Sq, 35%), and neuroendocrine-like (3%) [19]. Significant responses to atezolizumab were reported in the LumNS, LumU, and NE-like groups. Research suggests that these molecular classifications are predictive for immunotherapeutic response, although further study is necessary.

Molecular and Genomic Testing

Molecular and genomic testing should be performed for prognostic stage groups IVA and IVB bladder cancer and may be considered for stage IIIB. Ideally, testing is performed early after advanced bladder cancer diagnosis, to facilitate appropriate treatment initiation and avoid delays in administering later lines of therapy. In addition, testing may be used to screen for clinical trial eligibility (NCCN guideline).

The most commonly identified clinically relevant genetic alterations are cyclin-dependent kinase inhibitor 2A (CDKN2A, 34%), FGFR3 (21%), phosphatidylinositol 3-kinase catalytic subunit alpha (PIK3CA, 20%), and ERBB2 (17%) [25].

Pathology Reporting

As described above, bladder cancer reports should include the specimen type, anatomic location of the tumor, tumor size and number, histologic subtype, histologic grade, surgical margin status, treatment effect, any other intraepithelial lesions, lymph node involvement with the number of positive lymph nodes, largest metastatic tumor size, and the presence or absence of extranodal extension. In biopsy and TURBT specimens, some of the above information may not be reported or may be modified due to the nature of the specimen itself. A synopsis of the formats for biopsy and cystectomy cancer specimen reports are provided in Table 17.1.

References

1. Lopez-Beltran A, Bassi PF, Pavone-Macaluso M, Montironi R, European Society of U, Uropathology Working G. Handling and pathology reporting of specimens with carcinoma of the urinary bladder, ureter, and renal pelvis. A joint proposal of the European society of uropathology and the uropathology working group. Virchows Arch. 2004;445(2):103–10.
2. Chandra A, Griffiths D, McWilliam LJ. Best practice: gross examination and sampling of surgical specimens from the urinary bladder. J Clin Pathol. 2010;63(6):475–9.
3. International Agency for Research on C, Moch H. *WHO classification of tumours of the urinary system and male genital organs.* Lyon: International Agency for Research on Cancer; 2016
4. Amin MB, McKenney JK, Paner GP, et al. ICUD-EAU international consultation on bladder cancer 2012: pathology. Eur Urol. 2013;63(1):16–35.
5. American Joint Committee on Cancer. AJCC cancer staging manual. 8th ed. New York: Springer; 2017.
6. Lopez-Beltran A, Algaba F, Berney DM, et al. Handling and reporting of transurethral resection specimens of the bladder in Europe: a web-based survey by the European network of Uropathology (ENUP). Histopathology. 2011;58(4):579–85.
7. Lopez-Beltran A, Bassi P, Pavone-Macaluso M, Montironi R. Handling and pathology reporting of specimens with carcinoma of the urinary bladder, ureter, and renal pelvis. Eur Urol. 2004;45(3):257–66.
8. Cheng L, Montironi R, Davidson DD, Lopez-Beltran A. Staging and reporting of urothelial carcinoma of the urinary bladder. Mod Pathol. 2009;22(Suppl 2):S70–95.

9. Rastogi V, Puri N, Arora S, Kaur G, Yadav L, Sharma R. Artefacts: a diagnostic dilemma – a review. J Clin Diagn Res. 2013;7(10):2408–13.
10. Kamat AM, Hahn NM, Efstathiou JA, et al. Bladder cancer. Lancet. 2016;388(10061):2796–810.
11. Ro JY, Ayala AG, el-Naggar A. Muscularis mucosa of urinary bladder. Importance for staging and treatment. Am J Surg Pathol. 1987;11(9):668–73.
12. Philip AT, Amin MB, Tamboli P, Lee TJ, Hill CE, Ro JY. Intravesical adipose tissue: a quantitative study of its presence and location with implications for therapy and prognosis. Am J Surg Pathol. 2000;24(9):1286–90.
13. Magers MJ, Lopez-Beltran A, Montironi R, Williamson SR, Kaimakliotis HZ, Cheng L. Staging of bladder cancer. Histopathology. 2019;74(1):112–34.
14. Rosenblatt R, Sherif A, Rintala E, et al. Pathologic downstaging is a surrogate marker for efficacy and increased survival following neoadjuvant chemotherapy and radical cystectomy for muscle-invasive urothelial bladder cancer. Eur Urol. 2012;61(6):1229–38.
15. Van Allen EM, Mouw KW, Kim P, et al. Somatic ERCC2 mutations correlate with cisplatin sensitivity in muscle-invasive urothelial carcinoma. Cancer Discov. 2014;4(10):1140–53.
16. Liu D, Plimack ER, Hoffman-Censits J, et al. Clinical validation of chemotherapy response biomarker ERCC2 in muscle-invasive urothelial bladder carcinoma. JAMA Oncol. 2016;2(8):1094–6.
17. Groenendijk FH, de Jong J, van de Putte EE F, et al. ERBB2 mutations characterize a subgroup of muscle-invasive bladder cancers with excellent response to neoadjuvant chemotherapy. Eur Urol. 2016;69(3):384–8.
18. Plimack ER, Dunbrack RL, Brennan TA, et al. Defects in DNA repair genes predict response to neoadjuvant cisplatin-based chemotherapy in muscle-invasive bladder cancer. Eur Urol. 2015;68(6):959–67.
19. Kamoun A, de Reynies A, Allory Y, et al. A consensus molecular classification of muscle-invasive bladder cancer. Eur Urol. 2019;77(4):420–33.
20. Arora S, Velichinskii R, Lesh RW, et al. Existing and emerging biomarkers for immune checkpoint immunotherapy in solid tumors. Adv Ther. 2019;36(10):2638–78.
21. Yarchoan M, Albacker LA, Hopkins AC, et al. PD-L1 expression and tumor mutational burden are independent biomarkers in most cancers. JCI Insight. 2019;4(6):e126908. https://doi.org/10.1172/jci.insight.126908.
22. Lattanzi M, Balar AV. Current status and future direction of immunotherapy in urothelial carcinoma. Curr Oncol Rep. 2019;21(3):24.
23. Eckstein M, Cimadamore A, Hartmann A, et al. PD-L1 assessment in urothelial carcinoma: a practical approach. Ann Transl Med. 2019;7(22):690.
24. Prasad V, Kaestner V, Mailankody S. Cancer drugs approved based on biomarkers and not tumor type-FDA approval of Pembrolizumab for mismatch repair-deficient solid cancers. JAMA Oncol. 2018;4(2):157–8.
25. Ross JS, Wang K, Khaira D, et al. Comprehensive genomic profiling of 295 cases of clinically advanced urothelial carcinoma of the urinary bladder reveals a high frequency of clinically relevant genomic alterations. Cancer. 2016;122(5):702–11.

AJCC Staging of Bladder Cancers 18

Euno Choi, Sanghui Park, and Jae Y. Ro

Introduction

Bladder cancer is one of the major causes of cancer morbidity and mortality in men, accounting for an estimated 80,470 new cases and 17,670 cancer deaths in the United States in 2019 [1]. Among many prognostic determinants, pathologic stage is the most crucial factor in risk stratification, management, and surveillance follow-up for bladder cancer [2–6]. As with other hollow visceral organs, bladder tumor (T) stage categories are defined by the depth of invasion (extent of wall invasion). However, assigning pT stage category is sometimes problematic due to regional and individual histoanatomic variation. An ideal and uniform staging system would permit accurate reflection of the natural history of cancer, the extent of disease spread, the stratification of prognostic groups and comparison of therapeutic interventions among different hospitals. Staging guidelines from the International Union Against Cancer (UICC) were released in 2016 [7, 8], and on January 1, 2018, utilization of the eighth edition of the AJCC staging manual was implemented [9]. However, the UICC failed to incorporate new data considered in the new eighth edition of AJCC, and there are many differences between the staging recommendations of recent UICC and AJCC staging systems. Thus, this chapter will discuss the current staging recommendations of the AJCC staging manual eighth edition.

E. Choi · S. Park (✉)
Department of Pathology, Ewha Womans University/Mok-dong Hospital, Seoul, South Korea
e-mail: spark0430@ewha.ac.kr

J. Y. Ro
Department of Pathology and Genomic Medicine, Weill Medical College of Cornell University/Houston Methodist Hospital, Houston, TX, USA
e-mail: jaero@houstonmethodist.org

Stage pT0 Carcinoma

Stage pT0 carcinoma is assigned when there is no evidence of residual urothelial carcinoma in the cystectomy specimen, according to the eighth AJCC staging system [9]. The incidence of stage pT0 carcinoma is approximately 10% [10–15]. Recently, the incidence of pT0 carcinoma has been increasing due to the use of neoadjuvant chemotherapy [16–18]. The presence of variant histology is associated with a decreased rate of complete pathologic response (ypT0) [19]. The clinical outcome of patients with ypT0 carcinoma is variable. The 5-year recurrence-free, cancer-specific, and overall survival rates were 84%, 88% and 84%, respectively [11]. In one study, the presence of lymphovascular invasion and concomitant carcinoma in situ in the transurethral resection (TUR) specimen were the only significant prognostic factors associated with shorter overall

H. Zhou et al. (eds.), *Urinary Bladder Pathology*, https://doi.org/10.1007/978-3-030-71509-0_18

survival and recurrence-free survival in patients with ypT0 carcinoma [11]. The incidence of lymph node metastasis of patients with ypT0 carcinoma was 3–7% [12, 14].

Stage pTa Carcinoma

There are two types of noninvasive carcinomas with one pTa and the other with pTis. Stage pTa carcinoma is defined as noninvasive papillary carcinoma that lacks invasion, according to the eighth AJCC staging system [9]. pTa carcinoma should be distinguished from pT1 carcinoma by the absence of lamina propria or submucosal invasion.

Stage pTis Carcinoma

Stage pTis carcinoma is assigned when urothelial carcinoma in situ without stromal invasion is present in the cystectomy specimen, according to the eighth AJCC staging system (Fig. 18.1) [9]. pTis carcinoma is often associated with concurrent invasive urothelial carcinoma, but it can be present alone in about 10% of cystectomy specimens [20].

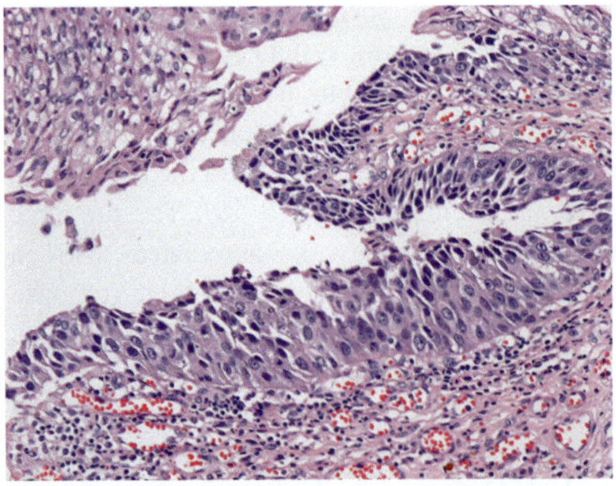

Fig. 18.1 Urothelial carcinoma in situ. Flat proliferation of urothelial cells characterized by loss of polarity, marked nuclear enlargement, irregularity, and hyperchromasia with full-thickness involvement of the urothelium. Mitoses are frequently observed

Stage pT1 Carcinoma

pT1 carcinoma is defined when a tumor invades the lamina propria/submucosa but not the proper muscle layer, according to the eighth AJCC staging system [9].

Topographic Variation of the Lamina Propria (Submucosa, Submucosal Connective Tissue Layer)

The lamina propria/submucosa (LP/SM) is composed predominantly of loose connective tissue stroma with a collection of thin smooth muscle fibers, vascular plexuses, nerves, and occasional adipose tissue between the mucosa and muscularis propria (MP) layer [21]. In the bladder, LP and SM are interchangeably used; however, the proper designation of LP and SM is available when muscularis mucosae (MM) is present: LP is the layer above MM, and SM is the layer below MM. Therefore, the proper term in the bladder is submucosal connective layer over LP or SM. In this chapter the term LP is used. The LP depth is more pronounced at the dome (0.98–3.07 mm), similar at the anterior, posterior, and lateral walls and relatively thinner at the bladder neck and trigone (0.46–1.58 mm) (Fig. 18.2) [21]. The mean tumor depth of pT1 carcinoma is 1.1–1.5 mm (range, 0.1–5 mm) [22, 23].

The MM in the urinary bladder LP layer was first described by Dixon and Gosling [24] in 1983, and Ro et al. later underlined its importance in the pathologic staging of bladder cancer [25]. The MM is usually at about the mid- to upper LP and forms a discernible layer in up to 40% of cystectomy specimens, varying by region but more common in the dome (75%) and less common in the trigone (~10%) [21]. Typically, the MM forms individual or small groups of slender and wavy fascicles or wispy fibers with (a) dispersed/scattered (71%), (b) discontinuous/interrupted (20%), or (c) continuous (3%) muscle layers (Fig. 18.3) [25]. The MM also has a focal to rarely extensive hyperplastic appearance with

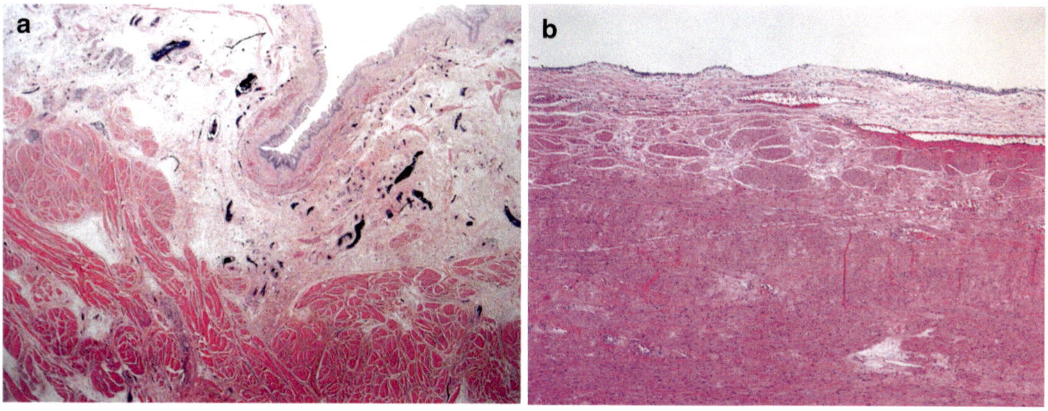

Fig. 18.2 Variable thickness of the lamina propria based on anatomical location. The lamina propria is more prominent in the dome (**a**) than in the trigone (**b**)

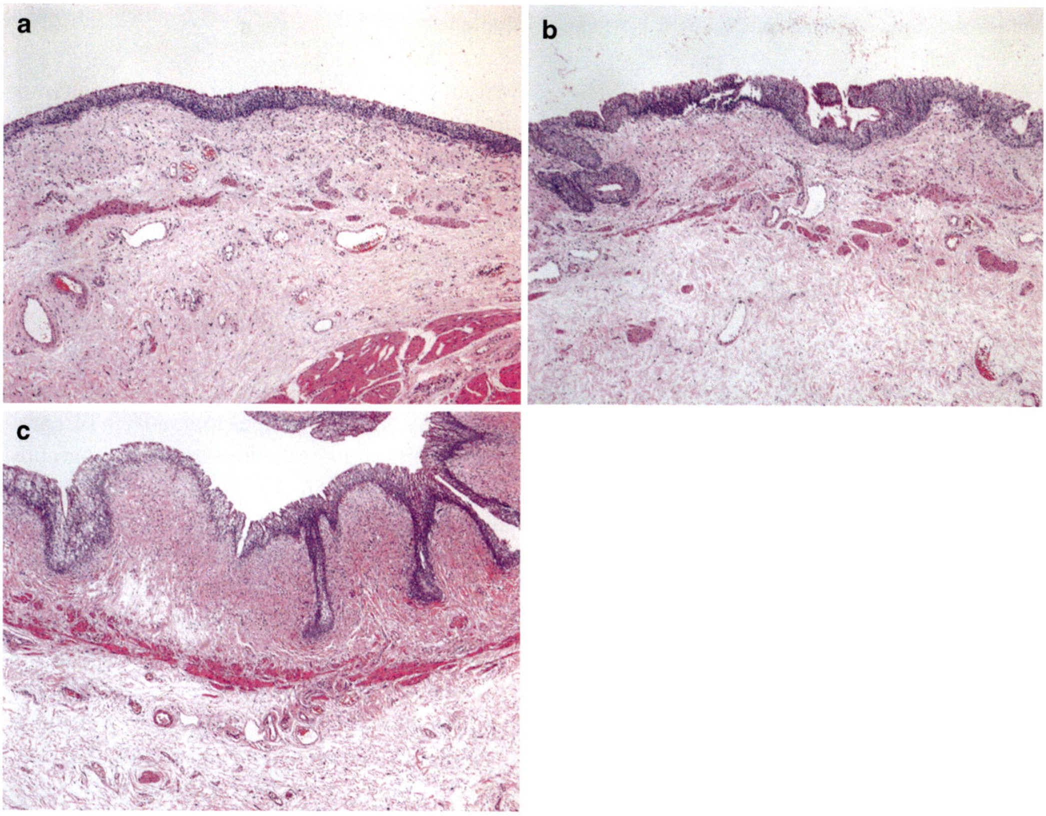

Fig. 18.3 The muscularis mucosae is composed of individual or small groups of slender and wavy fascicles or wispy fibers with variable patterns as follows: (**a**) dispersed/scattered, (**b**) discontinuous/interrupted, (**c**) continuous

two recognizable patterns of aggregates of hyperplastic MM with haphazard outlines and hyperplastic compact MM with parallel muscle fibers and a regular outline arranged singly or in small groups that sometimes mimics the muscularis propria (MP) (Fig. 18.4) [21]. Hyperplastic MM is relatively more common in the dome and less frequent in the trigone [21]. Awareness of

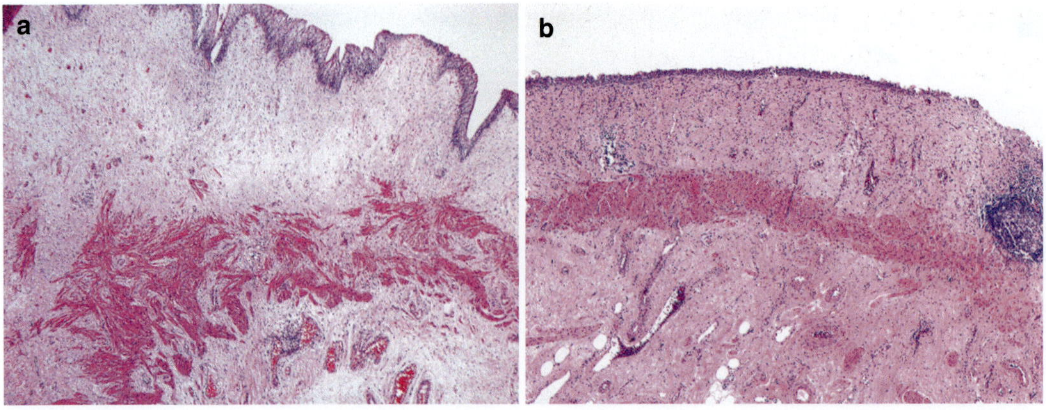

Fig. 18.4 The muscularis mucosae shows a variable hyperplastic appearance ranging from focal to rarely extensive with two discernible patterns: (**a**) haphazardly arranged hyperplastic muscularis mucosae with irregular outlines and (**b**) hyperplastic compact muscularis mucosae with parallel muscle fibers and regular outline arranged singly or in small groups. This pattern of the muscularis mucosae should be distinguished from the muscularis propria, especially in transurethral resection specimens

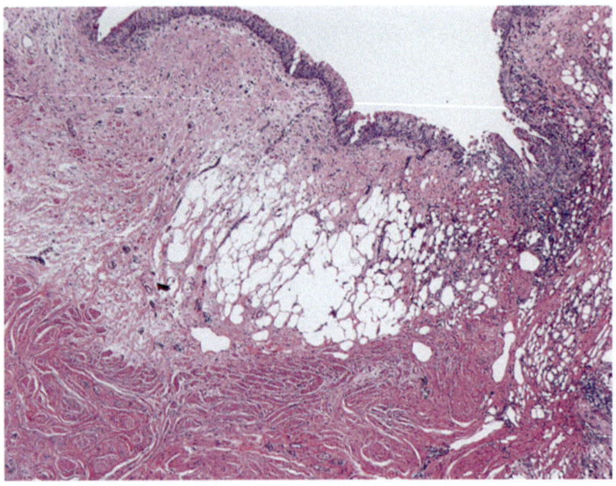

Fig. 18.5 Adipose tissue within the lamina propria. Adipose tissue is seen in the deep aspect of the lamina propria, which faces the superficial border of the muscularis propria. The presence of adipose tissue can be often misinterpreted as perivesical soft tissue in transurethral resection specimens, resulting in unnecessary overtreatment

these occasional hyperplastic MM patterns and distributions of hyperplastic MM is crucial to avoid overstaging of bladder cancer.

Adipose tissue within the LP is seen in about 50% of cystectomy specimens and typically located at the deep aspect near the superficial border of the MP (Fig. 18.5) [21, 26]. It is more often focal (35%), mostly situated in the dome (32%), and rare in the trigone (5%) [21]. Considering the high frequency of adipose tissue within the LP, care should be taken to avoid misinterpretation of pT1 carcinoma as perivesical soft tissue involvement (pT3 carcinoma) in TUR specimens to prevent inappropriate aggressive treatment.

Substaging of pT1 Bladder Carcinoma

A reproducible, easy-to-use, and accurate substaging system is essential to stratify pT1 carcinomas into prognostically distinct subgroups. There are two main approaches: histoanatomic and micrometric substaging. Histoanatomic substaging using the MM and/or vascular plexus as histologic landmarks is the most studied approach for pT1 carcinomas. Both two-tiered and three-tiered systems have been utilized. However, the size and distribution of the MM varies depending on anatomical location. Micrometric substaging of pT1 carcinoma involves measuring the depth of invasion from the mucosal basement membrane using an ocular micrometer with different linear cut-offs. However, the LP depth varies depending on location. The eighth edition of the AJCC staging manual recommends subcategorization of pT1, but no specific methods have been endorsed yet [9], and pT1 substages are not currently recommended to officially implement to use.

Histoanatomical Substaging

This method uses the MM and/or vascular plexus as landmarks to divide the extent of LP invasion [27–30]. The MM is usually at about the mid- to upper LP and disperses or forms a discernable layer as a discontinuous or infrequently near-continuous layer in only about 40% of cystectomy sections [21]. In cases that lack the MM, the vascular plexus has been proposed as a surrogate, because it is typically situated at about the same level of the accompanying MM. However, the location of the vascular plexus sporadically varies from the suburothelial to the deep LP region, being above, below, and/or at the plane of the MM [21]. Therefore, some cases cannot be properly staged using this method because of absent or incomplete MM and variable locations of the vascular plexus either above or below the MM [21].

These problems may cause concern about the feasibility of pT1 substaging. However, many studies have applied histoanatomical staging in pT1 carcinomas in relation to the MM and/or vascular plexus using either the three-tiered [above (T1a), into (T1b), and below (T1c)] or a two-tiered [above and into (T1a) and below (T1b)] approach, and substaging was feasible in 43–100% (median, 93%) of the tumors [22, 23, 27, 29–56].

Micrometric Substaging

Substaging pT1 carcinoma can also be carried out by measuring the depth of invasion using an ocular micrometer, and measurement of the depth of invasion from the mucosal basement membrane in biopsy specimens correlates well with the final pathologic stage at cystectomy [57, 58]. The most studied method uses a 0.5 mm (1 high power field) cut-off to divide pT1 into pT1m (microinvasive) and pT1e (extensive) [28, 56, 59]. In contrast to the histoanatomical method, micrometric pT1 substaging using a 0.5 mm cut-off was feasible in all (100%) tumors studied [29, 34, 35, 55, 56, 59]. Other studies have also proposed different cut-offs to divide pT1, including 1 mm, 1.5 mm, 3 mm, and 6 mm [22, 23, 29, 35]. Several studies have also suggested that measuring the aggregate linear length of invasive carcinoma in TUR fragments is a superior quantification approach for pT1 substaging [60, 61].

Microinvasive Carcinoma

Microinvasive carcinoma was originally defined as tumor extending up to 5 mm from the basement membrane (Fig. 18.6) [62]. Since then, several criteria has been proposed to define microinvasive carcinoma, and the cut-off has been lowered to the proposed 0.5 mm [59]. Alternatively, Lopez-Beltran et al. suggested using 20 infiltrating tumor cells within the LP as the cut-off rather than a linear measurement [63]. The 0.5 mm cut-off is currently proposed in pT1 substaging because it has been shown to be widely attainable and correlates with outcome in the majority of studies [29, 34, 35, 55, 56, 59]. Lawless et al. compared tumors with stalk-only invasion, base-focal invasion, and base-extensive invasion and suggested that patients with base-extensive invasion had worse prognosis [64]. They proposed that the site as well as the extent of the LP invasion matters in patient stratification for risk of progression [64].

Diagnostic Pitfalls

Factors in Superficially or Focally Invasive pT1 Carcinomas

Because pT1 carcinomas often invade the LP as single cells or irregularly shaped small nests, the identification of pT1 carcinoma can be sometimes challenging when problems are encoun-

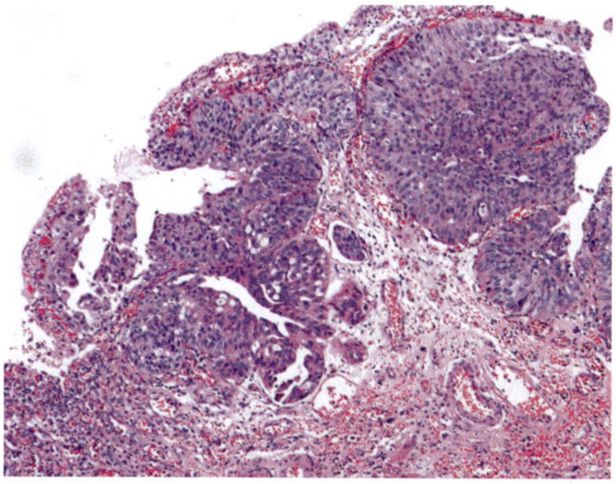

Fig. 18.6 Microinvasive carcinoma. Tumor cells microscopically invade the lamina propria with a depth less than 0.5 mm

tered such as improper tissue embedding (tangential cut or poor orientation), procedural artifacts (thermal injury or cautery artifact), or tumoral responses (obscuring due to inflammation) [65].

Bland Cytology and von Brunn Nests

Some variant histology such as nested variants show deceptively bland cytology, and florid von Brunn nests mimic invasion (Fig. 18.7) [65]. Tumor cells involving von Brunn nests either by pagetoid spread or direct extension from the adjacent tumor can be confusing and especially problematic when the involved von Brunn nests are distorted by inflammation or cautery artifact [66]. True LP invasion can be distinguished from pseudoinvasion of von Brunn nests by identifying the smooth linear contour of the basement membrane (Fig. 18.8).

Helpful Histological Features in Identifying Invasive Carcinoma

Histological features that can be helpful in identification of LP invasion include identifying single cells or irregularly shaped small nests, absence of parallel arrays of thin-walled vessels that often line the basement membrane of noninvasive nests, presence of retraction artifacts, stromal reaction, and paradoxical maturation, where invasive tumor cells obtain abundant eosinophilic cytoplasm [66]. Retraction is a helpful clue, but it sometimes mimics lymphovascular invasion, which can be distinguished from true lymphovascular invasion using immunohistochemical stains (CD34, CD31, and D2–40) [66, 67]. A stromal reaction may be helpful in identifying invasion but is not always present [68]. It may be hypocellular with myxoid background, cellular with spindle-shaped fibroblasts and variable collagenization, pseudosarcomatous, desmoplastic, or inflammatory (Fig. 18.9) [66, 67].

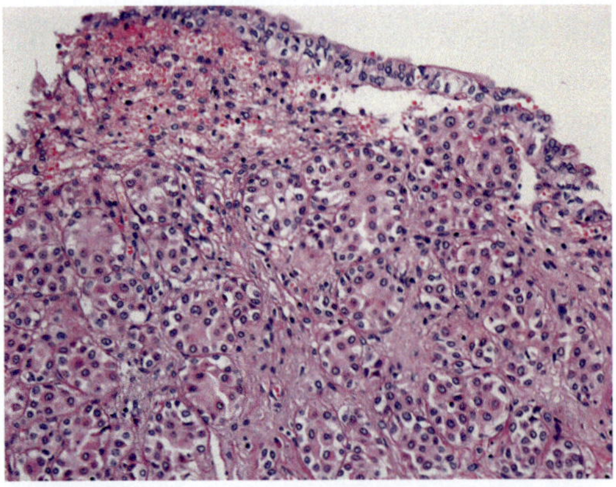

Fig. 18.7 Nested variant urothelial carcinoma. Tumor cells are arranged in tightly packed nests separated by fine collagenous stroma. Tumor cells exhibit deceptively bland cytology that often makes it difficult to distinguish nested variant urothelial carcinoma from florid von Brunn's nests

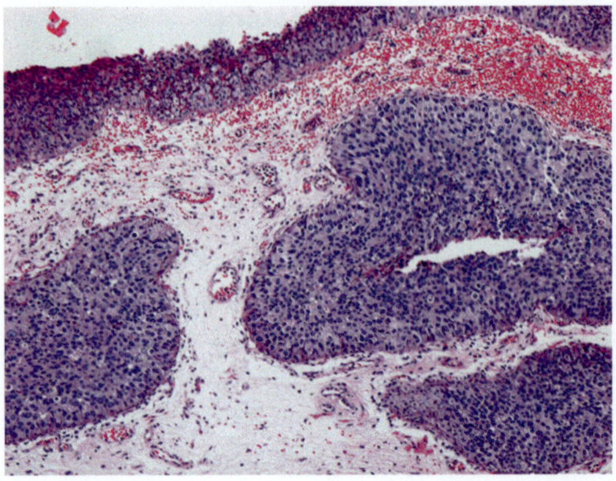

Fig. 18.8 Urothelial carcinoma in situ involving von Brunn's nests, which should not be misinterpreted as invasive carcinoma nests

Early Cystectomy

Proper muscle invasion in TUR specimens is the major indication for more aggressive treatment (radical cystectomy with bilateral pelvic lymphadenectomy, neoadjuvant chemotherapy or chemoradiation). However, early radical cystectomy can be considered when pT1 carcinoma is associated with other high-risk features such as concurrent carcinoma in situ, multiple or large tumor size (>3 cm), and repeated pT1 on re-TUR and variant histologies, particularly for micropapillary carcinoma [3, 5].

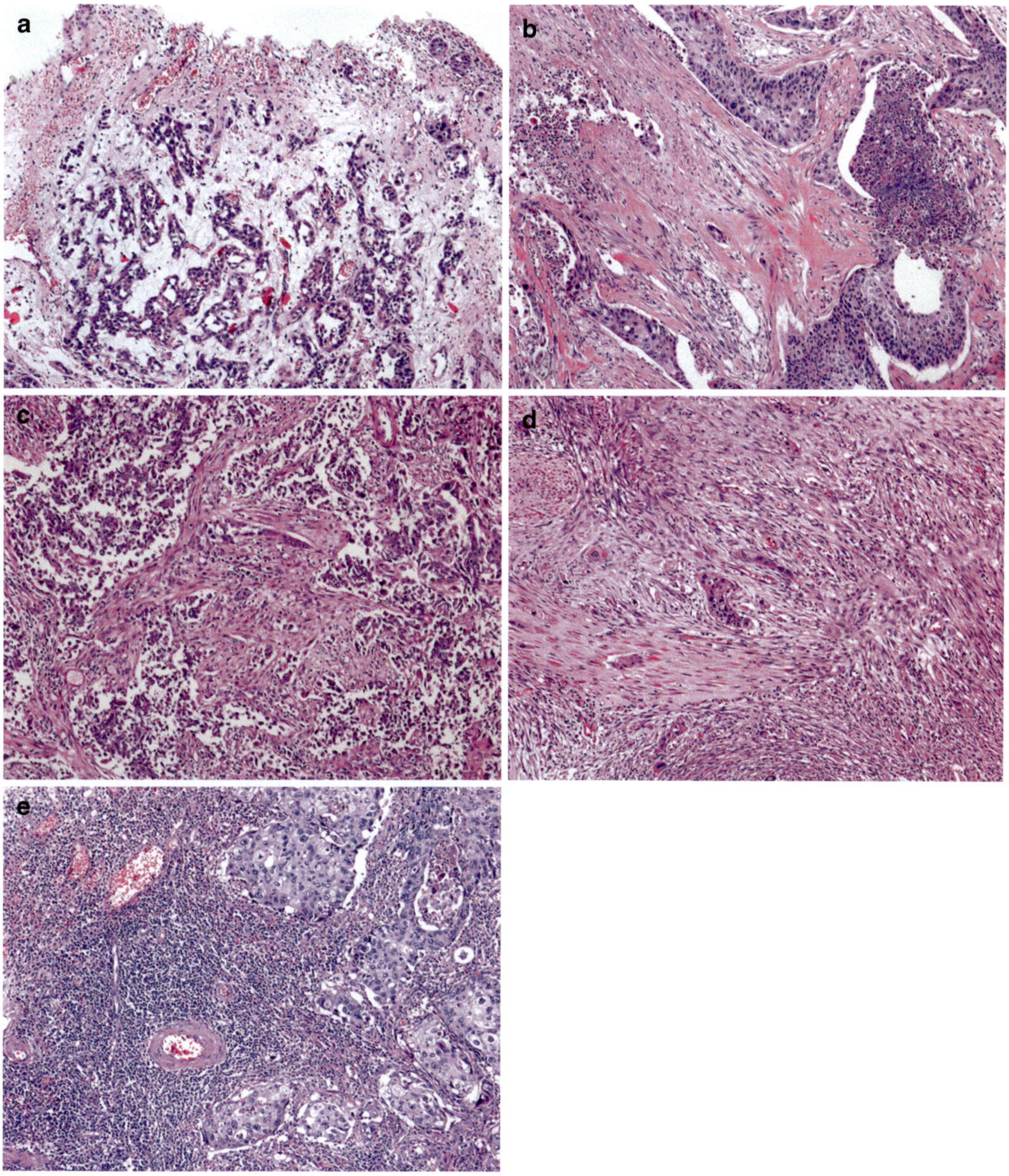

Fig. 18.9 Diverse stromal reaction seen in urothelial carcinomas. (**a**) Tumor cells infiltrate into hypocellular and loose stroma with a myxoid background. (**b**) Tumor cells are surrounded by cellular stroma composed of an admixture of spindle-shaped fibroblasts and variable collagenization. (**c**) Tumor cells are intermingled with fibrous stroma containing atypical spindle cells and lacking overt malignant histological features (i.e., increased mitotic activity, necrosis). (**d**) Tumor cells infiltrate in cords and single cells with abundant fibrous stroma. (**e**) Tumor cells are embedded in a rich inflammatory stroma with variable inflammatory cells, including lymphocytes, plasma cells, neutrophils, and eosinophils

Stage pT2 Carcinoma

Stage pT2 carcinoma is defined as tumor extending into the MP. The urinary bladder MP serves as a key anatomic landmark in the evaluation of depth of invasion and is most often the critical intersection between conservative and aggressive treatment. Diagnosing pT2 carcinomas in TUR specimens is essential for aggressive treatment, including radical cystectomy. Therefore, distinction between the MM and MP invasion is mandatory. The MP layer is composed predominantly of smooth muscle bundles, fibroconnective tissue, adipose tissue, and vessels in between the muscle bundles. A definite pT2 carcinoma is defined by infiltration into MP muscle bundles, but tumors situated in between MP muscle bundles within the MP layer are also typically staged as pT2 carcinoma [6].

Helpful Morphologic Features in Diagnosing pT2 Carcinoma

Hyperplastic MM

The MM is occasionally hyperplastic and could mimic the MP, obscuring pT1/pT2 [21, 28]. Helpful morphologic clues for the MM include thin and slender muscle bundles, superficial location, nonjuxtaposition to adipose tissue, closeness to the surface epithelium, or association with the vascular plexus [28].

LP-Inner MP Boundary and MP-Perivesical Boundary

The inner boundary of the MP can be irregular due to disconnected muscle bundles that vary in size. Therefore, the principle of defining the LP-inner MP boundary (junction of pT1 vs. pT2) is not clear. Traditionally, the outermost extent of the MP was considered the boundary distinguishing the outer MP from perivesical tissue. However, the criteria defining the outer boundary of the MP is unclear due to no clear defined boundary and aggregates of adipose tissue randomly separating MP bundles without a clear demarcation line and is different among expert pathologists. It is reasonable to follow the common approach in defining the outer MP-perivesical tissue boundary [28, 69]. A common criterion in defining the inner and outer boundary of the MP can be used. In a recent study, three general methods were reviewed by expert genitourinary pathologists without consensus, although one method (multiple boundary lines between variable outer bands of the MP) resulted in the highest level of interobserver reproducibility [69].

Staging pT2 Carcinoma in TUR Specimens

Definite pT2 carcinoma can be diagnosed by identifying tumor infiltrating into MP muscle bundles. Therefore, MP presence is considered a surrogate marker for good TUR quality [70–73]. In contrast to cystectomy specimens, the clear line of demarcation of the LP-inner MP boundary cannot be drawn in TUR specimens, where tissue fragmentation is common. Therefore, the diagnosis of pT2 carcinoma in TUR specimens is generally recommended to be restricted to cases where definite muscle invasion is present (Fig. 18.10). However, the MP can be often fractured and separated by carcinomas into small muscle bundles, masquerading pT1 carcinoma invading into the MM. Diagnosis of pT2 carcinoma is preferred when invasive carcinoma nests are surrounded by MP muscle bundles or invasive carcinoma nests are surrounding an MP muscle bundle, even without direct MP muscle invasion (Fig. 18.11) [6]. The diagnosis of pT3 carcinoma in TUR specimens is generally not recommended, because adipose tissue in the MP layer may be mistakenly considered to be perivesical adipose tissue (Fig. 18.12), complicating the distinction between pT2b and pT3a disease.

Substaging of pT2 Bladder Carcinoma

pT2 carcinoma is subdivided into tumor extending into the superficial (i.e., inner half) MP (pT2a) and tumor extending into the deep (i.e., outer half) MP (pT2b). The clinical implication of this substaging is still uncertain [66], although several recent large studies have shown the clinical utility of this approach [74–77]. Using the

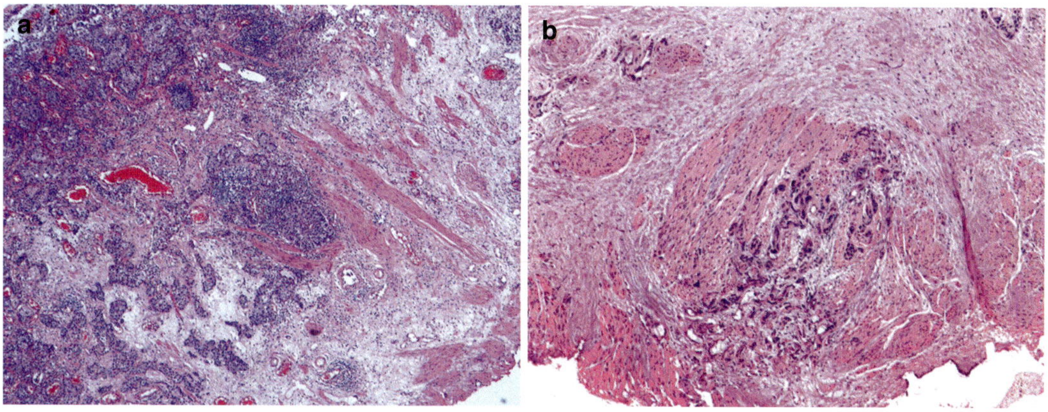

Fig. 18.10 Distinguishing between hypertrophic muscularis mucosae and muscularis propria can be problematic in transurethral resection specimens. (**a**) Tumor cell nests infiltrate into hypertrophic muscularis mucosae composed of thin and slender smooth muscle fibers (pT1). (**b**) Tumor cell nests invade into aggregates of thick muscular bundles (pT2)

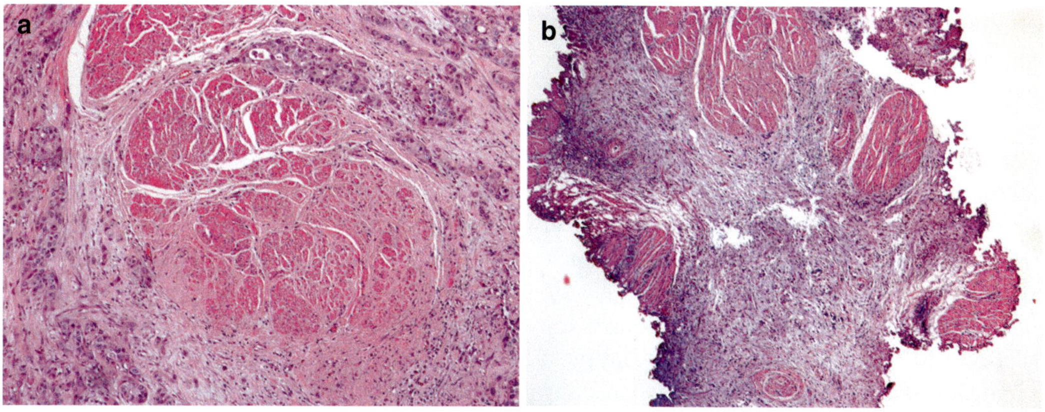

Fig. 18.11 Staging pT2 carcinoma in transurethral resection specimens. The diagnosis of pT2 urothelial carcinoma is favored when tumor cells surround some muscle bundles of the muscularis propria (**a**) or tumor cells are surrounded by muscle bundles of the muscularis propria (**b**) in transurethral resection specimens

middle of the MP as the cut-off seems to be profitable in pT2 substaging [67]. However, this substage is not recommended on TUR specimens.

Stage pT3 Carcinoma

pT3 carcinoma is defined by tumor extending into perivesical soft tissue. The outer boundary of the MP is not well delineated, confounding the distinction between T2b and T3a carcinomas. However, distinguishing pT2b from pT3a disease is critical, because pT3 disease is usually treated with adjuvant chemotherapy [69, 78, 79]. Subclassification of muscle invasive tumors (>pT2) should be made only in cystectomy specimens. It is usually not feasible to document pT3a carcinoma in biopsy or TUR specimens because the outer MP boundary is irregular, with discontinuous MP muscle bundles separated by adipose tissue or fibroconnective tissue [26].

The MP outer boundary is irregular due to discrete muscle bundles that vary in size. Therefore,

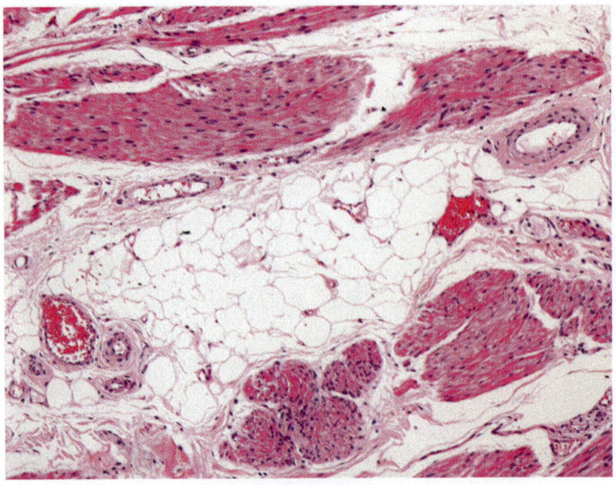

Fig. 18.12 Adipose tissue within the muscularis propria. Adipose tissue is frequently detected between the layers of the muscularis propria

the clear line of demarcation of the outer MP boundary (junction of pT2b vs. pT3a) cannot be delineated, and the criteria of definition vary among expert pathologists. In an interobserver study tasked to assign stage on equivocal cases, three categories for delineating the outer MP boundary were used as follows: (1) drawing a straight horizontal line using the outermost MP bundle edges as reference for the MP-perivesical tissue boundary, (2) drawing multiple discontinuous lines between the outermost MP bundle edges, and (3) making a curved line along every outermost MP muscle bundle edges. The most commonly used approach was by interconnecting the outermost MP bundles edges with multiple straight lines [69]. The presence of lymphovascular invasion alone in perivesical soft tissue should not be considered pT3a, although this is not mentioned in the eighth edition of AJCC TNM staging manual [9, 67].

Substaging of pT3 Bladder Carcinoma

pT3 carcinoma is subdivided further into pT3a (i.e., microscopic invasion of perivesical soft tissue) and pT3b (i.e., macroscopic invasion of perivesical soft tissue). To date, pT3 substaging counts entirely on meticulous gross examination of perivesical soft tissue. Even in a tertiary institution, the presence or absence of macroscopic perivesical soft tissue involvement was not documented in 17% of pT3 cystectomy specimens [80]. Moreover, there is considerable debate about the prognostic significance of pT3 substaging [81–86]. However, it was adopted for use in the AJCC 2010 system [87]. An alternative approach has also been proposed to subdivide pT3 by measuring the depth of invasion into the perivesical soft tissue from the base of the MP (>4.5 mm) [88], but this approach remains to be clarified due to inconsistency in defining the MP base (outer boundary of the MP) [69].

Stage pT4 Carcinoma

pT4 carcinoma is defined as extravesical tumor directly invading adjacent organs or structures and is subcategorized into pT4a (direct invasion into the prostatic stroma, uterus, or vagina) and pT4b (direct invasion into the pelvic or abdominal wall) [9]. Overall, 11.7–19.2% and 1.9–4.4% of patients with radical cystectomy harbor pT4a or pT4b disease, respectively, according to recent studies [89, 90].

Substaging of pT4 Bladder Carcinoma

Prostatic Stromal Invasion

Prostatic stromal invasion by bladder cancer may occur by transmural extravesical, transmural bladder neck, and superficially intraurethral invasion [91–93]. Among these routes, transmural direct invasion of the prostatic stroma through extravesical fat or the bladder neck merits classification as pT4a. However, the third pathway of invasion of the prostate, superficially intraurethral invasion, has been a matter of debate. Cases with superficially intraurethral invasion of the prostatic stroma are not as aggressive as a true pattern of transmural invasion [92, 94–98]. Thus, the prior 2010 AJCC staging manual excluded intraurethral spread from pT4a [87], and Patel et al. validated this revision by showing that cases with subepithelial prostatic stromal invasion had more favorable outcomes compared to transmu-

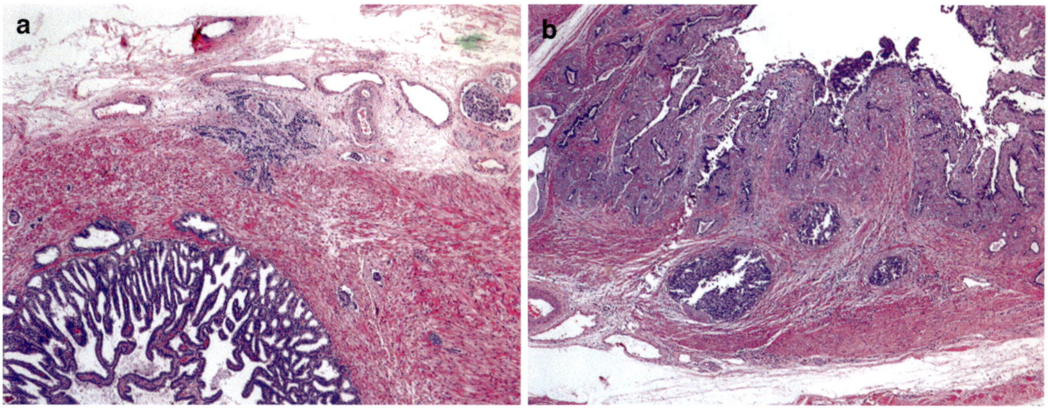

Fig. 18.13 Two distinct patterns of seminal vesicle involvement. (**a**) Direct perivesical tumor extension into the seminal vesicle. (**b**) Intramucosal pagetoid spread of urothelial carcinoma in situ

ral pT4a disease [99]. Because of the ambiguity of defining prostatic stromal invasion in the previous AJCC staging manual [87], the new eighth edition AJCC staging manual clarified that intraurethral spread of urothelial carcinoma with prostatic stromal invasion should be assigned as pT2 according to urethral cancer staging and not bladder cancer staging, and the bladder tumor should be staged separately per bladder cancer staging [9]. Therefore, providing two separate pT stages is advocated. In cases of prostatic TUR specimens, rendering a definite pT stage is not recommended. In the absence of direct prostatic stromal invasion, explanatory comments should be given and the tumor staged at least as pT2 unless otherwise specified.

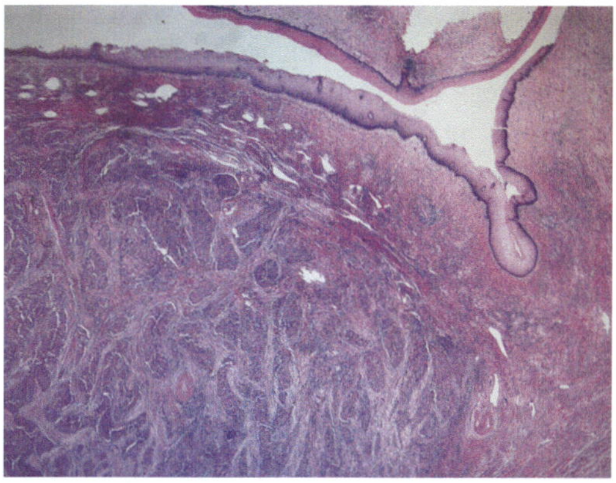

Fig. 18.14 Vaginal invasion of urothelial carcinoma. Tumor cell nests extend into the muscular layer of the vaginal wall

Seminal Vesicle Invasion

Seminal vesicle invasion may occur via direct bladder transmural perivesical soft tissue or intraepithelial extension from the prostate, and both have similarly poor prognosis (Fig. 18.13) [100]. However, the significance of seminal vesicle invasion through an intraurethral prostatic route is uncertain [101]. Direct seminal vesicle invasion is staged as pT4 according to the current eighth AJCC staging manual, but there is no further subclassification [9]. Studies demonstrate that seminal vesicle invasion has a more unfavorable effect on survival than prostatic stromal invasion alone and argue a prognosis comparable with pT4b tumor [100, 102, 103].

Gynecological Tract Invasion

Direct invasion of the uterus or vagina by bladder cancer is regarded as stage pT4a (Fig. 18.14) [9], and the incidence is relatively rare (3–6% of female cystectomy specimens) compared to prostatic stromal invasion (7–38% of male cystoprostatectomy specimens) [91–97, 104–110]. The involvement of urothelial carcinoma in the female gynecological tract either via pagetoid or metastatic spread would not be considered stage pT4a [9].

Pelvic or Abdominal Wall Invasion

Direct invasion of urinary bladder carcinoma into the pelvic or abdominal wall is assigned as stage pT4b [9]. Stage pT4b is uncommon due to the limited number of patients with this stage disease, constituting only 1.9–4.4% of all patients with radical cystectomy [89, 90].

Regional Nodal Staging (N Staging)

In the AJCC staging manual eighth edition, regional nodal staging in bladder cancer is determined by the number and location of positive lymph nodes, not by the number and size of positive lymph nodes [9]. In the previous edition, regional lymph nodes included the obturator, iliac (internal and external), sacral (lateral and sacral promontory), and common iliac lymph nodes [87]. In the current AJCC staging manual, perivesical lymph nodes are included as formal regional lymph nodes [9]. Regional nodal staging is classified as follows: (1) lymph nodes cannot be assessed (pNX); no lymph node metastasis (pN0); single regional lymph node metastasis in the true pelvis (pN1); multiple regional lymph node metastasis in the true pelvis (pN2); and metastasis to common iliac lymph nodes (pN3) [9]. Although reporting perinodal extension is not included in the AJCC staging manual eighth edition, it is recommended to report the presence or absence of extranodal extension as well as the total number of lymph nodes examined [9]. However, the minimum number of lymph nodes necessary to determine adequate pN staging has not been clarified yet for bladder cancer.

M Staging

Stage pM1 was previously designated for both non-regional lymph node metastasis and distant non-lymph node metastasis (Fig. 18.15) [87]. However, stage pM1 is now subdivided into non-regional lymph node metastasis (pM1a) and distant non-lymph node metastasis (pM1b) in the AJCC staging manual eighth edition [9] because patients with non-regional lymph node metastasis (pM1a) have a better clinical outcome than patients with distant non-lymph node metastasis (pM1b) [111].

Staging of Bladder Carcinoma Arising in a Diverticulum

The AJCC staging manual eighth edition provides formal recommendations regarding tumors arising in a diverticulum (Fig. 18.16). Most bladder diverticula are acquired and lack an MP layer [112]. Thus, the tumor moves directly from pT1 carcinoma into pT3 carcinoma without invading the MP [112–117]. The AJCC staging manual eighth edition advises skipping the pT2 stage [9].

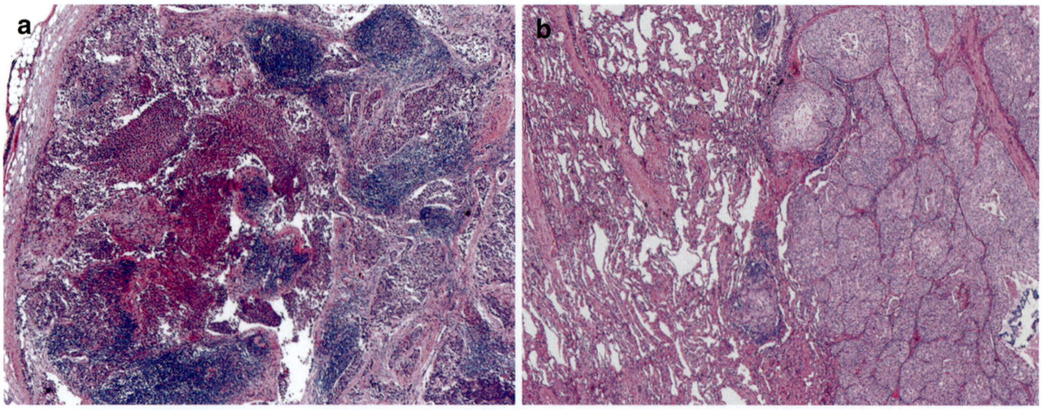

Fig. 18.15 Distant metastasis of urothelial carcinoma. (**a**) Non-regional lymph node metastasis. (**b**) Distant non-lymph node metastasis (lung metastasis)

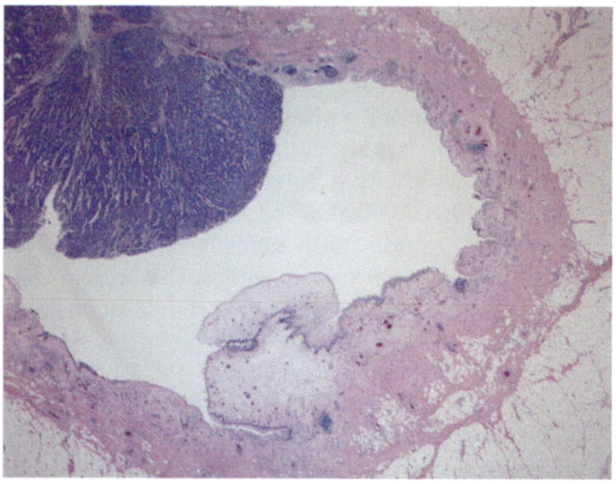

Fig. 18.16 Urothelial carcinoma arising from a diverticulum of the urinary bladder. The diverticulum, a mucosal outpouching without a muscle layer, is in direct contact with perivesical soft tissue in the deep portion. Infiltrating urothelial carcinoma that developed in a diverticulum invades into subepithelial connective tissue. Squamous metaplasia is noted in the non-tumoral epithelium within the diverticulum

In conclusion, this chapter provides a comprehensive review with regard to bladder cancer staging including a reliable substaging method of each stage based on histoanatomic characteristics. In addition, confounding factors or diagnostic pitfalls in the staging of bladder cancer were discussed. The accurate staging is crucial to determine the prognosis and the prompt treatment option of bladder cancer patients. This chapter will offer a standardized guideline for bladder cancer staging to reduce disagreement in staging among pathologists and to define the optimal treatment for bladder cancer patients.

References

1. Siegel RL, Miller KD, Jemal A. Cancer statistics, 2019. CA Cancer J Clin. 2019;69(1):7–34. https://doi.org/10.3322/caac.21551.
2. Alfred Witjes J, Lebret T, Comperat EM, Cowan NC, De Santis M, Bruins HM, Hernandez V, Espinos EL, Dunn J, Rouanne M, Neuzillet Y, Veskimae E, van der Heijden AG, Gakis G, Ribal MJ. Updated 2016 EAU guidelines on muscle-invasive and metastatic bladder Cancer. Eur Urol. 2017;71(3):462–75. https://doi.org/10.1016/j.eururo.2016.06.020.
3. Babjuk M, Bohle A, Burger M, Capoun O, Cohen D, Comperat EM, Hernandez V, Kaasinen E, Palou J, Roupret M, van Rhijn BW, Shariat SF, Soukup V, Sylvester RJ, Zigeuner R. EAU guidelines on non-muscle-invasive urothelial carcinoma of the bladder: update 2016. Eur Urol. 2017;71(3):447–61. https://doi.org/10.1016/j.eururo.2016.05.041.
4. Chang SS, Bochner BH, Chou R, Dreicer R, Kamat AM, Lerner SP, Lotan Y, Meeks JJ, Michalski JM, Morgan TM, Quale DZ, Rosenberg JE, Zietman AL, Holzbeierlein JM. Treatment of non-metastatic muscle-invasive bladder cancer: AUA/ASCO/ASTRO/SUO guideline. J Urol. 2017;198(3):552–9. https://doi.org/10.1016/j.juro.2017.04.086.
5. Chang SS, Boorjian SA, Chou R, Clark PE, Daneshmand S, Konety BR, Pruthi R, Quale DZ, Ritch CR, Seigne JD, Skinner EC, Smith ND, McKiernan JM. Diagnosis and treatment of non-muscle invasive bladder Cancer: AUA/SUO guideline. J Urol. 2016;196(4):1021–9. https://doi.org/10.1016/j.juro.2016.06.049.
6. Gallan AJ, Choy B, Paner GP. Contemporary grading and staging of urothelial neoplasms of the urinary bladder: new concepts and approaches to challenging scenarios. Surg Pathol Clin. 2018;11(4):775–95. https://doi.org/10.1016/j.path.2018.07.006.
7. Brierley JGM, Wittekind C. TNM classification of malignant tumours. 8th ed. Chichester: John Wiley & Sons Inc; 2017.
8. Delahunt B, Egevad L, Samaratunga H, Varma M, Verrill C, Cheville J, Kristiansen G, Corbishley C, Berney DM. UICC drops the ball in the 8th edition TNM staging of urological cancers. Histopathology. 2017;71(1):5–11. https://doi.org/10.1111/his.13200.
9. Amin MBES, Greene FL, et al. AJCC cancer staging manual. 8th ed. Chicago: Springer; 2016.
10. Dalbagni G, Genega E, Hashibe M, Zhang ZF, Russo P, Herr H, Reuter V. Cystectomy for bladder cancer: a contemporary series. J Urol. 2001;165(4):1111–6.
11. Kassouf W, Spiess PE, Brown GA, Munsell MF, Grossman HB, Siefker-Radtke A, Dinney CP, Kamat AM. P0 stage at radical cystectomy for bladder cancer is associated with improved outcome independent of traditional clinical risk factors. Eur Urol. 2007;52(3):769–74. https://doi.org/10.1016/j.eururo.2007.03.086.
12. Palapattu GS, Shariat SF, Karakiewicz PI, Bastian PJ, Rogers CG, Amiel G, Lotan Y, Vazina A, Gupta A, Sagalowsky AI, Lerner SP, Schoenberg MP. Cancer specific outcomes in patients with pT0 disease following radical cystectomy. J Urol. 2006;175(5):1645–9.; discussion 1649. https://doi.org/10.1016/s0022-5347(05)00995-x.
13. Thrasher JB, Frazier HA, Robertson JE, Paulson DF. Does of stage pT0 cystectomy specimen confer a survival advantage in patients with minimally invasive bladder cancer? J Urol. 1994;152(2 Pt 1):393–6. https://doi.org/10.1016/s0022-5347(17)32746-5.
14. Volkmer BG, Kuefer R, Bartsch G Jr, Straub M, de Petriconi R, Gschwend JE, Hautmann RE. Effect of

a pT0 cystectomy specimen without neoadjuvant therapy on survival. Cancer. 2005;104(11):2384–91. https://doi.org/10.1002/cncr.21475.
15. Yiou R, Patard JJ, Benhard H, Abbou CC, Chopin DK. Outcome of radical cystectomy for bladder cancer according to the disease type at presentation. BJU Int. 2002;89(4):374–8. https://doi.org/10.1046/j.1464-4096.2001.001020.x.
16. Kim HS, Jeong CW, Kwak C, Kim HH, Ku JH. Pathological T0 following cisplatin-based neoadjuvant chemotherapy for muscle-invasive bladder cancer: a network meta-analysis. Clin Cancer Res. 2016;22(5):1086–94. https://doi.org/10.1158/1078-0432.Ccr-15-1208.
17. Lavery HJ, Stensland KD, Niegisch G, Albers P, Droller MJ. Pathological T0 following radical cystectomy with or without neoadjuvant chemotherapy: a useful surrogate. J Urol. 2014;191(4):898–906. https://doi.org/10.1016/j.juro.2013.10.142.
18. Petrelli F, Coinu A, Cabiddu M, Ghilardi M, Vavassori I, Barni S. Correlation of pathologic complete response with survival after neoadjuvant chemotherapy in bladder cancer treated with cystectomy: a meta-analysis. Eur Urol. 2014;65(2):350–7. https://doi.org/10.1016/j.eururo.2013.06.049.
19. Pokuri VK, Syed JR, Yang Z, Field EP, Cyriac S, Pili R, Levine EG, Azabdaftari G, Trump DL, Guru K, George S. Predictors of complete pathologic response (pT0) to neoadjuvant chemotherapy in muscle-invasive bladder carcinoma. Clin Genitourin Cancer. 2016;14(1):e59–65. https://doi.org/10.1016/j.clgc.2015.09.013.
20. Shariat SF, Karakiewicz PI, Palapattu GS, Lotan Y, Rogers CG, Amiel GE, Vazina A, Gupta A, Bastian PJ, Sagalowsky AI, Schoenberg MP, Lerner SP. Outcomes of radical cystectomy for transitional cell carcinoma of the bladder: a contemporary series from the bladder Cancer research consortium. J Urol. 2006;176(6 Pt 1):2414–22.; discussion 2422. https://doi.org/10.1016/j.juro.2006.08.004.
21. Paner GP, Ro JY, Wojcik EM, Venkataraman G, Datta MW, Amin MB. Further characterization of the muscle layers and lamina propria of the urinary bladder by systematic histologic mapping: implications for pathologic staging of invasive urothelial carcinoma. Am J Surg Pathol. 2007;31(9):1420–9. https://doi.org/10.1097/PAS.0b013e3180588283.
22. Brimo F, Wu C, Zeizafoun N, Tanguay S, Aprikian A, Mansure JJ, Kassouf W. Prognostic factors in T1 bladder urothelial carcinoma: the value of recording millimetric depth of invasion, diameter of invasive carcinoma, and muscularis mucosa invasion. Hum Pathol. 2013;44(1):95–102. https://doi.org/10.1016/j.humpath.2012.04.020.
23. Cheng L, Neumann RM, Weaver AL, Spotts BE, Bostwick DG. Predicting cancer progression in patients with stage T1 bladder carcinoma. J Clin Oncol Off J Am Soc Clin Oncol. 1999;17(10):3182–7. https://doi.org/10.1200/jco.1999.17.10.3182.
24. Dixon JS, Gosling JA. Histology and fine structure of the muscularis mucosae of the human urinary bladder. J Anat. 1983;136(Pt 2):265–71.
25. Ro JY, Ayala AG, el-Naggar A (1987) Muscularis mucosa of urinary bladder. Importance for staging and treatment. Am J Surg Pathol 11(9):668–673. https://doi.org/10.1097/00000478-198709000-00002.
26. Philip AT, Amin MB, Tamboli P, Lee TJ, Hill CE, Ro JY. Intravesical adipose tissue: a quantitative study of its presence and location with implications for therapy and prognosis. Am J Surg Pathol. 2000;24(9):1286–90. https://doi.org/10.1097/00000478-200009000-00013.
27. Orsola A, Werner L, de Torres I, Martin-Doyle W, Raventos CX, Lozano F, Mullane SA, Leow JJ, Barletta JA, Bellmunt J, Morote J. Reexamining treatment of high-grade T1 bladder cancer according to depth of lamina propria invasion: a prospective trial of 200 patients. Br J Cancer. 2015;112(3):468–74. https://doi.org/10.1038/bjc.2014.633.
28. Paner GP, Montironi R, Amin MB. Challenges in pathologic staging of bladder cancer: proposals for fresh approaches of assessing pathologic stage in light of recent studies and observations pertaining to bladder Histoanatomic variances. Adv Anat Pathol. 2017;24(3):113–27. https://doi.org/10.1097/pap.0000000000000152.
29. Patriarca C, Hurle R, Moschini M, Freschi M, Colombo P, Colecchia M, Ferrari L, Guazzoni G, Conti A, Conti G, Luciano R, Magnani T, Colombo R. Usefulness of pT1 substaging in papillary urothelial bladder carcinoma. Diagn Pathol. 2016;11:6. https://doi.org/10.1186/s13000-016-0466-6.
30. Roupret M, Seisen T, Comperat E, Larre S, Mazerolles C, Gobet F, Fetissof F, Fromont G, Safsaf A, d'Arcier BF, Celhay O, Validire P, Rozet F, Irani J, Soulie M, Pfister C. Prognostic interest in discriminating muscularis mucosa invasion (T1a vs T1b) in nonmuscle invasive bladder carcinoma: French national multicenter study with central pathology review. J Urol. 2013;189(6):2069–76. https://doi.org/10.1016/j.juro.2012.11.120.
31. Andius P, Johansson SL, Holmang S. Prognostic factors in stage T1 bladder cancer: tumor pattern (solid or papillary) and vascular invasion more important than depth of invasion. Urology. 2007;70(4):758–62. https://doi.org/10.1016/j.urology.2007.06.638.
32. Angulo JC, Lopez JI, Grignon DJ, Sanchez-Chapado M. Muscularis mucosa differentiates two populations with different prognosis in stage T1 bladder cancer. Urology. 1995;45(1):47–53. https://doi.org/10.1016/s0090-4295(95)96490-8.
33. Bernardini S, Billerey C, Martin M, Adessi GL, Wallerand H, Bittard H. The predictive value of muscularis mucosae invasion and p53 over expression on progression of stage T1 bladder carcinoma. J Urol. 2001;165(1):42–6.; discussion 46. https://doi.org/10.1097/00005392-200101000-00011.
34. Bertz S, Denzinger S, Otto W, Wieland WF, Stoehr R, Hofstaedter F, Hartmann A. Substaging by esti-

mating the size of invasive tumour can improve risk stratification in pT1 urothelial bladder cancer-evaluation of a large hospital-based single-Centre series. Histopathology. 2011;59(4):722–32. https://doi.org/10.1111/j.1365-2559.2011.03989.x.
35. Chang WC, Chang YH, Pan CC. Prognostic significance in substaging of T1 urinary bladder urothelial carcinoma on transurethral resection. Am J Surg Pathol. 2012;36(3):454–61. https://doi.org/10.1097/PAS.0b013e31823dafd3.
36. Faivre d'Arcier B, Celhay O, Safsaf A, Zairi A, Pfister C, Soulie M, Rozet F, Roupret M, Fromont G, Mazerolles C, Gobet F, Fetissof F, Irani J. T1 bladder carcinoma: prognostic value of the muscularis mucosae invasion (T1a/T1b). A multicenter study by the French urological association (CCAFU). Prog Urol. 2010;20(6):440–9. https://doi.org/10.1016/j.purol.2010.02.002.
37. Fransen van de Putte EE, Behrendt MA, Pigot GL, van der Kwast TH, van Rhijn BW. Prognostic significance of substage and WHO classification systems in T1 urothelial carcinoma of the bladder. Curr Opin Urol. 2015;25(5):427–35. https://doi.org/10.1097/mou.0000000000000202.
38. Hasui Y, Osada Y, Kitada S, Nishi S. Significance of invasion to the muscularis mucosae on the progression of superficial bladder cancer. Urology. 1994;43(6):782–6. https://doi.org/10.1016/0090-4295(94)90134-1.
39. Hermann GG, Horn T, Steven K. The influence of the level of lamina propria invasion and the prevalence of p53 nuclear accumulation on survival in stage T1 transitional cell bladder cancer. J Urol. 1998;159(1):91–4. https://doi.org/10.1016/s0022-5347(01)64021-7.
40. Holmang S, Hedelin H, Anderstrom C, Holmberg E, Johansson SL. The importance of the depth of invasion in stage T1 bladder carcinoma: a prospective cohort study. J Urol. 1997;157(3):800–3.; discussion 804. https://doi.org/10.1016/s0022-5347(01)65044-4.
41. Kondylis FI, Demirci S, Ladaga L, Kolm P, Schellhammer PF. Outcomes after intravesical bacillus Calmette-Guerin are not affected by substaging of high grade T1 transitional cell carcinoma. J Urol. 2000;163(4):1120–3.
42. Lee JY, Joo HJ, Cho DS, Kim SI, Ahn HS, Kim SJ. Prognostic significance of substaging according to the depth of Lamina Propria invasion in primary T1 transitional cell carcinoma of the bladder. Korean J Urol. 2012;53(5):317–23. https://doi.org/10.4111/kju.2012.53.5.317.
43. Mhawech-Fauceglia P, Fischer G, Alvarez V Jr, Ahmed A, Herrmann FR. Predicting outcome in minimally invasive (T1a and T1b) urothelial bladder carcinoma using a panel of biomarkers: a high throughput tissue microarray analysis. BJU Int. 2007;100(5):1182–7. https://doi.org/10.1111/j.1464-410X.2007.07090.x.
44. Nguyen-Huu Y, Delorme G, Lillaz J, Bedgedjian I, Le Ray-Ferrieres I, Chabannes E, Bernardini S, Guichard G, Bittard H, Kleinclauss F. Muscularis mucosae invasion: prognostic factor for intravesical BCG immunotherapy failure for T1 bladder carcinoma. Prog Urol. 2012;22(5):284–90. https://doi.org/10.1016/j.purol.2011.10.002.
45. Olsson H, Hultman P, Rosell J, Jahnson S. Population-based study on prognostic factors for recurrence and progression in primary stage T1 bladder tumours. Scand J Urol. 2013;47(3):188–95. https://doi.org/10.3109/00365599.2012.719539.
46. Orsola A, Cecchini L, Raventos CX, Trilla E, Planas J, Landolfi S, de Torres I, Morote J. Risk factors for positive findings in patients with high-grade T1 bladder cancer treated with transurethral resection of bladder tumour (TUR) and bacille Calmette-Guerin therapy and the decision for a repeat TUR. BJU Int. 2010;105(2):202–7. https://doi.org/10.1111/j.1464-410X.2009.08694.x.
47. Orsola A, Trias I, Raventos CX, Espanol I, Cecchini L, Bucar S, Salinas D, Orsola I. Initial high-grade T1 urothelial cell carcinoma: feasibility and prognostic significance of lamina propria invasion microstaging (T1a/b/c) in BCG-treated and BCG-non-treated patients. Eur Urol. 2005;48(2):231–8.; discussion 238. https://doi.org/10.1016/j.eururo.2005.04.013.
48. Palou J, Sylvester RJ, Faba OR, Parada R, Pena JA, Algaba F, Villavicencio H. Female gender and carcinoma in situ in the prostatic urethra are prognostic factors for recurrence, progression, and disease-specific mortality in T1G3 bladder cancer patients treated with bacillus Calmette-Guerin. Eur Urol. 2012;62(1):118–25. https://doi.org/10.1016/j.eururo.2011.10.029.
49. Patschan O, Sjodahl G, Chebil G, Lovgren K, Lauss M, Gudjonsson S, Kollberg P, Eriksson P, Aine M, Mansson W, Ferno M, Liedberg F, Hoglund M. A molecular pathologic framework for risk stratification of stage T1 urothelial carcinoma. Eur Urol. 2015;68(5):824–32.; discussion 835-826. https://doi.org/10.1016/j.eururo.2015.02.021.
50. Platz CE, Cohen MB, Jones MP, Olson DB, Lynch CF. Is microstaging of early invasive cancer of the urinary bladder possible or useful? Modern pathology: an official journal of the United States and canadian academy of pathology. Inc. 1996;9(11):1035–9.
51. Shariat SF, Weizer AZ, Green A, Laucirica R, Frolov A, Wheeler TM, Lerner SP. Prognostic value of P53 nuclear accumulation and histopathologic features in T1 transitional cell carcinoma of the urinary bladder. Urology. 2000;56(5):735–40. https://doi.org/10.1016/s0090-4295(00)00756-1.
52. Smits G, Schaafsma E, Kiemeney L, Caris C, Debruyne F, Witjes JA. Microstaging of pT1 transitional cell carcinoma of the bladder: identification of subgroups with distinct risks of progression. Urology. 1998;52(6):1009–13.; discussion 1013-1004. https://doi.org/10.1016/s0090-4295(98)00374-4.

53. Soukup V, Duskova J, Pesl M, Capoun O, Feherova Z, Zamecnik L, Hanus T, Babjuk M. The prognostic value of T1 bladder cancer substaging: a single institution retrospective study. Urol Int. 2014;92(2):150–6. https://doi.org/10.1159/000355358.
54. Sozen S, Akbal C, Sokmensuer C, Ekici S, Ozen H. Microstaging of pT1 transitional cell carcinoma of the bladder. Does it really differentiate two populations with different prognoses? (pT1 subcategory). Urol Int. 2002;69(3):200–6. https://doi.org/10.1159/000063941.
55. De Marco V, Cerruto MA, D'Elia C, Brunelli M, Otte O, Minja A, Luchini C, Novella G, Cavalleri S, Martignoni G, Artibani W. Prognostic role of substaging in T1G3 transitional cell carcinoma of the urinary bladder. Mol Clin Oncol. 2014;2(4):575–80. https://doi.org/10.3892/mco.2014.290.
56. van Rhijn BW, van der Kwast TH, Alkhateeb SS, Fleshner NE, van Leenders GJ, Bostrom PJ, van der Aa MN, Kakiashvili DM, Bangma CH, Jewett MA, Zlotta AR. A new and highly prognostic system to discern T1 bladder cancer substage. Eur Urol. 2012;61(2):378–84. https://doi.org/10.1016/j.eururo.2011.10.026.
57. Cheng L, Weaver AL, Bostwick DG. Predicting extravesical extension of bladder carcinoma: a novel method based on micrometer measurement of the depth of invasion in transurethral resection specimens. Urology. 2000;55(5):668–72. https://doi.org/10.1016/s0090-4295(99)00595-6.
58. Cheng L, Weaver AL, Neumann RM, Scherer BG, Bostwick DG. Substaging of T1 bladder carcinoma based on the depth of invasion as measured by micrometer: a new proposal. Cancer. 1999;86(6):1035–43. https://doi.org/10.1002/(sici)1097-0142(19990915)86:6<1035::aid-cncr20>3.0.co;2-d.
59. van der Aa MN, van Leenders GJ, Steyerberg EW, van Rhijn BW, Jobsis AC, Zwarthoff EC, van der Kwast TH. A new system for substaging pT1 papillary bladder cancer: a prognostic evaluation. Hum Pathol. 2005;36(9):981–6. https://doi.org/10.1016/j.humpath.2005.06.017.
60. Hu Z, Mudaliar K, Quek ML, Paner GP, Barkan GA. Measuring the dimension of invasive component in pT1 urothelial carcinoma in transurethral resection specimens can predict time to recurrence. Ann Diagn Pathol. 2014;18(2):49–52. https://doi.org/10.1016/j.anndiagpath.2013.11.002.
61. Leivo MZ, Sahoo D, Hamilton Z, Mirsadraei L, Shabaik A, Parsons JK, Kader AK, Derweesh I, Kane C, Hansel DE. Analysis of T1 bladder cancer on biopsy and transurethral resection specimens: comparison and ranking of T1 quantification approaches to predict progression to Muscularis Propria invasion. Am J Surg Pathol. 2018;42(1):e1–e10. https://doi.org/10.1097/pas.0000000000000964.
62. Farrow GM, Utz DC, Rife CC. Morphological and clinical observations of patients with early bladder cancer treated with total cystectomy. Cancer Res. 1976;36(7 pt 2):2495–501.
63. Lopez-Beltran A, Cheng L, Andersson L, Brausi M, de Matteis A, Montironi R, Sesterhenn I, van det Kwast KT, Mazerolles C. Preneoplastic non-papillary lesions and conditions of the urinary bladder: an update based on the Ancona international consultation. Virchows Arch. 2002;440(1):3–11. https://doi.org/10.1007/s00428-001-0577-6.
64. Lawless M, Gulati R, Tretiakova M. Stalk versus base invasion in pT1 papillary cancers of the bladder: improved substaging system predicting the risk of progression. Histopathology. 2017;71(3):406–14. https://doi.org/10.1111/his.13247.
65. Lopez-Beltran A, Cheng L. Stage pT1 bladder carcinoma: diagnostic criteria, pitfalls and prognostic significance. Pathology. 2003;35(6):484–91. https://doi.org/10.1080/00313020310001619127.
66. Cheng L, Montironi R, Davidson DD, Lopez-Beltran A. Staging and reporting of urothelial carcinoma of the urinary bladder. Mod Pathol 2009;22 Suppl 2:S70–95. https://doi.org/10.1038/modpathol.2009.1.
67. Magers MJ, Lopez-Beltran A, Montironi R, Williamson SR, Kaimakliotis HZ, Cheng L. Staging of bladder cancer. Histopathology. 2019;74(1):112–34. https://doi.org/10.1111/his.13734.
68. Jimenez RE, Keane TE, Hardy HT, Amin MB. pT1 urothelial carcinoma of the bladder: criteria for diagnosis, pitfalls, and clinical implications. Adv Anat Pathol. 2000;7(1):13–25.
69. Ananthanarayanan V, Pan Y, Tretiakova M, Amin MB, Cheng L, Epstein JI, Grignon DJ, Hansel DE, Jimenez RE, McKenney JK, Montironi R, Oliva E, Osunkoya AO, Rao P, Reuter VE, Ro JY, Shen SS, Srigley JR, Tsuzuki T, Yao JL, Antic T, Haber M, Taxy JB, Paner GP. Influence of histologic criteria and confounding factors in staging equivocal cases for microscopic perivesical tissue invasion (pT3a): an interobserver study among genitourinary pathologists. Am J Surg Pathol. 2014;38(2):167–75. https://doi.org/10.1097/pas.0000000000000096.
70. Huang J, Fu J, Zhan H, Xie K, Liu B, Yang F, Lu Y, Zhou X. Analysis of the absence of the detrusor muscle in initial transurethral resected specimens and the presence of residual tumor tissue. Urol Int. 2012;89(3):319–25. https://doi.org/10.1159/000341103.
71. Mariappan P, Finney SM, Head E, Somani BK, Zachou A, Smith G, Mishriki SF, N'Dow J, Grigor KM. Good quality white-light transurethral resection of bladder tumours (GQ-WLTURBT) with experienced surgeons performing complete resections and obtaining detrusor muscle reduces early recurrence in new non-muscle-invasive bladder cancer: validation across time and place and recommendation for benchmarking. BJU Int. 2012;109(11):1666–73. https://doi.org/10.1111/j.1464-410X.2011.10571.x.

72. Mariappan P, Zachou A, Grigor KM. Detrusor muscle in the first, apparently complete transurethral resection of bladder tumour specimen is a surrogate marker of resection quality, predicts risk of early recurrence, and is dependent on operator experience. Eur Urol. 2010;57(5):843–9. https://doi.org/10.1016/j.eururo.2009.05.047.
73. Shoshany O, Mano R, Margel D, Baniel J, Yossepowitch O. Presence of detrusor muscle in bladder tumor specimens--predictors and effect on outcome as a measure of resection quality. Urol Oncol. 2014;32(1):40.e17-22. https://doi.org/10.1016/j.urolonc.2013.04.009.
74. Gakis G, Schilling D, Renninger M, Seibold J, Sievert KD, Stenzl A. Comparison of the new American joint committee on cancer substratification in node-negative pT2 urothelial carcinoma of the bladder: analysis of patient outcomes in a contemporary series. BJU Int. 2011;107(6):919–23. https://doi.org/10.1111/j.1464-410X.2010.09548.x.
75. Ghoneim MA, Abdel-Latif M, el-Mekresh M, Abol-Enein H, Mosbah A, Ashamallah A, el-Baz MA. Radical cystectomy for carcinoma of the bladder: 2,720 consecutive cases 5 years later. J Urol. 2008;180(1):121–7. https://doi.org/10.1016/j.juro.2008.03.024.
76. Sonpavde G, Khan MM, Svatek RS, Lee R, Novara G, Tilki D, Lerner SP, Amiel GE, Skinner E, Karakiewicz PI, Bastian PJ, Kassouf W, Fritsche HM, Izawa JI, Ficarra V, Dinney CP, Lotan Y, Fradet Y, Shariat SF. Prognostic risk stratification of pathological stage T2N0 bladder cancer after radical cystectomy. BJU Int. 2011;108(5):687–92. https://doi.org/10.1111/j.1464-410X.2010.09902.x.
77. Tilki D, Reich O, Karakiewicz PI, Novara G, Kassouf W, Ergun S, Fradet Y, Ficarra V, Sonpavde G, Stief CG, Skinner E, Svatek RS, Lotan Y, Sagalowsky AI, Shariat SF. Validation of the AJCC TNM substaging of pT2 bladder cancer: deep muscle invasion is associated with significantly worse outcome. Eur Urol. 2010;58(1):112–7. https://doi.org/10.1016/j.eururo.2010.01.015.
78. Milowsky MI, Rumble RB, Booth CM, Gilligan T, Eapen LJ, Hauke RJ, Boumansour P, Lee CT. Guideline on muscle-invasive and metastatic bladder cancer (European Association of Urology guideline): American society of clinical oncology clinical practice guideline endorsement. J Clin Oncol Off J Am Soc Clin Oncol. 2016;34(16):1945–52. https://doi.org/10.1200/jco.2015.65.9797.
79. Witjes JA, Comperat E, Cowan NC, De Santis M, Gakis G, Lebret T, Ribal MJ, Van der Heijden AG, Sherif A. EAU guidelines on muscle-invasive and metastatic bladder cancer: summary of the 2013 guidelines. Eur Urol. 2014;65(4):778–92. https://doi.org/10.1016/j.eururo.2013.11.046.
80. Tretter EM, Ebel JJ, Pohar KS, Zynger DL. Does the gross prosector impact pT3 subclassification or lymph node counts in bladder cancer? Hum Pathol. 2017;61:190–8. https://doi.org/10.1016/j.humpath.2016.12.009.
81. Boudreaux KJ Jr, Chang SS, Lowrance WT, Rumohr JA, Barocas DA, Cookson MS, Smith JA Jr, Clark PE. Comparison of American joint committee on Cancer pathologic stage T3a versus T3b urothelial carcinoma: analysis of patient outcomes. Cancer. 2009;115(4):770–5. https://doi.org/10.1002/cncr.24110.
82. Quek ML, Stein JP, Clark PE, Daneshmand S, Miranda G, Cai J, Groshen S, Cote RJ, Lieskovsky G, Quinn DI, Skinner DG. Microscopic and gross extravesical extension in pathological staging of bladder cancer. J Urol. 2004;171(2 Pt 1):640–5. https://doi.org/10.1097/01.ju.0000108664.39035.51.
83. Quek ML, Stein JP, Clark PE, Daneshmand S, Miranda G, Cai J, Groshen S, Lieskovsky G, Quinn DI, Raghavan D, Skinner DG. Natural history of surgically treated bladder carcinoma with extravesical tumor extension. Cancer. 2003;98(5):955–61. https://doi.org/10.1002/cncr.11569.
84. Scosyrev E, Yao J, Messing E. Microscopic invasion of perivesical fat by urothelial carcinoma: implications for prognosis and pathology practice. Urology. 2010;76(4):908–13.; discussion 914. https://doi.org/10.1016/j.urology.2010.02.073.
85. Stein JP, Lieskovsky G, Cote R, Groshen S, Feng AC, Boyd S, Skinner E, Bochner B, Thangathurai D, Mikhail M, Raghavan D, Skinner DG. Radical cystectomy in the treatment of invasive bladder cancer: long-term results in 1,054 patients. J Clin Oncol Off J Am Soc Clin Oncol. 2001;19(3):666–75. https://doi.org/10.1200/jco.2001.19.3.666.
86. Tilki D, Svatek RS, Karakiewicz PI, Novara G, Seitz M, Sonpavde G, Gupta A, Kassouf W, Fradet Y, Ficarra V, Skinner E, Lotan Y, Sagalowsky AI, Stief CG, Reich O, Shariat SF. pT3 substaging is a prognostic indicator for lymph node negative urothelial carcinoma of the bladder. J Urol. 2010;184(2):470–4. https://doi.org/10.1016/j.juro.2010.04.007.
87. Edge SBBD, Compton CC. AJCC cancer staging manual. 7th ed. New York: Springer; 2010.
88. Zarei S, Frank I, Boorjian SA, Thompson RH, Kim S, Weight C, Tarrell R, Thapa P, Cheville JC. Prognostic significance of measured depth of invasion of urothelial carcinoma of the bladder compared to the 2010 American joint committee on Cancer pT2 and pT3 classifications. J Urol. 2012;188(5):1706–11. https://doi.org/10.1016/j.juro.2012.07.035.
89. Moschini M, Zamboni S, Mattei A, Baumeister P, Di Bona C, Cornelius J, Shariat SF, Freschi M, Zaffuto E, Salonia A, Montorsi F, Briganti A, Colombo R, Gallina A. Radical cystectomy in pathological T4a and T4b bladder cancer patients: is there any space for sub stratification? Urol Int. 2019;102(3):269–76. https://doi.org/10.1159/000493899.
90. Tilki D, Svatek RS, Karakiewicz PI, Isbarn H, Reich O, Kassouf W, Fradet Y, Novara G, Fritsche HM,

Bastian PJ, Izawa JI, Stief CG, Ficarra V, Lerner SP, Schoenberg M, Dinney CP, Skinner E, Lotan Y, Sagalowsky AI, Shariat SF. Characteristics and outcomes of patients with pT4 urothelial carcinoma at radical cystectomy: a retrospective international study of 583 patients. J Urol. 2010;183(1):87–93. https://doi.org/10.1016/j.juro.2009.08.145.

91. Donat SM, Genega EM, Herr HW, Reuter VE. Mechanisms of prostatic stromal invasion in patients with bladder cancer: clinical significance. J Urol. 2001;165(4):1117–20.
92. Esrig D, Freeman JA, Elmajian DA, Stein JP, Chen SC, Groshen S, Simoneau A, Skinner EC, Lieskovsky G, Boyd SD, Cote RJ, Skinner DG. Transitional cell carcinoma involving the prostate with a proposed staging classification for stromal invasion. J Urol. 1996;156(3):1071–6.
93. Montironi R, Cheng L, Mazzucchelli R, Scarpelli M, Kirkali Z, Montorsi F, Lopez-Beltran A. Critical evaluation of the prostate from cystoprostatectomies for bladder cancer: insights from a complete sampling with the whole mount technique. Eur Urol. 2009;55(6):1305–9. https://doi.org/10.1016/j.eururo.2008.10.032.
94. Ayyathurai R, Gomez P, Luongo T, Soloway MS, Manoharan M. Prostatic involvement by urothelial carcinoma of the bladder: clinicopathological features and outcome after radical cystectomy. BJU Int. 2007;100(5):1021–5. https://doi.org/10.1111/j.1464-410X.2007.07171.x.
95. Knoedler JJ, Boorjian SA, Tollefson MK, Cheville JC, Thapa P, Tarrell RF, Frank I. Urothelial carcinoma involving the prostate: the association of revised tumour stage and coexistent bladder cancer with survival after radical cystectomy. BJU Int. 2014;114(6):832–6. https://doi.org/10.1111/bju.12486.
96. Njinou Ngninkeu B, Lorge F, Moulin P, Jamart J, Van Cangh PJ. Transitional cell carcinoma involving the prostate: a clinicopathological retrospective study of 76 cases. J Urol. 2003;169(1):149–52. https://doi.org/10.1097/01.ju.0000042810.43380.36.
97. Pagano F, Bassi P, Ferrante GL, Piazza N, Abatangelo G, Pappagallo GL, Garbeglio A. Is stage pT4a (D1) reliable in assessing transitional cell carcinoma involvement of the prostate in patients with a concurrent bladder cancer? A necessary distinction for contiguous or noncontiguous involvement. J Urol. 1996;155(1):244–7.
98. Vallo S, Gilfrich C, Burger M, Volkmer B, Boehm K, Rink M, Chun FK, Roghmann F, Novotny V, Mani J, Brisuda A, Mayr R, Stredele R, Noldus J, Schnabel M, May M, Fritsche HM, Pycha A, Martini T, Wirth M, Roigas J, Bastian PJ, Nuhn P, Dahlem R, Haferkamp A, Fisch M, Aziz A. Comparative analysis of the effect of prostatic invasion patterns on cancer-specific mortality after radical cystectomy in pT4a urothelial carcinoma of the bladder. Urol Oncol. 2016;34(10):432.e431-438. https://doi.org/10.1016/j.urolonc.2016.05.008.
99. Patel AR, Cohn JA, Abd El Latif A, Miocinovic R, Steinberg GD, Paner GP, Hansel DE. Validation of new AJCC exclusion criteria for subepithelial prostatic stromal invasion from pT4a bladder urothelial carcinoma. J Urol. 2013;189(1):53–8. https://doi.org/10.1016/j.juro.2012.09.006.
100. Daneshmand S, Stein JP, Lesser T, Quek ML, Nichols PW, Miranda G, Cai J, Groshen S, Skinner EC, Skinner DG. Prognosis of seminal vesicle involvement by transitional cell carcinoma of the bladder. J Urol. 2004;172(1):81–4. https://doi.org/10.1097/01.ju.0000132131.64727.ff.
101. Murphy WM, Crissman JD, Johansson SL, Ayala AG. Recommendations for the reporting of urinary bladder specimens that contain bladder neoplasms. Mod Pathol. 1996;9(7):796–8.
102. May M, Brookman-May S, Burger M, Gilfrich C, Fritsche HM, Rink M, Chun F, Fisch M, Roghmann F, Noldus J, Mayr R, Pycha A, Novotny V, Wirth M, Vallo S, Haferkamp A, Roigas J, Brisuda A, Stredele R, Volkmer B, Dechet C, Schnabel M, Denzinger S, Stief CG, Bastian PJ, Aziz A. Concomitant seminal vesicle invasion in pT4a urothelial carcinoma of the bladder with contiguous prostatic infiltration is an adverse prognosticator for cancer-specific survival after radical cystectomy. Ann Surg Oncol. 2014;21(12):4034–40. https://doi.org/10.1245/s10434-014-3827-y.
103. You D, Kim SC, Jeong IG, Hong JH, Ro JY, Ahn H, Kim CS. Urothelial carcinoma of the bladder with seminal vesicle invasion: prognostic significance. BJU Int. 2010;106(11):1657–61. https://doi.org/10.1111/j.1464-410X.2010.09494.x.
104. Ali-El-Dein B, Abdel-Latif M, Mosbah A, Eraky I, Shaaban AA, Taha NM, Ghoneim MA. Secondary malignant involvement of gynecologic organs in radical cystectomy specimens in women: is it mandatory to remove these organs routinely? J Urol. 2004;172(3):885–7. https://doi.org/10.1097/01.ju.0000133986.29257.bf.
105. Barocas DA, Patel SG, Chang SS, Clark PE, Smith JA Jr, Cookson MS. Outcomes of patients undergoing radical cystoprostatectomy for bladder cancer with prostatic involvement on final pathology. BJU Int. 2009;104(8):1091–7. https://doi.org/10.1111/j.1464-410X.2009.08558.x.
106. Chen ME, Pisters LL, Malpica A, Pettaway CA, Dinney CP. Risk of urethral, vaginal and cervical involvement in patients undergoing radical cystectomy for bladder cancer: results of a contemporary cystectomy series from M.D. Anderson Cancer Center. J Urol. 1997;157(6):2120–3.
107. Groutz A, Gillon G, Konichezky M, Shimonov M, Winkler H, Livne PM, Baniel J. Involvement of internal genitalia in female patients undergoing radical cystectomy for bladder cancer: a clinicopathologic study of 37 cases. Int J Gynecol Cancer. 1999;9(4):302–6. https://doi.org/10.1046/j.1525-1438.1999.99039.x.

108. Salem H, El-Mazny A. A clinicopathologic study of gynecologic organ involvement at radical cystectomy for bladder cancer. Int J Gynaecol Obstet. 2011;115(2):188–90. https://doi.org/10.1016/j.ijgo.2011.05.026.
109. Shen SS, Lerner SP, Muezzinoglu B, Truong LD, Amiel G, Wheeler TM. Prostatic involvement by transitional cell carcinoma in patients with bladder cancer and its prognostic significance. Hum Pathol. 2006;37(6):726–34. https://doi.org/10.1016/j.humpath.2006.01.027.
110. Varkarakis IM, Pinggera G, Antoniou N, Constantinides K, Chrisofos M, Deliveliotis C. Pathological review of internal genitalia after anterior exenteration for bladder cancer in women. Evaluating risk factors for female organ involvement. Int Urol Nephrol. 2007;39(4):1015–21. https://doi.org/10.1007/s11255-006-9158-6.
111. Galsky MD, Moshier E, Krege S, Lin CC, Hahn N, Ecke T, Sonpavde G, Godbold J, Oh WK, Bamias A. Nomogram for predicting survival in patients with unresectable and/or metastatic urothelial cancer who are treated with cisplatin-based chemotherapy. Cancer. 2013;119(16):3012–9. https://doi.org/10.1002/cncr.28146.
112. Hansel DE, Paner GP, Nese N, Amin MB. Limited smoothelin expression within the muscularis mucosae: validation in bladder diverticula. Hum Pathol. 2011;42(11):1770–6. https://doi.org/10.1016/j.humpath.2011.02.022.
113. Golijanin D, Yossepowitch O, Beck SD, Sogani P, Dalbagni G. Carcinoma in a bladder diverticulum: presentation and treatment outcome. J Urol. 2003;170(5):1761–4. https://doi.org/10.1097/01.ju.0000091800.15071.52.
114. Hu B, Satkunasivam R, Schuckman A, Miranda G, Cai J, Daneshmand S. Urothelial carcinoma in bladder diverticula: outcomes after radical cystectomy. World J Urol. 2015;33(10):1397–402. https://doi.org/10.1007/s00345-014-1472-5.
115. Idrees MT, Alexander RE, Kum JB, Cheng L. The spectrum of histopathologic findings in vesical diverticulum: implications for pathogenesis and staging. Hum Pathol. 2013;44(7):1223–32. https://doi.org/10.1016/j.humpath.2012.11.005.
116. Tamas EF, Stephenson AJ, Campbell SC, Montague DK, Trusty DC, Hansel DE. Histopathologic features and clinical outcomes in 71 cases of bladder diverticula. Arch Pathol Lab Med. 2009;133(5):791–6. https://doi.org/10.1043/1543-2165-133.5.791.
117. Walker NF, Gan C, Olsburgh J, Khan MS. Diagnosis and management of intradiverticular bladder tumours. Nat Rev Urol. 2014;11(7):383–90. https://doi.org/10.1038/nrurol.2014.131.

Conclusion and Remarks

19

Haijun Zhou, Charles C. Guo, and Jae Y. Ro

High Prevalence of Bladder Cancer

Bladder cancer is one of the most common cancers in the world, and it is especially prevalent in males [1]. The lifetime risk worldwide of developing urinary bladder cancer is 1.1% for males and 0.27% for females [2]. Globally, approximately 550,000 new cases were diagnosed in 2018 (approximately 425,000 males and 125,000 females) [2]. The survival rate of bladder cancer patients is also relatively high. In the United States, the 5-year relative survival rate for all bladder cancer patients is 77%. Of the 81,400 new cases of bladder cancer projected to be diagnosed in 2020 in the United States, 17,980 people will die from the disease [3]. The high survival rate is largely because of the diagnosis of non-muscle-invasive bladder cancers (NMIBC) in approximately 70–80% of new patients, including noninvasive papillary tumor (pTa), carcinoma in situ (CIS; pTis), or early invasive tumor (non-muscle-invasive; pT1). These tumors can be managed locally with transurethral resection of bladder tumor (TURBT) and intravesical chemotherapy or Bacillus Calmette-Guérin (BCG) treatment. The 5-year survival rate of pTa and pTis patients is reported to be 96% [3]. Approximately 10–20% of NMIBCs progress to muscle-invasive bladder cancer (MIBC). Characteristically, 50–70% of these cases recur [4, 5]; thus, the volume of bladder cancer surveillance cases is considerable. With increasing levels of treatment development and improved health care, bladder cancer survival rates are expected to increase, leading to a subsequent increase in the prevalence of bladder cancer [1].

The average age for an initial diagnosis of bladder cancer is 65–70 years. Global population growth and aging will increase the number of bladder cancer cases. The United Nations has reported that the world population is expected to increase from an estimated 7.7 billion people worldwide in 2019 to around 8.5 billion people in 2030 and then to 9.7 billion people in 2050 [6]. The number of persons more than 60 years of age is expected to double by 2050 to a projected 2.1 billion people [7]. With continuing population growth and aging, more bladder cancer cases are expected to be diagnosed. Pathologists are expected to see a high volume of bladder cancer cases, and bladder pathology will continue to be a common practice field.

H. Zhou (✉) · J. Y. Ro
Department of Pathology and Genomic Medicine, Weill Medical College of Cornell University/Houston Methodist Hospital, Houston, TX, USA
e-mail: hzhou@houstonmethodist.org; JaeRo@houstonmethodist.org

C. C. Guo
Department of Pathology, The University of Texas MD Anderson Cancer Center, Houston, TX, USA
e-mail: ccguo@mdanderson.org

H. Zhou et al. (eds.), *Urinary Bladder Pathology*, https://doi.org/10.1007/978-3-030-71509-0_19

Diagnostic Challenges and Clinical Management of Bladder Cancer

Cystoscopy with biopsy or TURBT requires the pathological evaluation of muscle invasiveness. T1 tumors invade lamina propria but are not muscle-invasive, and their clinical course and treatment are more like Ta tumors. Ta and T1 tumors are grouped as non-muscle-invasive tumors and are usually treated locally. Treatment of muscle-invasive tumors often involves a radical cystectomy, if operable. During microscopic evaluation, the presence or absence of muscularis propria should be documented. Hyperplastic muscularis mucosa can mimic the thick muscle bundles of the muscularis propria [8, 9], and sometimes a repeat biopsy or further studies with immunostains may be required.

Histological variants account for approximately 25% of bladder cancer cases, which poses a challenge for the practice of bladder pathology. The identification of these histological variants has important diagnostic, prognostic, and therapeutic implications [10]. The recognition of non-muscle-invasive micropapillary urothelial carcinoma warrants an early radical cystectomy in most medical centers because of its aggressive behavior [11]. The presence of sarcomatoid urothelial carcinoma suggests a poor prognosis: one large series study showed that median survival was only 18.4 month following diagnosis [12]. Plasmacytoid feature is an independent prognostic factor for overall survival for plasmacytoid urothelial carcinoma, which is associated with adverse clinicopathological features and worse overall mortality compared to the conventional urothelial carcinoma [13, 14]. Besides urothelial carcinoma variants and other non-urothelial type primary carcinoma, secondary malignancies can occur in the bladder from metastasis or local extension. Recognizing these uncommon entities determines appropriate clinical management.

With the prolonged survival of bladder cancer patients, thanks to early detection and advances in treatment regimens, surveillance biopsy plays a critical role in monitoring patients local resection, intravesical treatment, and chemotherapy or radiation therapy. Pathological challenges include differentiating recurrent tumoral lesions from metaplastic changes that may happen frequently after variable treatments on bladder mucosa and differentiating tumoral lesions from reactive changes such as post-biopsy reparative changes, hemorrhagic cystitis, or radiation cystitis. Stromal changes may mimic mesenchymal sarcoma which can happen de novo or post-radiation. Morphologic diagnosis, therefore, is critically important for patient management, and pathologists must be familiar with all aspects of bladder pathology.

Pathological Diagnosis and Clinical and Radiological Findings of Bladder Cancer

The diagnosis of bladder cancer should never happen in a black box. Microscopic findings should be correlated with clinical pictures. The patient's clinical presentation, urine analysis, cytology, systemic review, and past medical history can all aid in the accurate evaluation of histologic tissue.

Cystoscopy is important and necessary for the diagnosis of bladder cancer. Pertinent gross features of the tumor (location, size, number, and most importantly, flat or papillary appearances) and other mucosal abnormalities can be ascertained during cystoscopy. Therefore, cystoscopic images and reports are extremely helpful for pathologic evaluation.

Imaging studies are not often used as the first modality to evaluate bladder cancer. However, both computerized tomography (CT) and magnetic resonance imaging (MRI) may be used for assessment of local invasion, primarily to detect T3b disease or higher. Recent studies have also shown that MRI combined with diffusion-weighted imaging can differentiate T1 or less tumors from T2 or greater tumors before surgery with a 91% sensitivity and 96% specificity [15]. CT and MRI detection of regional lymph node metastasis has low sensitivity and specificity. Staging for distal metastases can best be done with CT [16, 17]. Imaging studies can also help with the diagnosis of bladder mesenchymal tumors when bladder mucosal change is nonexistent or minimal. Adjacent organ abnormalities from the bladder (prostate, rectum, uterus, etc.) can also be visualized with CT or MRI and can broaden the differential diagnosis when pathologists are evaluating tissue procured from the bladder when the diagnosis of a secondary tumor is considered.

Molecular Pathology of Bladder Tumors

Despite the prevalence of bladder cancer worldwide, few advances have been made in the clinical management of bladder cancer in recent years, largely due to the poor understanding of its molecular signatures. Bladder cancer is pathologically and molecularly heterogeneous, and molecular profiling studies and whole genomic sequencing have helped to categorize bladder cancer into subtypes that are associated with different prognoses and responses to therapies [18]. These details have been discussed in depth in Chap. 14. These molecular advances have already helped to shift pathology practice forward. With sound molecular techniques, pathologists can now provide more accurate information for tumor prognosis, help to design appropriate treatment regimens, and predict treatment efficacy. With the development of molecular pathology, urologists and urological oncologists have many more options to provide tailored precision medicine for bladder cancer patients with molecularly defined tumor subtypes.

Digital Pathology and the Use of Artificial Intelligence in Bladder Cancers

Because of the rapid development of computer technology and Internet innovations, digital pathology, including the use of digitized whole-slide images for computational analysis aided by artificial intelligence (AI), has advanced greatly in recent years [19]. AI-based approaches for the detection, segmentation, diagnosis, and analysis of digitized images were first compared with conventional microscopy in 2018 in a large-scale multicenter comprehensive study [20] that demonstrated that the diagnostic performance of WSI was comparable to that of traditional microscopy-based approaches. With deep learning approaches, AI-based analyses have a similar level of accuracy to that of expert pathologists [21–23].

Computer engineers and data scientists have focused on the development of new AI-based image analysis approaches in pathology and oncology to improve diagnostic accuracy and to identify novel biomarker for precision medicine. As end users, pathologists need efficient digital slide scanners, cloud-based database, and appropriate AI algorithms to instantly share images with AI-based predictions worldwide. A detailed discussion of these technologies is beyond the scope of this book, but to learn more, readers can refer to other recent publications [19].

With the continuing expansion of computer science and AI, remote online pathology practice with the aid of advanced internet technology is a very promising development for pathologists to embrace in the near future.

Remarks

This book has extensively summarized recently published data about urothelial carcinomas and other bladder lesions. However, due to the rapid evolution of our understanding of bladder cancer and numerous recent publications, there are omissions in this book for newly published papers. This book is a summary of the authors' knowledge, expert understanding of these diseases, and the best angles of approach for diagnosis in bladder pathology. Numerous other professional books, including pathology books, have been published regarding bladder cancer. Our book will serve as an addition to the collective knowledge regarding bladder cancer, particularly in its pathological diagnosis. It is our hope that readers will benefit from our book and that practicing pathologists and pathology trainees will maximize their diagnostic ability aided by the guidance of this and other related books.

References

1. Richters A, Aben KKH, Kiemeney L. The global burden of urinary bladder cancer: an update. World J Urol. 2020;38(8):1895–1904
2. Global cancer observatory: cancer today. International agency for research on cancer. Available from: https://gco.iarc.fr/today. Cited 01 May 2020.
3. Cancer Facts and Statistics. American cancer society Atlanta, GA: American cancer society; 2020.
4. Babjuk M, Burger M, Zigeuner R, Shariat SF, van Rhijn BW, Comperat E, et al. EAU guidelines on non-muscle-invasive urothelial carcinoma of the bladder: update 2013. Eur Urol. 2013;64(4):639–53.
5. Moch H. HPA, Ulbright T.M., Reuter V.E. WHO Classification of Tumours of the Urinary System and Male Genital Organs. 4th ed. Lyon, France: IARC Press; 2016.
6. World Population Prospects 2019: Highlights (ST/ESA/SER.A/423). . United Nations, Department of Economic and Social Affairs, Population Division 2019.
7. World Population Ageing 2017 - Highlights (ST/ESA/SER.A/397). United Nations, Department of Economic and Social Affairs, Population Division 2017.
8. Vakar-Lopez F, Shen SS, Zhang S, Tamboli P, Ayala AG, Ro JY. Muscularis mucosae of the urinary bladder revisited with emphasis on its hyperplastic patterns: a study of a large series of cystectomy specimens. Ann Diagn Pathol. 2007;11(6):395–401.
9. Paner GP, Ro JY, Wojcik EM, Venkataraman G, Datta MW, Amin MB. Further characterization of the muscle layers and lamina propria of the urinary bladder by systematic histologic mapping: implications for pathologic staging of invasive urothelial carcinoma. Am J Surg Pathol. 2007;31(9):1420–9.
10. Lobo N, Shariat SF, Guo CC, Fernandez MI, Kassouf W, Choudhury A, et al. What Is the Significance of Variant Histology in Urothelial Carcinoma? Eur Urol Focus. 2020;6(4):653–663.
11. Kamat AM, Dinney CP, Gee JR, Grossman HB, Siefker-Radtke AO, Tamboli P, et al. Micropapillary bladder cancer: a review of the University of Texas M. D. Anderson Cancer Center experience with 100 consecutive patients. Cancer. 2007;110(1):62–7.
12. Sui W, Matulay JT, Onyeji IC, Theofanides MC, James MB, RoyChoudhury A, et al. Contemporary treatment patterns and outcomes of sarcomatoid bladder cancer. World J Urol. 2017;35(7):1055–61.
13. Kim DK, Kim JW, Ro JY, Lee HS, Park JY, Ahn HK, et al. Plasmacytoid Variant Urothelial Carcinoma of the Bladder: A Systematic Review and Meta-analysis of the Clinicopathological Features and Survival Outcomes. J Urol. 2020;204(2):215–223
14. Ro JY, Shen SS, Lee HI, Hong EK, Lee YH, Cho NH, et al. Plasmacytoid transitional cell carcinoma of urinary bladder: a clinicopathologic study of 9 cases. Am J Surg Pathol. 2008;32(5):752–7.
15. Huang L, Kong Q, Liu Z, Wang J, Kang Z, Zhu Y. The Diagnostic Value of MR Imaging in Differentiating T Staging of Bladder Cancer: A Meta-Analysis. Radiology. 2018;286(2):502–11.
16. Heidenreich A, Albers P, Classen J, Graefen M, Gschwend J, Kotzerke J, et al. Imaging studies in metastatic urogenital cancer patients undergoing systemic therapy: recommendations of a multidisciplinary consensus meeting of the Association of Urological Oncology of the German Cancer Society. Urol Int. 2010;85(1):1–10.
17. Witjes JA, Bruins HM, Cathomas R, Comperat EM, Cowan NC, Gakis G, et al. European Association of Urology Guidelines on Muscle-invasive and Metastatic Bladder Cancer: Summary of the 2020 Guidelines. Eur Urol. 2021;79(1):82–104.
18. Inamura K. Bladder Cancer: New Insights into Its Molecular Pathology. Cancers (Basel). 2018;10(4).
19. Bera K, Schalper KA, Rimm DL, Velcheti V, Madabhushi A. Artificial intelligence in digital pathology - new tools for diagnosis and precision oncology. Nat Rev Clin Oncol. 2019;16(11):703–15.
20. Mukhopadhyay S, Feldman MD, Abels E, Ashfaq R, Beltaifa S, Cacciabeve NG, et al. Whole Slide Imaging Versus Microscopy for Primary Diagnosis in Surgical Pathology: A Multicenter Blinded Randomized Noninferiority Study of 1992 Cases (Pivotal Study). Am J Surg Pathol. 2018;42(1):39–52.
21. Ehteshami Bejnordi B, Veta M, Johannes van Diest P, van Ginneken B, Karssemeijer N, Litjens G, et al. Diagnostic Assessment of Deep Learning Algorithms for Detection of Lymph Node Metastases in Women With Breast Cancer. Jama. 2017;318(22):2199–210.
22. Nagpal K, Foote D, Liu Y, Chen PC, Wulczyn E, Tan F, et al. Development and validation of a deep learning algorithm for improving Gleason scoring of prostate cancer. NPJ Digit Med. 2019;2:48.
23. Bychkov D, Linder N, Turkki R, Nordling S, Kovanen PE, Verrill C, et al. Deep learning based tissue analysis predicts outcome in colorectal cancer. Sci Rep. 2018;8(1):3395.

Index

A
Acute leukemia
  bladder's blood vessels, 133, 136
  extravascular infiltration of myeloid blasts, 133, 136
  myeloid sarcoma, 133, 137
Adenocarcinoma, 88, 154
  primary adenocarcinoma, 88
  secondary adenocarcinoma, 90
  urachal adenocarcinoma, 90–93
Adipose tissue within lamina propria, 232
Alpha-methyl acyl-coenzyme A racemase (AMACR), 161
Alternaria, 150
American Joint Committee on Cancer (AJCC), 216–218
American Joint Committee on Cancer (AJCC) staging of bladder cancers
  bladder diverticula, 240, 241
  M staging, 240
  pT1 carcinoma
    bland cytology and von Brunn nests, 234
    diverse stromal reaction, 235
    early cystectomy, 234
    factors in superficially/focally invasive, 233, 234
    histoanatomical substaging, 233
    histological features in invasive carcinoma identification, 234
    lamina propria/submucosa, 230–232
    microinvasive carcinoma, 233
    micrometric substaging, 233
  pT2 carcinoma
    hyperplastic MM, 236
    LP-inner MP boundary and MP-peivesical boundary, 236
    substaging, 236, 237
    in TUR specimens, 236–238
  pT3 carcinoma, substaging, 238
  pT4 carcinoma
    gynecological tract invasion, 239
    pelvic/abdominal wall invasion, 239, 240
    prostatic stromal invasion, 238, 239
    seminal vesicle invasion, 239
  regional nodal staging (N staging), 240
  stage PTA carcinoma, 230
  stage pTis carcinoma, 230
American Society of Clinical Oncology (ASCO) Genitourinary Cancers Symposium 2020, 201
Anaplastic large cell lymphoma, 130
Anatomy and histology
  anatomic structure, 7–8
  bladder exstrophy, 12
  cystitis, 16
  cystitis glandularis, 14
  cystoprostatectomy, 9
  diverticulum, 12
  ectopic prostate tissue, 13
  fibroepithelial polyps, 17
  functional anatomy, 8
  gross evaluation, 8, 9
  handling of bladder specimens, 8
  Innervation, 8
  lamina propria, 10
  lymphatic drainage, 8
  malakoplakia, 17
  Mullerian lesions, 17
  muscularis mucosa, 11
  muscularis propria, 11
  nephrogenic adenoma, 15
  perivesical adipose tissue, 11
  polypoid cystitis, 17
  squamous metaplasia, 14
  urachal cyst, 12
  urachal remnants, 12
  urothelium, 9
  vascular supply, 8
  von Brunn nests, 13
APOBEC mutagenesis, 176
Artificial intelligence (AI), 251
Ataxia telangiectasia mutation (*ATM*), 176
Atypical urothelial cells (AUC), 149

B
Bacillus Calmette-Guerin (BCG), 150, 183
Bacterial cystitis, 150
Basal urothelial cells, 149
Benign superficial and intermediate urothelial cells, 149
BISCAY trial, 202
BK polyomavirus infection, 151

H. Zhou et al. (eds.), *Urinary Bladder Pathology*, https://doi.org/10.1007/978-3-030-71509-0

Bladder cancer
  artificial intelligence, 251
  clinical course and management, 3
  CT/MRI, 250, 251
  cystoscopy, 250
  diagnosis
    clinical history, 211
    CT/MRI scan, 212
    cystoscopic findings, 212, 213
    pathological examination history, 212
  diagnostic challenges and clinical management, 250
  digital pathology, 251
  epidemiology, 1–2
  high prevalence, 249
  molecular pathology, 251
  pathologic evaluation, 3
  surgical resection, 3
  urothelial carcinogenesis, 2
Bladder lymphomas
  CLL/SLL, 130, 131
  DLBCL, 133, 135
  FL cells, 131, 132
  high grade B cell lymphomas, 133
  lymphoepithelioma-like urothelial carcinoma, 133
  MALT lymphoma, 129
  MCL lymphoma, 131, 132
  non-specific urinary symptoms, 129
  plasmacytoid urothelial carcinoma, 138
  primary, 129
  secondary, 130
Breast cancer, 142
Burkitt's lymphoma, 130

C
Candida albicans, 150
CD138, 138
CD44, 161
CD56, 118
CDH1 mutations, 180
CDKN2A gene, 176–179, 181, 182
Cervical squamous cell carcinoma, 143
Chromatin-modifying genes (CMGs), 176
Chromogranin, 118
Chronic lymphocytic leukemia/small lymphocytic lymphoma (CLL/SLL), 130, 131
Cisplatin-based neoadjuvant chemotherapy, 199
CK20, 161
Clear cell carcinoma, 93–94
Clear cell renal cell carcinoma, 143
Colonic adenocarcinoma, 144
Columnar urothelial cells, 149
Continent urine diversion, 197
CREB-binding protein (*CREBBP*), 176
Cxbladder assay, 155
Cystitis cystica, 13, 150
Cystitis glandularis, 150
Cytokeratin, 160
Cytokeratin 20, 120
Cytomegalovirus (CMV), 151

D
Denonvilliers' fascia, 195
Diffuse large B cell lymphoma (DLBCL), 130, 133, 135
Digital rectal examination (DRE), 189
Diverticulum, of urinary bladder, 241
DNA damage response (DDR) gene, 183
Dovitinib (TKI258), 202
Dual-track molecular carcinogenesis theory, 2
Ductal type adenocarcinomas, 142
Dyscohesive high-grade urothelial carcinoma cells, 147

E
Endometrial neuroendocrine tumor, 144
Endometrial stromal sarcoma, 144
Enfortumab vedotin (EV), 200
Epithelial membrane antigen (EMA), 118
Epithelioid gastrointestinal stromal tumor, 144
ERBB2 amplification, 180
Erdafitinib, 202, 203
Extra-adrenal paraganglioma, 122
Extra-adrenal pheochromocytoma, *see* Extra-adrenal paraganglioma

F
FAT atypical cadherin 1 (*FAT1*), 176
Flat urothelial lesion, 21
  carcinoma in situ (CIS), 27–32
    definition, 27
    diagnosis, 30
    histological features, 27
    intravesical BCG, 32
    muscle-invasive urothelial carcinoma, 31
    neoplastic cells, 29
  cytologic features, 22
  diagnostic features, 22
  dysplasia, 26
  histologic features, 23
  hyperplasia, 24
  lesional biopsies, 21
  mucosal margins, 21
  normal urothelium, 22
  pathological diagnosis, 21
  radiation atypia, 25
  radiation cystitis, 26
  random biopsies, 21
  reactive atypia, 25–26
  TURBT, 21
  UAUS, 26
  UPUMP, 24–25
  urothelial dysplasia, 26
Follicular lymphoma (FL), 130

G
Gastrointestinal cancer, 144
GATA3, 120, 124, 142, 164
Gene expression signature, 226
Germinal center B-cell-like (GCB), 133

Glandular tumors of urachus, 92
Gleason score, 166
Gynecological malignancies, 143
Gynecological tract invasion, 239

H
Hematoxylin-eosin (H&E) stain, 159, 160, 163, 165
Hematuria, 117, 147
Hepatocyte nuclear factor-1β (HNF-1β), 169
High grade B cell lymphoma, 133, 135
High grade prostatic adenocarcinoma, 142
High grade serous carcinoma, 143
High-grade papillary Urothelial Carcinoma (HGPUC), 39, 40
High-grade serous carcinoma, 143
High-grade urothelial carcinoma (HGUC), 149, 152, 153
Homeobox B13 (HOXB13), 121
Human epidermal growth factor receptor 2 (HER2), 203
Hyperchromasia, 124
Hyperplastic muscularis mucosae, 220

I
ImmunoCyt/uCyt tests, 155
Immunohistochemistry in bladder cancer
  biomarkers development, 159
  differential diagnoses, 160
  economy, 161
  flat urothelial lesions, 162
    AMACR, 161
    CD44, 161
    CK20, 161
    Ki-67, 161
    P53, 161
  four issues, 160
  high-grade prostate adenocarcinoma *vs.* urothelial carcinoma, 165
    disadvantages, 167
    ERG, 166, 167
    histologic features, 165
    HMWCK antibody clone 34βE12, 167
    morphologic characteristics on H&E sections, 165
    NKX3.1, 166
    PSA and PSMA, 166
    selection of immunostain panel, 167
    thrombomodulin, 166
  histologic variants of infiltrating UC, 161
  invasive urothelial carcinoma, 163
  metastatic carcinoma to urinary bladder, 170
  NA (*see* Nephrogenic adenoma (NA))
  need for, 159, 160
  positive stain, 160
  primary adenocarcinoma and secondary adenocarcinoma, 170
  prognosis and molecular classification
    CK20, CD44, uroplakin, CK14, GATA3 and CK5/6, 171
    PD-L1, 171
  proper panel selection, 160
  in separating spindle cell neoplasms of bladder, 170, 171
  smoothelin, 163
  TURP specimens, 163
  urothelial linage and rule out metastasis
    GATA3, 163, 164
    p63, 164
    S100P, 164, 165
    Uroplakin II, 164
Incontinent urine diversion, 197
Indiana pouch, 197
Infigratinib (BGJ398), 203
Infiltrating urothelial carcinoma
  chordoid/myxoid/mucinous stroma, 77
  with divergent differentiation, 64
    glandular differentiation, 65
    squamous differentiation, 64
    trophoblastic differentiation, 66
  giant cell variant, 73
  glycogen-rich variant, 76
  histological variants, 63
  LELC variant, 71
  lipid-richvariant, 77
  microcystic variant, 68
  micropapillary variant, 69
  nested variant, 67
  osteoclast-rich undifferentiated carcinoma, 76
  plasmacytoid variant, 72
  pseudoangiosarcomatous variant, 77
  rhabdoid features, 77
  sarcomatoid variant, 74–75
Inflammatory myofibroblastic tumor (IMT), 106
  ALK-1 immunohistochemical stain, 108
  cytokeratin cocktail stain, 108
  differential diagnosis, 108
  Ki67 stain, 109
  occasional strap-shaped cells, 107
  spindle cells, 108
  transurethral resection, 108
  ulcerated masses, 106
Instrumented urine specimens, 148
Insulin-like growth factor–binding protein 3 (*IGFBP3*), 180
Insulinoma-associated protein 1 (INSM1), 118
International Consultation on Urologic Disease–European Association of Urology, 147
International Society of Urological Pathology (ISUP), 216
International Union Against Cancer (UICC), 216–218
Invasive urothelial carcinoma (UC), 45
  cancer invasion process, 45, 48
  diagnostic criteria, 46
  invasive bladder cancer, 54, 57
  lamina propria invasion, 48–49
  lymphovascular invasion, 53
  muscle-invasive bladder cancer, 45, 56
  muscularis mucosae, 51
  muscularis propria, 50
  prostate involvement, 52–53
  stroma
    exuberant fibrosis, 47
    inflammatory reaction, 47
  TURBT, 45, 51

K
Ki-67, 122, 161, 169
Koch ileocecal reservoirs, 197

L
Lamina propria/submucosa (LP/SM), 230
Langhans-type giant cells, 150
Large-cell neuroendocrine carcinoma (LCNEC)
  clinical features, 121
  epidemiology, 121
  immunohistochemical features, 121, 122
  pathologic features, 121
  PET/CT scans, 121
Lithiasis, 151
Long non-coding RNAs (lncRNAs), 183
Loss of heterozygosity (LOH), 2
Low-grade papillary urothelial carcinoma (LGPUC), 39
Low-grade urothelial neoplasm (LGUN), 149, 151, 152
Lymph nodes, 223, 224
Lymphoepithelial lesions, 129
Lymphoepithelioma-like urothelial carcinoma, 133
Lymphovascular invasion (LVI), 222
Lynch syndrome, 181
Lysine (K)–specific methyltransferase 2C (*KMT2C*), 176

M
Mainz pouch, 197
Makorin ring finger protein 2 (*MKRN2*), 176
Malignant carcinoid, 113
Malignant melanoma, 144, 145
Mammalian target of rapamycin (mTOR) inhibitors, 183
Mantle cell lymphoma (MCL), 130–132
Melamed-Wolinska bodies, 151
Mesenchymal tumors, 97
  benign stromal tumors, 101
    ganglioneuroma, 101
    gastrointestinal stromal tumor, 101
    granular cell tumor, 101
    lipomas, 101
    schwannoma, 101
  leiomyoma, 100
  malignant tumors, 101
    angiosarcoma, 104–105
    chondrosarcoma, 105
    leiomyosarcoma, 102
    rhabdomyosarcomas, 103
    sarcomas, 105
  myofibroblastic lesions, 106
    inflammatory myofibroblastic tumor, 106–108
    PSCN, 106
  neurofibroma, 101
  paragangliomas, 97
Metastatic breast cancer, 142
Metastatic lung squamous cell carcinoma, 145
Metastatic melanomas, 143, 144
Microinvasive carcinoma, 233
Micropapillary carcinoma (MPC), 141
Micropapillary urothelial carcinoma (MPUC), 180
Micro-RNA (miRNA), 181
Microsatellite instability (MSI)-high, 224, 225
Mismatch repair deficient (dMMR) tumors, 224, 225
Mitogen-activated protein kinase (MAPK), 183
Mixed-lineage leukemia 2 (*MLL2*) gene, 176
Molecular and genomic testing, 226
Monomethyl auristatin E (MMAE), 200
Mouse double minute 2 homolog (*MDM2*), 176–178
Mucosa-associated lymphoid tissue (MALT) lymphoma, 129, 130, 133
Muscle invasive bladder carcinoma (MIBC), 175
Muscularis mucosae (MM), 163, 230–232
Muscularis mucosae invasion vs. muscularis propria invasion, 50–52
Muscularis propria (MP), 114, 116, 118, 123, 163, 238
Mutation detection assays, 182
Myeloid sarcoma, 133

N
Necrotic urothelial cells, 151
Nectin-4, 200
Negative for high-grade urothelial carcinoma (NHGUC), 149
Neoadjuvant chemotherapy (NAC), 183
Nephrogenic adenoma (NA)
  AMACR, 168
  vs. clear cell adenocarcinoma of the bladder, 168, 169
  histologic patterns, 168
  irritative bladder symptoms, 167
  vs. papillary urothelial carcinoma, 169
  PAX2 or PAX-8, 168
  PAX-8 and AMACR, 168
  vs. prostate adenocarcinoma, 169
  urothelial carcinoma or prostate adenocarcinoma, 168
Nested variant of urothelial carcinoma, 181
Nested variant urothelial carcinoma, 234
Neuroendocrine tumors (NETs)
  clinical and pathologic features, 113–115
  LCNEC (*see* Large-cell neuroendocrine carcinoma (LCNEC))
  paraganglioma (*see* Paraganglioma)
  SCNEC (*see* Small cell neuroendocrine carcinoma (SCNEC))
  WDNETs (*see* Well-differentiated neuroendocrine tumors (WDNETs))
Non-bilharzial *vs*. bilharzial SCC, 84
Non-invasive versus invasive bladder cancer, 219, 220
Non-muscle-invasive bladder cancers (NMIBC), 175, 249
NOTCH1 gene, 175
Nuclear pleomorphism, 124

O
Oat cell carcinoma, *see* Small cell neuroendocrine carcinoma (SCNEC)

P
p53, 161, 169
Papillary urothelial hyperplasia, 38
Papillary urothelial neoplasm of low malignant potential (PUNLMP), 38

Papillary urothelial neoplasms, 35
benign papillary urothelial neoplasm
inverted urothelial papilloma, 37
squamous papilloma, 37
urothelial papilloma, 36
HGPUC, 39
inverted growth pattern, 41
LGPUC, 39
non-neoplastic papillary lesions, 41–42
PUNLMP, 38
UPUMP, 38
Paraganglioma, 143
clinical features, 122
CT and MRI scans, 122
epidemiology, 122
immunohistochemical features, 124
pathological features, 123
Paraneoplastic syndrome, 117
Paris System for Reporting Urinary Cytology, 147, 149
Partial cystectomy, 191, 215, 216
PAX8, 143, 169
Pelvic/abdominal wall invasion, 239, 240
Pelvic lymphadenectomy, 194, 195
Pemigatinib, 203
Peroxisome proliferator activated receptor gamma (*PPARG)*, 176
PIK3/AKT/MTOR pathway, 178, 179
Plasma cell neoplasms, 133, 138
Plasmacytoid urothelial carcinoma, 138, 180
Polyomavirus, 151
Polypoid/papillary cystitis, 42
Post-cystectomy ileal conduit/neobladder specimens, 148
Postoperative spindle cell nodule (PSCN), 106
Primary bladder lymphomas, 129
Primary lung squamous cell carcinoma, 145
Primary uterine carcinomas, 144
Programed death-ligand 1 (PD-L1), 171
Prophylactic antibiotics, 192
Prostate acid phosphatase (PAP), 117
Prostate cancers, 142
Prostatic adenocarcinoma, 142
Prostatic ductal adenocarcinoma, 142
Prostatic stromal invasion, 238, 239

R

Racemase, 160
Radical cystectomy, 192–194
female, 196
male, 195
RB1 mutation, 176–178, 180, 183
Receptor tyrosine kinase (RTK), 183
Regional nodal staging in bladder cancer, 240
Renal cell carcinoma (RCC), 142, 143
Re-staging transurethral resection (re-TUR), 191
Rogaratinib (BAY1163877), 203

S

Sacituzumab govitecan (SG), 201
Sarcomatoid urothelial carcinoma, 180
Schistosoma haematobium, 151, 153
Secondary bladder lymphomas, 129, 130
Secondary tumors
adenocarcinomas, 141
breast cancer, 142
gastrointestinal cancer, 144
gynecological malignancies, 143, 144
lungs, 145
malignant melanoma, 144, 145
micropapillary carcinoma, 141
prostate cancer, 142
renal cell carcinoma, 142, 143
Seminal vesicle invasion, 239
Sienna test, 155
Sirtratumab vedotin (SV), 201
Sloughed renal tubular cells, 150
Small cell neuroendocrine carcinoma (SCNEC)
clinical features, 117
cystectomy, 117
epidemiology, 117
immunohistochemical features, 118, 121
molecular genetics, 117, 118
pathologic features, 118
Small cell/neuroendocrine carcinoma of bladder (SmCC), 181
Smooth muscle of indeterminate type (SMIT), 52
Smoothelin, 163
Somatostatin receptors (SSTRs), 121
Specimen handling and reporting
biopsy and transurethral resection of bladder tumors, 213, 214
histologic tumor grade, 216
histologic tumor type, 216
immunohistochemical PD-L1 assays for bladder cancer, 225
lymph nodes and distant spread, 223, 224
lymphovascular invasion, 222
non-invasive vs. invasive bladder cancer, 219, 220
partial cystectomy, 215, 216
pathologic information, 217–218
pathologic stage classification of bladder cancer, 219
pathology reporting, 226
predictive tissue markers for immunotherapy, 224
gene expression signature, 226
mismatch repair deficient tumors, 224, 225
molecular and genomic testing, 226
PD-L1 immunohistochemistry, 224
tumor mutation burden, 225, 226
predictive tissue markers for neoadjuvant chemotherapy, 224
prostate involvement, 223
resection margins, 222
T1 stage versus T2 stage, 220, 221
T1 substaging, 220
T2 staging, 221, 222
T3 staging, 222
total cystectomy, radical cystoprostatectomy, and pelvic exenteration
dissection of specimens, 214
lymph nodes sampling, 215
margins sampling, 215

Specimen handling and reporting (*cont.*)
non-tumoral mucosa sampling, 215
orientation of specimens, 214
other organs sampling, 215
prostate gland sampling, 215
seminal vesicle sampling, 215
urothelial carcinoma in situ, 222
Spectrin alpha non-erythrocytic 1 (*SPTAN1*), 176
Squamous cell carcinoma (SCC), 83–87, 143, 153
basaloid SCC, 87
clinical features, 84–85
epidemiology, 83–84
etiology, 84
molecular and genetic aspects, 86–87
overview, 83
pathological features, 85–86
sarcomatoid SCC, 88
treatment and prognosis, 87
verrucous carcinoma, 87
Superficial squamous cells, 149
SurePath liquid preparations, 148
Surgical treatment in urinary bladder cancer
partial cystectomy, 191
pelvic lymphadenectomy, 194, 195
radical cystectomy, 192–194
female, 196
male, 195
TURBT
DRE, 189
obturator nerve, 190
re-TUR, 191
surgical skills, 190
urethrectomy, 196, 197
urinary diversion, 197
continent diversion, 197
incontinent urine diversion, 197
Suspicious for high-grade urothelial carcinoma (SHGUC), 149
Synaptophysin, 124

T
Targeted therapeutic strategies
TAAs using ADCs
characteristics, 201
nectin-4 with enfortumab vedotin, 200, 201
SLITRK6 with sirtratumab vedotin, 201
trop-2 with sacituzumab govitecan, 201
targeting FGFR with TKIs, 202
AZD4547, 202
dovitinib, 202
erdafitinib, 202, 203
infigratinib, 203
pemigatinib, 203
rogaratinib, 203
targeting HER2, 203
T cell lymphomas, 130
Telomerase reverse transcriptase (TERT), 176, 181
The Cancer Genom Atlas (TCGA) data, 175
The Paris System, 152
ThinPrep method, 148
Thrombomodulin, 166
Thyroid hurtle cell carcinoma, 145
TP53 gene, 176, 178
Transitional cell carcinomas (TCCs), 142
Transurethral resection of bladder tumor (TURBT), 45, 124
DRE, 189
obturator nerve, 190
re-TUR, 191
surgical skills, 190
Transurethral resection of prostate (TURP) specimens, 163
Treatment-related adverse events (TRAEs), 203
tRNA splicing endonuclease subunit 2 (*TSEN2*), 176
Trophoblast cell-surface antigen 2 (Trop-2), 201
TSC1 gene, 175
Tumor mutation burden (TMB), 225, 226
28-8 pharmDx (Nivolumab) assays, 224
22C3 pharmDx (Pembrolizumab), 224

U
Upper urinary tract (UUT), 147, 148
Urethrectomy, 196, 197
Urine cytology
ancillary tests, 154, 155
atypical category, 152
Bacillus Calmette-Guérin, 150
bacterial cystitis, 150
benign superficial and intermediate urothelial cells, 149
columnar urothelial cells, 149
cystoscopy and upper urinary tract, 147
degenerative changes, 151
direct extension and metastatic tumor to urinary bladder, 154
fungi, 150
hematuria, 147
high-grade urothelial carcinoma, 152, 153
instrumented urine specimens, 148
International Consultation on Urologic Disease–European Association of Urology, 147
intrinsic limitations, 148
lithiasis, 151
low-grade urothelial neoplasiaithiasis, 151, 152
necrosis, 151
NMP22, 155
Paris System for Reporting Urinary Cytology, 147
post-cystectomy ileal conduit/neobladder specimens, 148
primary non-urothelial tumor, 153, 154
sloughed renal tubular cells, 150
specimen adequacy, 148
superficial squamous cells, 149
suspicious category, 152
The Paris System, 149
viral infection, 151
voided urine and instrumental urine, 147
voided urine specimens, 148

Uroplakin II, 164
UroSEEK, 155, 182
Urothelial cancer (UC)
BCG responsiveness, 183
distant metastasis, 240
diverticulum of urinary bladder, 241
epigenetic alterations, 176, 177
high grade tumors
PIK3/AKT/MTOR Pathway, 178, 179
TP53/RB1 pathway, 178
inheritance, 181, 182
inverted urothelial papillomas, 179, 180
low grade tumors, FGFR3/RAS pathway, 178
micropapillary urothelial carcinoma, 180
micro-RNA, 181
molecular markers for treatment
DDR gene alterations and treatment, 183
FGFR3 inhibitors, 182, 183
lncRNAs, 183
mTOR inhibitors, 183
molecular pathways, 177, 178
mutation detection assays, 182
mutations
APOBEC, 176
FGFR3 gene, 176
FGFR3–TACC3 gene, 176
MLL2 gene, 176
TERT gene, 176
TP53 gene, 176
nested variant of urothelial carcinoma, 181
numerical chromosomal alterations, 175
plasmacytoid urothelial carcinoma, 180
sarcomatous and urothelial components, 180
small cell/neuroendocrine carcinoma of the bladder, 181
tumor progression, 179
UroSEEK, 182
urothelial carcinoma with divergent differentiation, 180
urothelial hyperplasia and dysplasia, 179
urothelial papilloma, 179
Urovysion assay, 182
vaginal invasion, 239
Urothelial carcinoma in situ, 222, 230
Urothelial dysplasia, 177
Urothelial hyperplasia, 179
Urothelial papilloma (UP), 179
Urothelial proliferation of uncertain malignant potential (UPUMP), 38, 41
Urovysion assay, 154, 155, 182

V
Ventana SP142 (Atezolizumab), 224
Voided urine specimens, 148
von Brunn's nests, 219, 234

W
Well-differentiated neuroendocrine tumors (WDNETs)
clinical features, 116
cystoscopic transurethral resection, 116
epidemiology, 113
immunohistochemical features, 117
insular growth pattern with fibrovascular stroma and artifactual stromal retraction, 116
pathologic features, 116

Z
Ziehl-Neelsen staining, 150

Printed by Printforce, the Netherlands